Psychodynamic Formulation

Psychodynamic Formulation

An Expanded Approach

The Psychodynamic Formulation Collective

WILEY Blackwell

Registered Office(s)

John Wiley & Sons, Inc., 111 River Street, Hoboken, NJ 07030, USA

John Wiley & Sons Ltd, The Atrium, Southern Gate, Chichester, West Sussex, PO19 8SQ, UK

Editorial Office

9600 Garsington Road, Oxford, OX4 2DQ, UK

For details of our global editorial offices, customer services, and more information about Wiley products visit us at www.wiley.com.

Wiley also publishes its books in a variety of electronic formats and by print-on-demand. Some content that appears in standard print versions of this book may not be available in other formats.

Library of Congress Cataloging-in-Publication Data applied for

Hardback: 9781119797265

Cover Design: Wiley

Cover Image: Courtesy of Deborah L. Cabanis

Set in 10/12pt, PalatinoLTStd by Straive, Pondicherry, India

SKY10074462_050324

To our patients

Table of Contents

Preface

The year 2020 was an exceptional one. To start, the COVID-19 pandemic brought significant individual, community, and societal changes as we all faced concerns about health and safety, while also renegotiating our engagement with one another. In the midst of these monumental changes, the United States was forced to reckon with long-standing issues of structural racism and racial injustice highlighted by the murders of George Floyd, Ahmaud Arbery, and Breonna Taylor at the hands of law enforcement. In this context, racial inequities were brought to the fore, highlighting staggering disparities not only in COVID deaths, but also in all areas of life including education, housing, economic opportunities, law enforcement encounters, the criminal justice system, and health care.

Systemic discrimination and implicit bias have left Blacks with inadequate access to health care and unequal healthcare treatment. Implicit and explicit biases have resulted in disparaged or ignored health determinants in minorities, leading to these being considered unworthy of study or omitted completely in research and clinical approaches.

Such biases have been reflected in prior editions of this book. They are embedded in the institutional and systemic racism present within our field of psychoanalysis and its psychodynamic psychotherapeutic treatments. We have undertaken this new edition to examine these biases within our profession; biases that have led not only to marginalization of our clinicians of color, but also to the prioritization of Whiteness, and to a lack of appropriately formulating the racial and ethnic contributions that are so important to the people we treat. Our patients come from rich and diverse backgrounds and bring so much that is not often reflected in psychodynamic and psychoanalytic formulation and treatment. Additionally, we have not adequately considered and formulated the trauma, discrimination, and systemic oppression that individuals from these backgrounds have experienced as a result of their racial backgrounds, and how that trauma affects their view of themselves, how others perceive them, and their presentation to mental health providers. In this edition, we have attempted to highlight these blind spots, to place their evaluation within our field and with our patients front and center, and to give equal and heavy consideration to the impact of these inequities in a new and expanded approach to psychodynamic formulation.

Here are the highlights of what's new in *Psychodynamic Formulation: An Expanded Approach*:

The effect of culture and society - We feel very strongly that psychodynamic formulations must be expanded to include the larger influences of society and culture on the development of the conscious and unconscious mind. People who have good early relationships can, when subject to trauma, disadvantage, discrimination, and systemic oppression, develop difficulties with domains such as trust, self-perception, relationships, and adapting. People who may be privileged or valued over others by society can develop a distorted sense of their abilities, leading to challenges in navigating stressors or adversity experienced in later life. We have integrated Bronfenbrenner's Ecological Systems model (Bronfenbrenner, 1977) into our organizing framework as a way of conceptualizing this, offering it as an idea about development on equal footing with other psychodynamic models. We can think of this as one way of addressing the biopsychosocial factors that shape the development of a mind. While this book has been written by authors who live and work in the United States, we hope that this approach may prompt readers to consider the unique effects of culture and society on persons in their location.

Diversity and inclusion - In this edition, we use non-binary pronouns, replacing "he/she" with "they" for the singular and plural. We have written inclusive vignettes, while following current guidelines to only include demographic identifiers that add to the significance of the examples. As such, the vignettes vary in length. Some focus on a very specific point. Others zoom out to consider the full lived and layered experience of the person. We recognize that all readers and clinicians will bring their own assumptions, positionality, and lived experience to the vignettes. We have chosen to use names rather than initials for the persons included in the vignettes to bring the examples to life. Some of the names used might reflect the diverse backgrounds of persons in the United States. We have updated sections on attachment to acknowledge the predominantly White and western bias of the original research in this area. Likewise, we have also updated sections on conflict and triadic relationships to acknowledge the often heteronormative bias of early ego psychological models.

Conscious and unconscious - We believe that psychodynamic formulations help us to form hypotheses about the entirety of a person's mind—conscious and unconscious. In this edition, we expand this formulation to discuss the development of both conscious and unconscious thoughts and feelings.

Lived experience - People can develop conscious and unconscious problems and patterns throughout life—not only during their early childhood. We have added more on the importance of lived experiences, with expanded sections on trauma and adulthood.

Bias - We have added sections that acknowledge and discuss how culture, identity, and the biases of the clinician affect the creation of psychodynamic formulations. We have added discussions in several sections—including those on trust, identity, and attachment—that address how traditional psychodynamic concepts may be inadequate when creating formulations about people from marginalized groups. Acknowledging the diversity of gender and sexual development, we have de-emphasized triadic (Oedipal) relationships in middle childhood and their role in adult psychopathology. At all points, we have tried to move away from White, heteronormative, and ableist expectations, while understanding, in the spirit of cultural humility, that there may be ways in which this continues to be present.

Identity - We have greatly expanded our discussion of identity in this edition, given that it is the part of self-experience that relates to how we see ourselves in relation to our culture and society.

Defenses - Starting from the idea that all defenses were adaptive at one point in life, we no longer label defenses along the "adaptive-maladaptive" continuum. Rather, we discuss the benefit and cost of defenses, noting that this balance can change over the lifespan.

Values - We have added "values" to our list of function domains. We call this domain "values" rather than "super-ego function" so as not to privilege ego psychology as the dominant psychodynamic model, to broadly address systems of right and wrong, and to include discussion of personal values.

The collaborative process - We create psychodynamic formulations *with* our patients, not about our patients. This edition emphasizes the collaborative nature of this process.

Expanded educators' guide and more suggested activities - Psychodynamic formulation must be learned actively. We have included suggested activities in each chapter so that learners can practice the concepts in real time. These activities can be performed by individual learners or in a classroom setting. We have also expanded our educators' guide to help instructors actively teach this important psychotherapeutic skill.

Whether you are learning psychodynamic formulation for the first time, or revisiting concepts that have become well-known, we hope that our journey of discovery may prompt you to expand that way you conceptualize your patients' development, and that, in some way, this contributes to diminishing the inequity in psychoanalysis, our healthcare system, and our world.

Reference

1. Bronfenbrenner, U. (1977). Toward an experimental ecology of human development. *American Psychologist*, 32(7), 513–531. https://doi.org/10.1037/0003-066x.32.7.513

Acknowledgments

In 2020, the tragic murders of Black men and women at the hands of the police, and the resulting social uprising were stark reminders that structural racism remains at the core of American society. The authors of *Psychodynamic Formulation* realized that it was also part of the way we conceptualize and treat patients. To study and address this, we needed new perspectives and expertise, so we created The Psychodynamic Formulation Collective. In the midst of the pandemic, this incredible group of thinkers, writers, and colleagues worked entirely remotely to transform this book and to expand the way we think about psychodynamic formulation. We are:

Shirin Ali, an assistant clinical professor of psychiatry at the Columbia University Vagelos College of Physicians and Surgeons. A graduate of the Columbia University Center for Psychoanalytic Training and Research, she enjoys teaching and supervising psychiatry residents in psychodynamic psychotherapy. In her clinical practice, she focuses on mood and anxiety disorders, psychosis, culture and identity, and emerging adulthood.

Deborah L. Cabaniss, a professor of clinical psychiatry at the Columbia University Vagelos College of Physicians and Surgeons, associate director of the Adult Psychiatry Residency Program in the Columbia University Department of Psychiatry, and a training and supervising analyst at the Columbia University Center for Psychoanalytic Training and Research. Her teaching and writing focus on psychotherapy education, and she practices psychiatry and psychoanalysis in New York City.

Sabrina Cherry, a clinical professor of psychiatry at Vagelos College of Physicians and Surgeons, Columbia University. She is also an associate director and training and supervising analyst at the Columbia Center for Psychoanalytic Training and Research where she teaches candidates and conducts research on psychoanalytic career development. She practices psychotherapy and psychoanalysis in New York City.

Angela Coombs, an associate medical director at Alameda County Behavioral Health, where she focuses on increasing access to county mental health services and supports clients in East Oakland, California. Her scholarly work focuses on mental health inequities facing Black American populations and other minoritized and/or marginalized groups.

Carolyn J. Douglas, an associate clinical professor of psychiatry at the Columbia University Vagelos College of Physicians and Surgeons and an adjunct associate professor of clinical psychiatry at Weill-Cornell Medical College. She has been closely involved in psychiatric residency training throughout her career, has published several articles about teaching psychodynamic psychotherapy, and has won teaching awards from residents in psychiatry both at Columbia and at Weill-Cornell for her didactic courses and supervision in supportive psychodynamic psychotherapy.

Jack Drescher, a distinguished life fellow of the American Psychiatric Association and a clinical professor of psychiatry at the Columbia University Vagelos College of Physicians and Surgeons. He is also an adjunct professor at New York University's Postdoctoral Program in Psychotherapy and Psychoanalysis and a training and supervising analyst at the William Alanson White Institute.

Ruth Graver, an assistant clinical professor of psychiatry at the Columbia University Vagelos College of Physicians and Surgeons. She teaches and supervises at the Columbia University Center for Psychoanalytic Teaching and Research where she is currently the co-chair of the Columbia Academy for Psychoanalytic Educators (CAPE), a new program designed to hone skills relevant to treating and supervising candidates. Her scholarly interests include clinical technique, attachment theory, and psychoanalytic writing. She conducts her clinical practice of psychotherapy and psychoanalysis in New York City

Sandra Park, a training and supervising analyst at the Columbia University Center for Psychoanalytic Training and Research and an assistant professor of psychiatry at the Weill Cornell Medical Center. She has a private practice in Manhattan, and she teaches and supervises at Columbia and Cornell.

Aaron Reliford, vice chair for diversity, equity and inclusion and an associate clinical professor of child and adolescent psychiatry at New York University. He is also the training director of NYU's Child and Adolescent Psychiatry Fellowship, and both the director of child and adolescent psychiatry and the associate medical director of Behavioral Health Sunset Terrace Family Health Center of NYU Langone Brooklyn. Dr. Reliford's clinical research interests include telepsychiatry, racial health disparities in pediatric mental health, cultural psychiatry, pediatric psychopharmacology, effects of early trauma on development of psychopathology, child parent psychotherapy, psychoanalysis, and dynamic/ insight oriented psychotherapy.

Anna Schwartz, a clinical assistant professor of psychiatry at the Columbia University Vagelos College of Physicians & Surgeons. She is also a faculty member of the Columbia University Center for Psychoanalytic Training and Research, where she has taught and supervised psychotherapy trainees for many years. She is in private practice in New York City.

Susan C. Vaughan, the Aaron R. Stern Professor of Psychodynamic Psychiatry at Cornell University. She also served as the Director of the Columbia University Center for Psychoanalytic Training and Research from 2017 to 2022. She has special interest in LGBTQ issues and teaches about sexuality, gender, and the intersections between psychotherapy and neuroscience.

Many thanks to Susan Vaughan for creating the Margaret Morgan Lawrence Fund at the Columbia University Center for Psychoanalytic Training and Research, which supports psychoanalytic and psychodynamic education for trainees from traditionally under-represented minorities and to which we are donating all royalties from this book. Thanks to Jake Opie and Monica Rogers, our team at Wiley, for your enthusiasm for this project. Thanks to Anna Ornstein for her reminder many years ago that we create formulations collaboratively with our patients. Thank you to our families for lending us out for nights and weekends. And to Thomas Cabaniss for once again reading every word.

Finally, thank you in advance to our readers. We hope that *Psychodynamic Formulation: An Expanded Approach* contributes to the way that psychodynamic thinkers and clinicians help patients in a changing world.

—The authors, January 2022

PART ONE: Introduction to the Psychodynamic Formulation

1 What Is a Psychodynamic Formulation?

Key concepts

A formulation is an explanation or hypothesis.

A psychodynamic formulation is a hypothesis about the way a person's conscious and unconscious thoughts and feelings

- may have developed
- may be causing or contributing to the difficulties that have led the person to treatment

Throughout our lives, biological, psychological, and social/cultural factors affect the development of our conscious and unconscious ways of thinking about ourselves, our relationships with others, and our world; thus, all should be included in a psychodynamic formulation.

Psychodynamic formulations do not offer definitive explanations; rather, they are hypotheses that can change over time.

Psychodynamic formulations can aid our work with all patients, not just those in psychodynamic psychotherapy.

What is a formulation?

Very nice history. Now can you formulate the case?

All mental health trainees have heard this, but what does it mean? What is a formulation? Why is it important?

Formulating means explaining (Eells, 2022), or better still, hypothesizing. All healthcare professionals create **formulations** all the time to understand their patients' problems. In mental health fields, the kinds of problems we try to understand involve

---

Psychodynamic Formulation: An Expanded Approach, First Edition. The Psychodynamic Formulation Collective.
© 2022 John Wiley & Sons Ltd. Published 2022 by John Wiley & Sons Ltd.

the way our patients think, feel, and behave. When we formulate, we think not only about *how* people think, feel, behave, but also *why* they do. For example,

> *Why is she behaving this way?*
>
> *Why does he think that about himself?*
>
> *Why are they responding to me like this?*
>
> *Why is that his way of dealing with stress?*
>
> *Why is she having difficulty working and enjoying time off?*
>
> *What is preventing them from living the life they want to lead?*

Different etiologies suggest different treatments; thus, having hypotheses about these questions is vital for recommending and conducting treatment.

What makes a formulation psychodynamic?

Many different kinds of formulations exist (Campbell & Rohrbaugh, 2006/2013; Eells, 2010; Wright et al., 2017). There are cognitive behavioral therapy formulations, psychopharmacologic formulations, and family systems formulations, just to name a few. Each type of formulation is based on a different idea about what causes the kinds of problems that bring people to mental health treatment.

A **psychodynamic frame of reference** suggests that these problems may be caused or contributed to by thoughts and feelings that are out of awareness—that is, that are **unconscious**. These unconscious thoughts and feelings affect the way we think about ourselves, other people, and our relationship to the world Thus, a **psychodynamic formulation** is a hypothesis about the way a person's conscious *and* unconscious thoughts and feelings

- may have developed
- may be causing or contributing to the difficulties that have brought the person to treatment

This is important to understand, as helping people become aware of their unconscious thoughts and feelings is an important psychodynamic technique.

Unconscious vs. implicit

According to social scientists, **implicit** mental processes are those that "occur outside conscious awareness" (Devos & Banaji, 2003). People may not be aware that they exist, or they may simply operate outside of conscious control (Devos & Banaji, 2003). When implicit processes influence our judgments—for example, about people on the basis of race or gender—we call this **implicit bias** (FitzGerald & Hurst, 2017). We can have these biases about ourselves, others, or society at large. In this book, we use the terms unconscious and implicit interchangeably to mean mental processes that operate out of awareness and that, once formed, automatically influence our thoughts, feelings, and behaviors.

A developmental process throughout life

It's well known that psychodynamically oriented mental health professionals are interested in their patients' childhoods. But why? One reason is that using psychodynamic technique is about more than just helping people become aware of their unconscious thoughts and feelings—it's also about trying to make sense of how and why those unconscious thoughts and feelings developed.

Although there are significant temporal windows early in life during which massive amounts of development occurs, conscious and unconscious thoughts and feelings change throughout life. Erikson's "Eight Ages of Man" (Erikson, 1968), which conceptualizes development as occurring throughout the life span, is a good place to begin, but today we must take this even further. Traumatic events that occured to parents before conception; maternal stress during pregnancy; discrimination, inequity, and systemic oppression during adulthood; and late-life loss may all contribute to the individual's mental life in the here and now. Thus, we aim to address the entirety of a person's lived experience in a psychodynamic formulation.

While that's all well and good, how can we learn about and try to make sense of developmental processes that have already occurred? Even with videos and scrapbooks, we can't go back in time to watch early development unfold. In this way, creating a psychodynamic formulation is a lot like being a detective trying to solve a mystery. Like the detective, we work retrospectively, first looking at our patients' problems and patterns and then scrolling back through their life stories to try to understand their development.

Biological, psychological, and social

So, how *do* our characteristic patterns of thinking, feeling, and behaving develop? John Locke said that each person is born as a blank slate—a *tabula rasa* (Locke, 1689/1975). E. O. Wilson argued that social behavior is shaped almost entirely by genetics (Wilson, 1975/2000). Nature—nurture: it isn't one or the other but both, with the relative contributions of each varying from person to person. Freud (1937/1964) called the nature part "constitutional" and the nurture part "accidental." However, you think about it, people come into the world with their inherited genetics and then continue to develop as they interact with their environment. The more we learn about the interrelationship between genes and environment, the clearer it is that our genetics shape our experience and vice versa; complex interactions between the two result in our characteristic views of ourselves, the way we relate to other people, and our patterns of adapting to stress. In thinking about how to understand and describe how we develop, we must consider genetics, intrauterine exposures, temperament—the

biological factors—as well as the environmental factors. They are all part of psychodynamic formulation.

Traditionally, psychoanalysts thought about the environmental part of the equation as related mostly to the effects of children's early interactions with the people in their immediate environment (e.g., primary caregivers and other family members). This immediate environment is sometimes called the person's **microsystem** (Bronfenbrenner, 1977). We often think of these early interactions as the **psychological** factors contributing to a person's development. But **culture and society** also affect the development of the conscious and unconscious ways we think about ourselves, other people, and our world (Fanon, 1952/2019). This includes both the person's communities (e.g., schools, religious groups, local organizations)—sometimes called the **mesosystem**—as well as society at large (e.g., laws, public policies, cultural values)—sometimes called the **macrosystem** (Bronfenbrenner, 1977). This is particularly pronounced when we are disadvantaged by what has been described as hierarchical **systems of oppression**, including racism, sexism, heterosexism, cisgenderism, ableism, classism, ageism, and religious or ethnic discrimination (Crenshaw, 2017; Hays, 2016). These systems affect us throughout our lives, and may powerfully and adversely affect our implicit mental processes even when our early experiences with caregivers were generally positive. In this edition, we expand the psychodynamic formulation to include the way that culture and society affect the development of conscious and unconscious ways of thinking about the self, others, and the world throughout life (see Chapter 20).

More than reporting

A news story gives a report of *what* happened; a psychodynamic formulation offers a hypothesis about *why* things happened. The following examples illustrate the difference.

Reporting

Nick, who is 32 years old and has been married for 10 years, presents because he needs to go on a business trip and is unable to be away from his wife for more than one night. He was born to a single teenage mother who had little support and who likely had postpartum depression. As a child, Nick had severe separation anxiety and spent long periods of time at home "sick."

Formulating

Nick, who is 32 years old and has been married for 10 years, presents because he needs to go on a business trip and is unable to be away from his wife for more than one night. He was born to a single teenage mother who had little support and who likely had postpartum depression. As a child, Nick had severe separation anxiety and spent long periods of time at home "sick." It is possible that his mother's depression affected his ability to develop a secure attachment, which makes it hard for him to think of himself as a separate person. It may have impeded his capacity to separate successfully from his mother. Now, it may be making it difficult for him to be apart from his wife for more than one night.

Although both vignettes tell a "story," only the second attempts to link the history and the problem to make an etiological hypothesis. A psychodynamic formulation is more than a story; it is a narrative that tries to explain how and why people think, feel, and behave the way they do based on their development and lived experience. In the above example, the sentences "It is possible . . ." and "This may have impeded . . ." suggest causative links between Nick's problem with separation and his history— links of which he is not aware and are, thus, unconscious. *These causative links make this a formulation rather than just a history.*

Different kinds of psychodynamic formulations

Psychodynamic formulations can explain one or many aspects of the way a person thinks, feels, or behaves. They can be based on a small amount of information (e.g., the history a clinician obtains during a single encounter in an emergency room), or an enormous amount of information (e.g., everything that a psychoanalyst learns about a patient during the course of a multi-year analysis). They can try to explain how someone behaves in a moment of therapy, during a discrete crisis, or over a lifetime. They can be used in any treatment setting, for brief or long-term treatments. If they are responses to questions about how people think, feel, and behave that consider the effect and development of conscious and unconscious thoughts and feelings, they are psychodynamic formulations.

Not a static process

It's important to remember that a psychodynamic formulation is just a hypothesis. As above, we can never really know what happened, but, in order to understand our patients better, we try to get an idea of what shaped the way they developed. Earlier in the history of psychoanalysis, the psychodynamic formulation was thought to be a definitive explanation of a person's development. Now, we understand that it is better conceptualized as a tool to improve our treatment methods and understanding of our patients.

Hypotheses are generated to be tested and revised. The same is true of psychodynamic formulations. The process of creating a psychodynamic formulation does not end when the clinician and patient first generate a hypothesis; rather, it continues for as long as they work together. The formulation represents an ever-changing, ever-growing understanding of the patient and their development. We can call this a **working psychodynamic formulation.** Over time, both patient and therapist learn about new patterns and new history. With this, new ways of thinking about development may become useful, and these can help generate new hypotheses. The process of describing patterns, reviewing the life story, and then linking the two using organizing ideas about development, is repeated again and again during the course of the treatment, shaping and honing both the therapist's and patient's understanding.

Formulating psychodynamically is ultimately a way of thinking

We think the best way to learn to formulate psychodynamically is to actually write a psychodynamic formulation. Taking the time to do this, as well as committing your ideas to paper (or screens), will help you to consolidate your ideas about a patient and to practice the skills you will learn in this book. However, not all formulations are written. Most, in fact, are not. We formulate psychodynamically all the time—when we listen to patients, when we think about patients, and when we decide what to say to patients. Ultimately, formulating psychodynamically is a way of thinking that happens constantly in a clinician's mind. Having a psychodynamic formulation—that is, having ideas about the development and workings of a patient's conscious and unconscious mind—can help you in many types of clinical situations, including acute care, inpatient units, medical settings, and primarily pharmacological treatments. Our hope is that you will use the skills you learn in this book to formulate psychodynamically all the time with *all* your patients, not just those in psychodynamic psychotherapy.

Now that we have introduced some basic concepts, let's move on to Chapter 2 to begin thinking about how we collaboratively create psychodynamic formulations.

Suggested activity

Can be done by individual learners or in a classroom setting.

Think about a recent moment you experienced with a patient in any clinical setting. Perhaps the patient was late, didn't want to speak to you, or had nothing to say. What do you think led the patient to react the way they did? Take a look at what you have written. Is it reporting or formulating? It is formulating if you have included a causative link—the reason you think this happened. Try to identify that link. If you are working in a classroom, you can do this in pairs.

References

1. Bronfenbrenner, U. (1977). Toward an experimental ecology of human development. *American Psychologist*, 32(7), 513–531. https://doi.org/10.1037/0003-066x.32.7.513
2. Campbell, W. H., & Rohrbaugh, R. M. (2013). *Biopsychosocial formulation manual: A guide for mental health professionals*. Routledge.
3. Crenshaw, K. (2017). *On intersectionality essential writings*. The New Press.
4. Devos, T., & Banaji, M. (2003). Implicit self and identity. *Annals of the New York Academy of Sciences*, 1001(1), 177–211. https://doi.org/10.1196/annals.1279.009
5. Eells, T. D. (2022). *Handbook of psychotherapy case formulation (3rd ed)*. Guilford.
6. Erikson, E. H. (1968). *Identity: Youth and crisis*. Faber & Faber.
7. Fanon, F. (2019). *Black skin, white masks*. Grove Press. (Originally published in 1952).
8. FitzGerald, C., & Hurst, S. (2017). Implicit bias in healthcare professionals: A systematic review. *BMC Medical Ethics*, 18(1). https://doi.org/10.1186/s12910-017-0179-8
9. Freud, S. (1964). Analysis terminable and interminable. In J. Strachey (Ed.), *The standard edition of the complete psychological works of Sigmund Freud, (1937–1939), volume XXIII* (pp. 209–254). Hogarth Press.
10. Hays, P. A. (2016). *Addressing cultural complexities in practice: Assessment, diagnosis, and therapy*. American Psychological Association.
11. Locke, J. (1975). In P. Nidditch (Ed.), *An essay concerning human understanding (Clarendon Edition of the Works of John Locke)*. Oxford University Press. (Original work published in 1689).
12. Wilson, E. O. (2000). *Sociobiology: A new synthesis*. Harvard University Press. (Originally published in 1975).
13. Wright, J. H., Brown, G. K., Thase, M. E., & Basco, M. R. (2017). *Learning cognitive-behavior therapy: An illustrated guide* (2nd ed). American Psychiatric Association Publishing.

2 How Do We Create a Psychodynamic Formulation?

> **Key concepts**
>
> When we create psychodynamic formulations, we
> - DESCRIBE the patient's primary problems and patterns.
> - REVIEW their life story
> - LINK problems and patterns to the life story using organizing ideas about development
>
> We co-create psychodynamic formulations with our patients.

How do we develop hypotheses to explain things we observe? It could be anything—a cultural trend, the relationship between two people, or a natural phenomenon. For example, let's say that people have a sense that there was less snowfall than usual in their town, and they want to know whether this will be a trend. First, they must define the phenomenon by using careful observation and measurement. Then, they must research the history of snowfall in the area. Once they've done this, they can use meteorological theories—for example, theories about global warming—to help them link their observations and the history to form a hypothesis about what's happening and what might happen in the future. They can then explain their hypotheses to others in a cogent way.

The three basic steps to creating a psychodynamic formulation

We follow the same steps when we create psychodynamic formulations to help us understand how and why people develop their characteristic patterns of thinking, feeling, and behaving. This process involves three basic steps:

- We DESCRIBE the primary problems and patterns
- We REVIEW the life story
- We LINK the problems and patterns to the life story using organizing ideas about development

Psychodynamic Formulation: An Expanded Approach, First Edition. The Psychodynamic Formulation Collective.
© 2022 John Wiley & Sons Ltd. Published 2022 by John Wiley & Sons Ltd.

Taken together, these three steps comprise the formulation. Each step is crucial to the process and is discussed at length in Parts Two–Four; we briefly outline them here by way of introduction.

DESCRIBE the primary patterns and problems

Before we think about *why* people developed their primary problems and patterns, we must be able to describe *what* they are. Here, we're not just talking about the chief complaint, but about the issues that underlie the person's predominant ways of thinking, feeling, and behaving. We can divide these into six basic areas of function:

- Self
- Relationships
- Adaptation
- Cognition
- Values
- Work and play

It is important to describe each of these areas in order to understand the way a person functions. To do this, we learn from what the patient *tells* us as well as from what the patient *shows* us. For example, a patient may say they get along well with others but then argue with the therapist throughout the first session. We have to use both sources of information when we describe their relationships with others. It's also essential to have more than just a surface description of each of these functions to really understand our patients. We will address all these areas and how to describe them in **Part Two**.

REVIEW the life story

When patients come to see us, we ask them about the events that led them to seek help. But to create a psychodynamic formulation, we need to do much more than that. Our goal is to learn everything we can about our patients in order to begin to create links between their life stories and the development of their primary problems and patterns. To do so, we must learn about how they **developed**. Their development begins before birth, with their family of origin, prenatal development, and genetic endowment; it includes every aspect of the first years of life, including attachment, early relationships with caregivers, and trauma; and then continues through later childhood, adolescence, and adulthood, until the present moment. Because we don't know why people develop their typical patterns, we must consider everything—we're interested in heredity and environmental factors and the relationship between the two. We want to understand periods of development that went well, as well as periods that were problematic. We need all the information we can get to begin to hypothesize causative links between the life story and the development of the patient's primary problems and patterns. Reviewing the patient's development throughout life is the subject of **Part Three**.

LINK the problems and patterns to the life story using organizing ideas about development

The final step in creating a psychodynamic formulation is linking the problems and patterns to the life story to form a longitudinal narrative that offers hypotheses about how and why patients developed their ways of thinking, feeling, and behaving. In doing this, we can be helped by **organizing ideas about development**. These organizing ideas offer different ways of conceptualizing and understanding our patients' developmental experiences. They help us think about how our patients' life stories could have led to their current problems and patterns. Different ideas may be more helpful in understanding different problems and patterns. The organizing ideas we discuss in **Part Four** address the way the following affect development:

- Trauma
- Early cognitive and emotional difficulties
- The effects of culture and society
- Conflict and defense
- Relationships with others
- The development of the self
- Attachment

Co-creating formulations—it takes two

As clinicians, we use everything we learn about our patients to consider hypotheses about the development of their conscious and unconscious mental processes. But we do not do this alone; rather, we do this collaboratively with our patients as part of the therapeutic process. We share our ideas as questions, clarifications, and ultimately interpretations, which our patients hear, reshape, and send back to us. This iterative process continues throughout treatment, helping the therapist and patient continuously deepen and enrich their understanding of the patient's mental life. Consider this collaboration between a patient and a therapist, who have been discussing the patient's anxiety during the therapist's vacation:

> Therapist: It sounds like you worried that I would never come back—even though you knew that I would. I wonder if that's the same kind of fear you had when your mother was in the hospital with postpartum depression after your brother was born—you worried she might never come home.

> Patient: Oh, interesting. You're right—of course, I knew you'd be back. I had it in my calendar and you've always come back before. But this time felt different—I was really worried. I guess that's what that dream was about. But, you know, during that time, it was my father I was worried about. I sat at the window every night, waiting for him to come home while the babysitter talked on the phone. I watched it get darker and darker and thought,' "maybe the next car will be his," and then it wasn't. And then when I saw the car turn into the driveway, I was so relieved. I'd forgotten all about that. I was probably five years old.

> Therapist— What a powerful memory. It's so helpful for us to understand.

In the previous example, the therapist has a hypothesis that the patient's current anxiety relates to an early experience. The therapist shares this idea with the patient as an interpretation. The patient hears the interpretation and uses it to access a memory with an alternative interpretation. The therapist can use this collaboration to understand more about the transference and to deepen their understanding of the patient's mind.

Once we begin to create a formulation, how do we use it? Learn more about it in Chapter 3.

Suggested activity
Can be done by individual learners or in a classroom setting

Working alone, write a short exchange between a patient and a therapist in which the patient helps to shape the therapist's understanding of a situation in therapy. Working in a group, role play this exchange.

3 How do We Use Psychodynamic Formulations?

> **Key concepts**
>
> A psychodynamic formulation is like a map—it guides every aspect of treatment.
> Having a working psychodynamic formulation enables us to
> - Make treatment recommendations and set goals
> - Understand what patients need developmentally
> - Develop therapeutic strategies and predict how patients will react in treatment
> - Construct meaningful interventions
> - Help our patients create cohesive life narratives

Formulation is our map

Having a working psychodynamic formulation means having continuously evolving ideas about the conscious and unconscious thoughts and feelings that affect our patients' ways of thinking, feeling, and behaving. But how do we learn about parts of the mind that are out of awareness? We **listen** carefully to what our patients say for clues that might guide us toward unconscious material, we **reflect** on what our patients say, and we **intervene** in ways that help them learn more about their minds (Cabaniss et al., 2017). In psychodynamic psychotherapy, we follow the patient's lead, but it does not mean we work without a map. That map is our psychodynamic formulation. When we have a sense of our patients' primary problems and patterns, their life stories, and how and why they are developing as they are, we listen to them, keeping our psychodynamic formulation in mind.

Using a psychodynamic formulation in treatment

To further explore this, consider Leila, a patient who seeks psychotherapy saying, "I'm worried my husband is going to leave me." Leila and her husband, who have been married for 15 years, are both first-generation Pakistani Americans. Leila says

---

Psychodynamic Formulation: An Expanded Approach, First Edition. The Psychodynamic Formulation Collective.
© 2022 John Wiley & Sons Ltd. Published 2022 by John Wiley & Sons Ltd.

that her husband is a "genius," and that she cannot understand why he wants to remain married to someone who just stays home and takes care of the children. She remarks

> I've become one of those boring housewives. The only thing I can talk about is the soccer schedule.

Making a treatment recommendation and setting goals

As the therapist learns about Leila, she notices that Leila is unable to say anything good about herself. The therapist also recognizes that Leila's self-effacement seems incongruous with her apparent abilities. The therapist begins to wonder why Leila has this view of herself. As the therapist listens to Leila's life story, she learns that Leila was a gifted painter who, feeling pressure from her parents and extended family to have what they called a "useful" career, gave up painting when she married. The therapist also learns that Leila's mother was a world-famous scientist who was critical of her daughter's complete lack of interest in science, preferring Leila's brother, who became a physicist. While Leila and her brother were good students, their mother pushed her brother to pursue a career in science. The therapist also asks about Leila's family's immigration history, the gender roles accepted by her family and childhood community, and the way in which self-esteem was supported and diminished in her family and culture. The therapist begins to consider an early **psychodynamic formulation** (i.e., hypothesis) that Leila has conscious and unconscious ways of perceiving herself and regulating her self-esteem that might have developed as a result of Leila's problematic relationship with her mother and comparisons with other women in her cultural community. Although the therapist knows there is much more to learn about Leila, she shares her preliminary formulation with Leila to make a **treatment recommendation** and to collaboratively **set early goals**, stating:

> It is clear to me that you are worried about your relationship with your husband. However, it also seems that you are overly tough on yourself, and that you do not allow yourself to do things that interest you. These difficulties could be related to longstanding feelings you have about yourself that may date back to your early relationship with your mother, and the ways you may have experienced yourself in your community. Exploring these feelings in a psychodynamic psychotherapy may help us understand why you are so unhappy in your current situation and help you improve both your relationships and feelings about yourself. Does that make sense to you?

Forming a therapeutic strategy

This makes sense to Leila, and she agrees to begin a twice-a-week psychodynamic psychotherapy. Beginning with the hypothesis that Leila was not able to develop an adequate sense of self, the therapist expands her early formulation to consider that Leila may have a **developmental need** to improve her self-perception and her capacity for self-esteem regulation. This forms the basis for the therapist's **therapeutic strategy**, where she will listen to everything Leila says, paying close attention to material that might relate to Leila's difficulties with her sense of self.

Conducting the treatment

For example, one year into the treatment, Leila tells her therapist,

> *You must be tired of me just talking about my problems day after day. You probably have other patients who need your help more than I do.*

The therapist uses her formulation to help Leila notice her problematic self-perception, stating,

> *I think that you presume that I, like your mother, will be disappointed in you and will be more interested in others.*

Creating a life narrative

Over time, Leila begins to believe that the therapist is, in fact, truly interested in her. Through her conversations with the therapist, she realizes that she had a distorted expectation that the therapist, like her mother, would find her dull and lacking. Together, they use this formulation to **create a life narrative** for Leila, which helps her to make sense of how she developed this problematic unconscious fantasy. In Leila's words,

> *I never realized how hurt I was that my mother wasn't as interested in me as she was in my brother. I also never understood the toll it took on the way I thought about myself, particularly as a woman. I'm now seeing that my husband isn't uninterested in me—I just presume that everyone is.*

As the treatment unfolds, Leila and her therapist deepen this formulation, and the therapist uses the evolving formulation to set goals, develop therapeutic strategies, listen to Leila, make interventions, and foster Leila's understanding of her life and how she sees herself with respect to her family, culture, and community. It will remain key to every part of the treatment, from beginning to end.

Suggested activity

Can be done by individual learners or in a classroom setting

Think about a patient with whom you are working. Write a few sentences about

- The goals toward which you and the patient are working in therapy
- Your therapeutic strategy (i.e., how you hope to achieve those goals)

How might you describe your therapeutic strategy to the patient? If you are working in a classroom setting, consider sharing in pairs or larger groups.

Reference

1. Cabaniss, D. L., Cherry, S., Douglas, C. J., & Schwartz, A. (2017). *Psychodynamic psychotherapy: A clinical manual.* Wiley Blackwell.

4 Psychodynamic Formulation and Bias

Key concepts

We have **bias** when we disproportionately favor an idea or thing, usually in a way that is closed-minded, prejudicial, or unfair. Bias that operates out of awareness is called **implicit bias**.

Psychodynamic formulations are inevitably influenced by the biases of the formulator.

Formulations can be damaging when influenced by harmful biases.

Therapists can provide more culturally informed care when they consider a patient's broader socio-cultural environment when formulating.

Like all people, therapists have internal lives and past experiences that shape the way they view the world. Furthermore, like all people, therapists have prejudices for or against certain ideas or people. These are known as their **biases**. When they operate out of our awareness, they are known as **implicit biases** (Banaji & Greenwald, 2016). These biases affect everything we do, including our work with patients, and thus affect the way we formulate psychodynamically.

Without the lab findings of medical formulations, psychodynamic formulations are inevitably subject to the biases of the formulator. Biased formulations have been, and continue to be, hurtful to patients. Having awareness of the historical context of psychodynamic formulation and our own theoretical biases can make our formulations more useful to our patients and their treatment.

The historical context

The history of psychodynamic formulations has too often been characterized by a tendency to fill in gaps in knowledge, including the lack of empirical data, with biases reflecting the belief system of the formulator. For example, consider the following formulation from 1938 of a patient with recurrent ulcers, which, at the time, were thought to be a psychosomatic illness:

> *This patient is a 41-year-old female attorney who came to analysis for recurrent duodenal ulcer, agoraphobia, handwriting difficulties, and a feeling of social maladjustment. This patient exhibited certain personality trends described as frequent in ulcer personalities. Specifically, I refer to the intense incorporating tendencies that are repressed and led to overcompensation through increased activity and ambitious effort in life. She is an aggressive, hard-working, efficient, and successful attorney (Wilson, 1938, pp. 23–24).*

Psychoanalytic literature abounds with cases formulating putative psychological causes of ulcers. Yet, in 1982, Barry Marshall and Robin Warren, two Australian gastro-enterologists, who would later win the Nobel Prize in medicine, discovered *Helicobacter pylori*, the bacterium found to cause gastric ulcers. Antibiotics now treat what was once considered a psychosomatic illness brought on by intrapsychic conflicts.

Ulcers were not the only symptoms subject to misuse by psychodynamic formulations. For many decades, male homosexuality was formulated as a psychological and behavioral problem arising from a man's early relationship with his mother. Consider this formulation from 1955:

> *The case demonstrates that the mother had long been unconsciously seductive with her son and that this parent's specific permissive impulse, communicated to the patient as an adolescent, induced his overt homosexual behavior. His father was obsessed with business and had little association with his wife and children. . ... His mother, who was still alive, dominated her children, especially the patient, with her ambivalent solicitude. . ... The patient made a strong, hostile, feminine identification with her (Kolb & Johnson, 1955, p. 508).*

To this date, the "causes" of homosexuality—or of heterosexuality, for that matter—remain unknown and a question of ongoing scientific interest (Bailey et al., 2016). While formulations like the one above with little scientific basis dominated psychodynamic thinking for much of the Twentieth century, in 1973 the American Psychiatric Association removed the diagnosis of homosexuality from its *Diagnostic and Statistical Manual of Mental Disorders* (DSM). In 1992, The World Health Organization (WHO) followed suit by removing the diagnosis from the International Classification of Diseases (ICD-10) (Bayer, 1981; Drescher, 2015). Nevertheless, it took several decades for psychoanalytic practitioners, deeply attached to their own formulations, to accept the growing consensus that homosexuality was a normal expression of human sexuality (Drescher, 2008).

Theoretical bias

Biases may also be related to the theoretical orientation of the clinician. There are many different "schools" of psychoanalysis (e.g., ego psychology, self-psychology, and object relations theory), each of which ascribes different meanings and importance to developmental milestones (Greenberg & Mitchell, 1983; Stepansky, 2009). Thus, psychodynamic formulations will differ depending on the theoretical orientation of the formulator. For example, one could imagine that the same problem formulated according to concepts of each of these theoreticians might place the formative years at diverse points in development:

Psychoanalytic Theoretician	Important Phase of Development
Melanie Klein (Klein, 1935)	1st year of life
Sigmund Freud (Freud, 1924/1961)	1st 3–4 years of life
Harry Stack Sullivan (Sullivan, 1956)	Pre-adolescence (ages 9–12)
Erik Erikson (Erikson, 1950/1995)	Vulnerable periods throughout the life cycle

Different theories will yield different formulations, and thus always using a single psychodynamic theory may introduce bias in our formulations.

The broad impact of the environment

As discussed in Chapter 1, psychodynamic formulations have always considered the way in which nature and nurture intersect. However, limiting our formulations to considerations of the impact of the immediate environment (primary caregivers) and leaving out the impact of culture and society at large can introduce bias to our formulations. Consider the following:

> *Robert is a 70-year-old African-American man who grew up in a low-income neighborhood of a large industrial northern U.S. city. His parents, the children of sharecroppers, were part of the "great migration" in the early part of the Twentieth century. Both died young, leaving Robert in the care of an aunt who had five children of her own. Robert did not finish high school and has had difficulty making ends meet throughout his life. He and his wife raised three boys, whom they have trained to be wary of White people and to "watch their backs" when in White neighborhoods. Having recently had cancer surgery, he is now depressed and seeks treatment in a local clinic. He is wary of his White therapist, who is also a psychiatry resident and who suggests medication. When discussing Robert with her supervisor, the therapist formulates Robert's "paranoia" about her as being largely secondary to his "abandonment at a young age," and his subsequent difficulty developing trust for his caregivers.*

Robert's immediate environment may have clearly had an impact on the development of his conscious and unconscious ways of thinking about himself and others. However the resident's formulation does not take into consideration that being a Black man in the United States, particularly one who is the son and grandson of people dramatically affected by racism, may have understandably led him to mistrust White people. This clear bias in the psychodynamic formulation will inevitably affect the treatment.

The humility of formulating

Psychodynamic formulations are useful clinical tools. However, formulations that do not take into account the prejudices and biases of the formulator and the patient's socio-cultural context will generally be less than ideal. We suggest approaching psychodynamic formulation with humility, an open mind, and a willingness to learn from our patients and from one another. In the next chapter, we will explore the ways that **cultural differences and similarities** between therapist and patient can also potentially introduce bias into the formulation.

Suggested activity
Can be done by individual learners or in a classroom setting

List two biases that might affect the way that you think about patients. These could relate to your own background and identity, or could relate to your theoretical perspective or training. In a class, consider discussing this in small groups.

References

1. Bailey, M.J., Vasey, P.L., Diamond, L.M., Breedlove, S.M., Vilain, E. & Epprecht, M. (2016). Sexual orientation, controversy and science. *Psychological Science in the Public Interest*, 17(2):45–101.
2. Banaji, M. R., & Greenwald, A. G. (2016). *Blindspot: Hidden biases of good people*. Bantam Books.
3. Bayer, R. (1981). *Homosexuality and American psychiatry*. Basic Books.
4. Drescher, J. (2008). A history of homosexuality and organized psychoanalysis. *The Journal of the American Academy of Psychoanalysis and Dynamic Psychiatry*, 36(3), 443–460. https://doi.org/10.1521/jaap.2008.36.3.443
5. Drescher, J. (2015). Out of DSM: Depathologizing homosexuality. *Behavioral Sciences*, 5(4), 565–575. https://doi.org/10.3390/bs5040565
6. Erikson, E. H. (1995). *Childhood and society*. Vintage. (Originally published in 1950).
7. Freud, S. (1961) The Dissolution of the Oedipus Complex. In J. Strachey (Ed). The Standard Edition of the Complete Psychological Works of Sigmund Freud, (1923–1925), Volume XIX (pp. 173–182). Hogarth Press. (Originally published in 1924).
8. Greenberg, J. R., & Mitchell, S. A. (1983). *Object relations in psychoanalytic theory*. Harvard University Press.
9. Klein, M. A. (1935). Contribution to the psychogenesis of manic-depressive states. *International Journal of Psychoanalysis*, 16, 145–174.
10. Kolb, L. C., & Johnson, A. M. (1955). *Etiology and therapy of overt homosexuality*. The *Psychoanalytic Quarterly*, 24(4), 506–515. https://doi.org/10.1080/21674086.1955.11926000
11. Stepansky, P. E. (2009). *Psychoanalysis at the margins*. Other Press.
12. Sullivan, H. S. (1956). *Clinical studies in psychiatry*. Norton.
13. Wilson, G. W. (1938). The transition from organ neurosis to conversion hysteria. *International Journal of Psychoanalysis*, 19, 23–40.

5 Who We Are Affects Our Formulations

Key concepts

Who we are as people affects every aspect of the treatments we conduct, including how we formulate. This encompasses how we feel about ourselves, our connections to our communities, and our relationship to society at large.

Every patient-therapist pair is unique, and thus every psychodynamic formulation is distinct and co-constructed.

The more we understand ourselves and our perspectives, the more we can appreciate how these perspectives shape the way we see our patients and conceptualize our formulations. We can use our feelings to help in doing so.

Being different from our patients presents certain challenges in terms of formulation, as does being similar to them. Therapists from marginalized groups may choose to discuss feelings about identity or racial differences with their patients as part of the collaborative process of formulation.

As therapists, we strive to maintain an open and neutral stance about our patients. Nevertheless, the way we formulate is invariably filtered through the lens of who we are as therapists and people. Our training as mental health professionals affects the way we think about our patients, as does our gender, race, sexual orientation, gender identity, age, gender expression, religion, abilities and disabilities, culture, education, socio-economics, appearance, trauma history, and individual psychology. For example, a White cisgender heterosexual, upper-middle-class, male therapist may need to reflect on his own privilege when treating a patient who may not have the same advantages as he. Our own experiences of privilege—of any type—might make it challenging for us to understand the disadvantages our patients who lack privilege may face (Tummala-Narra, 2021).

Every therapeutic pair is unique

When a patient and a therapist meet for a consultation or to begin treatment, it's a meeting of two distinct individuals. Each person comes to the meeting with their

Psychodynamic Formulation: An Expanded Approach, First Edition. The Psychodynamic Formulation Collective.
© 2022 John Wiley & Sons Ltd. Published 2022 by John Wiley & Sons Ltd.

own genetics and life story. No two patient-therapist pairings are alike. Thus, each treatment is different, and each collaboratively constructed psychodynamic formulation is unique. Of course, two therapists with very different life stories may notice similar themes as they relate to a patient, but differences will always be found. For example, a therapist who is a twin treating a patient who is also a twin will likely have a different experience of the patient than will a therapist who is not a twin— although both therapists may note the patient's wish to be someone's "one and only." Every treatment is unique with respect not only to the therapeutic pair, but also the historical, social, cultural, and systemic contexts in which the therapy takes place (Bonovitz, 2005). Our understanding of our patients may be enriched or clouded by our life experience. The aim is not to eliminate the effects of our individuality, which is actually impossible and unhelpful. Rather, it is to be as aware of our perspectives as possible, so we can use them to understand our patients and ourselves.

When we are different from our patients

When treating people whose backgrounds are different or unfamiliar to us, we may feel uncomfortable with not knowing, we may avoid topics related to the difference, or we may be overly curious in ways that serve our curiosity rather than the patients' needs. Sometimes, we may even have conscious or unconscious ideas about our patients that reflect our own implicit biases. The more we can be aware of our biases, the more we will be able to understand our patients' experiences and collaboratively create useful psychodynamic formulations. Consider the following:

A 50-year-old White female therapist has been treating Christine, a 45-year-old Taiwanese American woman who was born and raised in the United States in a middle-class, predominantly White community. In the course of their two-year psychotherapy, the patient focused on her relationships and career. The therapist never asked directly about the patient's race, and the patient never spontaneously discussed it. The therapist did not make much of the absence of this discussion, as she had not reflected on her own feelings about her race or Whiteness, and she followed Christine's lead in not discussing race.

In the wake of the rise of anti-Asian hate and violence during the COVID-19 pandemic, Christine began exploring her feelings about being Asian. In particular, she expressed fears about the safety of her family members and herself. She also felt angry and distraught that despite being an American, she would be seen by some as a perpetual foreigner because of her appearance. As the therapist listened to Christine, she wondered about why Christine's race was never discussed in therapy. The therapist speculated that her avoidance of the topic was related to the fact of her being White. After empathizing with Christine's anger and confusion about the rise in overt racism in America, the therapist said, "I realize that race is a central part of your experience, and I wonder how it feels to talk about this with me since I am White." Christine then acknowledged that this was a difficult subject because she feared the therapist would not be able to understand her. They then talked about how not feeling fully understood is central to Christine's experience in many relationships, and how feeling different has permeated her life.

When we are similar to our patients

Similarity to our patients can facilitate our understanding, but it can also lead us to miss areas where our stories do not align (Comas-Diaz & Jacobsen, 1991), as in the following:

> *A 55-year-old African-American female therapist is treating Frances, a 50-year-old African American woman from a similar background. Frances, a health professional, has not been able to work for years. Although the therapeutic relationship seemed positive, the therapist noticed that Frances was failing to move forward in her life but not addressing this in sessions. Instead, Frances often shared stories about how she hoped to get her life back on track, but inevitably something would get in the way. The therapist found Frances to be a compelling patient and wanted to believe that Frances would eventually succeed despite evidence to the contrary. At the same time, because the therapist had the lingering concern that Frances was not advancing in treatment or in life, she decided to talk about Frances in a peer supervision group. It was immediately apparent that the members of the supervision group felt that Frances was flailing and in denial of her difficulties. They also wondered whether she might be more limited than she presented herself to be. Reflecting on this different perspective, the therapist realized that she had failed to fully see Frances' difficulties because of their shared racial and professional backgrounds. The similarities between them served to preserve a friendly repartee that originally may have facilitated an alliance, but over time prevented the therapist from addressing Frances' problems. With this realization, the therapist was able to reformulate the struggles in Frances' career as related to her difficulty in acknowledging personal limitations.*

How to be aware of the way that our similarities to and differences from our patients affects formulation

As we work with patients, continuously learning about our identities and feelings about our patients helps us to mitigate potential biases and deepen our work.

Learning about our identities and how they affect our formulations

Being aware of our own identities and the way they affect our work as therapists is facilitated by regularly asking ourselves questions like the following:

> *How do I understand my various identities (e.g., gender, race, sexual orientation, gender identity, class, ability status, age, religion, socio-economics, professional)?*
>
> *How might my privilege be contributing to blindspots when formulating?*
>
> *What assumptions am I making about myself, patients, and treatment based on my identities and training?*
>
> *How do my assumptions inform how I understand and formulate my clinical work?*

Learning about our feelings about patients and how this affects our formulations

Similarly, being aware of our feelings about our patients and how they affect our formulation is facilitated by regularly asking ourselves questions like the following:

How does this patient make me feel?

What is happening in the treatment to make me feel this way?

How are these feelings related to issues with myself or with the patient, and what is happening between us?

Could these feelings be related to something that was said, done, or unspoken?

Now that I can identify my feelings about the patient, how can I use them to formulate about what is happening with the patient or in the treatment?

Having reviewed this introductory material about formulations, let's move on to **Part Two: DESCRIBE**, the first step of psychodynamic formulation.

Suggested activity

Can be done by individual learners or in a classroom setting

Think about a patient who you think is similar to you. Write a few sentences about the way that you think the similarities are affecting the treatment. Then, think about a patient who you think is different from you. Write a few sentences about the way that you think the differences are affecting the treatment. If you are working in a classroom, consider sharing these impressions in groups.

References

1. Bonovitz, C. (2005). Locating culture in the psychic field: Transference and countertransference as cultural products. *Contemporary Psychoanalysis, 41*(1), 55–76.
2. Comas-Diaz, L., & Jacobsen, F. M. (1991). Ethnocultural transference and countertransference in the therapeutic dyad. *American Journal of Orthopsychiatry, 61*(3), 392–402.
3. Tummala-Narra, P. (2021). Racial trauma and dissociated worlds within psychotherapy: A discussion of "Racial difference, rupture, and repair: A view from the couch and back". *Psychoanalytic Dialogues, 30*(6), 732–741.

PART TWO: Describe

Introduction

When we think about how something **functions**, we consider whether it does what it was designed to do. A refrigerator is designed to keep food at a low temperature, so if the milk is cold, it is functioning well, and if the milk is warm, it is functioning poorly. A car is designed to transport people from place to place, so if it reliably allows us to get around, it is functioning well, and if it is always in the shop, it is functioning poorly. Things that are designed to have multiple functions can sometimes work well in one way but not another. For example, if a desk chair that is meant to be both comfortable and stylish creates a sleek look in an office but leaves workers with backaches, it is fulfilling one function but not the other.

While it's easy to know the intended function of a refrigerator or a chair, it's much harder to know what a person is supposed to be able to do. For example, should all people work? Get married? Have children? Belong to a religious organization? Be altruistic? As mental health professionals, it is not our job to make those kinds of judgments. On the contrary, we know that there are as many ways to live as there are people on Earth. However, when people **suffer**, it suggests that their functioning may be faltering in some way.

Before explaining, first describe!

We create formulations to try to explain how and why people function the way they do. We must be able to describe their function before we can explain it. We can do this by describing both the **problem** and the **person**.

Describing the problem

We can define the **problem** as what is giving the person the most difficulty *right now*. It is generally, but not always, the reason they give for consulting a mental health professional. Sometimes we agree with patients about the primary problem, and sometimes we don't. Either way, we must acknowledge and address their concerns. Here are a few examples of problems that bring people to psychotherapy:

> *I need help understanding my teenage daughter.*
>
> *I need help figuring out whether or not I should get divorced.*
>
> *I need help because I am so anxious at work.*
>
> *I feel alienated from my community.*
>
> *My doctor thinks I should see a therapist to get back on my feet after being fired.*
>
> *I want to figure out why I can't seem to have a romantic relationship.*

Of course, many patients have more than one problem. They might have depression and ongoing difficulty with a spouse, or they might drink too much and have an ailing parent. Nevertheless, to focus the formulation, it is important to be able to identify and describe what is most troubling the person *right now*. Challenge yourself to answer the question, "Why did this person come to see me *now*?" and you are likely to identify the primary problem.

It is important to get all the details about the problem, whether it is an interpersonal difficulty or symptoms of a mood or anxiety disorder. Carefully diagnosing our patients' cognitive and emotional difficulties (e.g., attention deficit disorder, eating disorders, anxiety and mood disorders, etc.) is critical to understanding their conscious and unconscious thoughts, feelings, and behaviors.

Describing the person

We have defined the **problem** as what is giving the patient the most difficulty *right now*. But to fully understand the way someone functions, we also must be able to describe the way they *generally* think, feel, and behave. We call this describing the **person**. To consider the differences between the **problem** and the **person**, consider Kate and Millie, two people in their thirties who have recently been left by their respective long-term partners. Although they have the same problem, they are experiencing it very differently:

Kate—I feel desperate and alone. I have no one else. I call my partner every day, begging her to come home. Last night, I said that I'd cut myself if she didn't come home. I feel completely unlovable—I'll never be able to have another relationship. Who will help me with the children?

Millie—I'd be lying if I said that I wasn't shocked and upset. I am. But my friends and family have been amazing—calling and helping out with the kids. I feel so lucky. I'm trying to focus on the kids so their lives will be minimally disrupted. I'm not ready to date, but that will come in time, too.

It's likely that Kate and Millie reacted differently to a similar problem because they generally functioned differently before the problem arose. This general, ongoing functioning is what we refer to as the **person**; thus, we have to know who the person is as well as the problem that they have.

Describing patterns helps us to describe the person

We can describe the **person** by describing their characteristic ways of thinking, feeling, and behaving. We can call these their characteristic **patterns**. By the time they are adults, people develop characteristic patterns in several aspects of their lives. Throughout the ages, observers of human behavior have used different methods to describe people's characteristic ways of functioning. Some of these methods have attempted to place these people with differing characteristics into **categories**, based on their certain shared features. Hippocrates categorized people according to their balance of four essential bodily fluids (Arikha, 2007), Freud grouped people according to their fixations along a psychosexual developmental pathway Freud (1905/1953), and the *Diagnostic and Statistical Manual of Mental Disorders* (DSM) categorizes people using lists of shared characteristics (American Psychiatric Association, 2022). However, more and more researchers in this area advocate describing people's characteristic patterns of thinking and behaving using a set of **dimensions** (Cloninger, 2000; Widiger, 2005). In this book, we take this dimensional approach, using six basic areas of function:

- Self
- Relationships
- Adapting
- Cognition
- Values
- Work and play

We describe each area in more depth using a series of **variables**. Learning about and being able to describe every patient's functioning in each of these areas is essential to learning about them as a person. How and why a person develops one pattern versus another is an important aspect of what we want to try to understand using our psychodynamic formulation. In Chapters 6–11, we describe each of these areas, including the basics of the area, common patterns in that area, and ways to assess the area.

Strengths and difficulties

People are complex, and even within one area of function, they may have strengths and difficulties. Some people function very well in one area but have more difficulty in another. Consider a person who has never had a long-term romantic relationship, but who has many close friends with whom they socialize and confide. Or consider a person who is an excellent manager and businessperson but is extremely anxious in social situations and hides out at home on weekends. Like most people, these individuals are **mosaics**, with good function in one area and more difficulty in another.

Sometimes, as mental health professionals, we focus exclusively on problems and neglect areas of strength and resilience. However, we need to rely on our patients' strengths to help them build new, more beneficial ways of functioning. Describing our patients' strengths and difficulties allows us to hypothesize about both in our psychodynamic formulations.

Conscious and unconscious patterns

People are aware of some, but not all, of the ways they think, feel, and behave. Consider the way two people present to a therapist:

> I have so much trouble feeling good about myself. I've always been like that, ever since I was a child. It's something I'd like to work on.

> My partner said that it was either therapy or separation. That I don't listen to him. Why should I? He drones on all the time about work—accounting—what could be more boring? By the way, you need a new receptionist. Yours mispronounced my name twice—not too bright.

Both people seem to have difficulty with self-esteem. However, this is conscious for the first person, while it emerges in the behavior of the second. When we think psychodynamically, we are interested in both conscious and unconscious patterns.

To learn about patients, ask about stories

To collaboratively create psychodynamic formulations, we must help our patients tell us about their inner lives. A good way to do this is to ask them to tell us stories about themselves. These could be stories about long ago or stories about yesterday.

Stories about friends, family, wishes, fears, and dreams help us to understand the richness of our patients' conscious and unconscious minds. A good way to ask about stories is to first ask an opening question, and then to ask for a story. For example:

> *Therapist: Do you have someone who you consider to be your best friend?*
>
> *Patient: Yes*
>
> *Therapist: What's that person's first name?*
>
> *Patient: Jeanine*
>
> *Therapist: What's Jeanine like? Can you tell me about something that you and Jeanine did recently that really meant a lot to you?*

Asking for a first name brings the patient's friend to life. Suddenly, there's a real person in the room. Then, asking for a story brings their personal relationship to life.

At the end of each section in this part of the book, we suggest questions that can help us to describe our patients. We find that using these as opening questions, followed by requests for stories, aids our patients in telling us about their inner lives.

Looking ahead

Each area of function is important, and allowing ourselves to learn about them all is essential to describing our patients. Let's move on to Chapter 6 and patterns related to the **self**.

References

1. American Psychiatric Association. (2022). *Diagnostic and statistical manual of mental disorders* (5th ed.). American Psychiatric Press.
2. Arikha, N. (2007). *Passions and tempers*. HarperCollins.
3. Cloninger, C. R. (2000). Biology of personality dimensions. *Current Opinion in Psychiatry*, *13*(6), 611–616.
4. Freud, S. (1953). Three essays on the theory of sexuality. In J. Strachey (Ed.), *The standard edition of the complete psychological works of Sigmund Freud, volume VII (1901–1905): A case of hysteria, three essays on sexuality and other works*. Hogarth Press. (Originally published in 1905).
5. Widiger, T. A. (2005). Five factor model of personality disorder: integrating science and practice. *Journal of Research in Personality*, *39*(1), 67–83.

6 Self

Key concepts

By the time we are adults, we develop characteristic patterns of experiencing ourselves. We can describe these patterns using the following variables:

- Self-perception
  - Identity
  - Fantasies about the self
- Self-esteem regulation, including the following:
  - Vulnerability to self-esteem threats
  - Use of others to help regulate self-esteem
  - Internal response to self-esteem threats
  - External effects on self-esteem

Failed exams, breakups, job loss, discrimination, bullying, medical illness—life is full of experiences that threaten our sense of who we are and our ability to feel good about ourselves. Why do some people cope with these situations without a loss of self-esteem, while others are devastated? In order to form hypotheses about this, we must be able to describe the characteristic ways people experience their sense of **self** (Kohut, 1977).

Defining the area: self

When we write "identifying information" about people in a psychological or medical history, we usually start with a sentence that outlines certain things about them, such as their age, gender, sexuality, relationship status, racial/cultural group, and employment. When we think about people's self-experiences in a psychodynamic formulation, however, we must consider not only their demographics but also their conscious and unconscious thoughts and feelings about themselves.

Psychodynamic Formulation: An Expanded Approach, First Edition. The Psychodynamic Formulation Collective.
© 2022 John Wiley & Sons Ltd. Published 2022 by John Wiley & Sons Ltd.

Variables for describing patterns related to the self

We can describe a person's self-experience using two major variables:

- Self-perception
- Self-esteem regulation

Self-perception

Everything we do in life, from having relationships with others to choosing what we do for work and play, relates to how we think about ourselves—it is our **self-perception**. Having a realistic idea of what we can do and what we like to do helps us choose relationships and activities that bring us satisfaction and pleasure, and helps us maintain good feelings about ourselves even in the face of adversity. Thus, our self-experience is central to the way we function.

Variables for describing self-perception

We can describe self-perception using two **variables:**

- Identity
- Fantasies about the self

Identity

Identity is the part of self-perception that specifically includes a person's relation to their surrounding culture (Auchincloss & Samberg, 2012). We have individual identities (i.e., our sense of ourselves as unique), group identities (i.e., our sense of ourselves in relation to others), and universal identities (i.e., our sense of ourselves as part of the human race) (Sue et al., 2019). Group identities are based on variables, such as race and ethnicity, gender, sexual orientation, gender identity, religion, age, abilities and disabilities, and profession. Our sense of belonging to groups can be based on shared values, ways in which we are seen, and/or common experiences. Group identities can fluctuate and develop over time, have varying levels of importance throughout our lives, and are more in the forefront of our minds when they involve differences that can be seen by others. Adults have varying ability to readily access different parts of themselves across time and in different situations (Bromberg, 1998). For example, consider two people who've left their out-of-the-home jobs when they had children. One says, "Even though I miss my job as a music teacher, I am excited to teach my daughter to enjoy music," while the other says, "Ever since I stopped working, I feel lost and don't know who I am." The first person can maintain a professional identity while also enjoying an identity as a parent, yet the second cannot. The ability to access multiple identities simultaneously can help people feel whole and satisfied as their lives change over time.

Fantasies about the self

At all stages of life, **fantasies about the self** are narratives that structure how we live—for example, a student imagines being praised by a teacher for a well-done assignment, a teenager imagines going on a date with someone whom they like, a scientist imagines winning a Nobel Prize, and a retired person imagines being a beloved grandparent. These fantasies can provide us with comfort, goals, and escapes (Blos, 1972; Freud, 1914/1966) and can also help us move forward, strive, and achieve. Those of us who have fantasies about the self which are accurately attuned to our talents and limitations are more likely to feel good about ourselves than those of us who cling to personal goals that are not consonant with our abilities (Kohut & Wolff, 1978).

We have both conscious and unconscious fantasies about ourselves. While patients may be able to tell us their conscious fantasies, we must learn about their unconscious fantasies in other ways—for example, by listening to dreams and noticing behaviors. For example, consider the unmarried sister of a bride who says, "I don't know why I was upset after her wedding. I never wanted to get married, and I gave the best toast." Although she consciously experiences herself as the perennial bridesmaid, her feelings after her sister's wedding, as well as what sounds like a wish to have "stolen the show," suggests that she may have unconscious fantasies about taking center stage as a bride herself.

Self-esteem regulation

Esteem is respect or admiration, so self-esteem is the respect or admiration we have for ourselves. We develop self-esteem by feeling valued by ourselves or others, or by feeling connected to those we admire. Most of us begin life excited by our abilities— think of the joy on babies' faces when they say their first words or take their first steps. But maintaining self-esteem in the face of everything that happens to us during life can sometimes feel like a never-ending obstacle course. The ability to pick oneself up after disappointments or slights is called **self-esteem regulation** and is an important part of how people function in the world (Reich, 1960; Sandler et al., 1963).

Variables for describing self-regulation

Anything that imperils good feelings about oneself is a **self-esteem threat** (sometimes called a **narcissistic injury**) (Kohut, 1972). Because people vary in the way they perceive and respond to self-esteem threats, we can use the following **variables** to describe individual patterns of self-esteem regulation:

- Vulnerability to self-esteem threats
- Internal response to self-esteem threats
- Use of others to help regulate self-esteem
- Responses to external effects on self-esteem

Vulnerability to self-esteem threats

Some people can maintain their positive self-regard in the face of massive emotional injuries, such as severe medical illness or job loss, while others crumble if someone looks at them the wrong way. An individual's vulnerability to self-esteem threats may vary across situations. For example, a person might be able to handle criticism from people at work but be very sensitive to criticism from a partner.

Self-esteem vulnerability is often apparent in the way someone reacts to being compared with others. Some of us have no difficulty maintaining good feelings about ourselves when we lack something others have, while others find this intolerable. When people are so unable to tolerate this situation that they need to destroy what others have, we say they are **envious**; if they just want to be on par with others, we say they are **jealous** (Neubauer, 1982). Consider two people who admire the outfit of an acquaintance at a party; one mocks it as "garish" to a gathered group, while the other makes a mental note of it for later purchase. Envy leads to the wish to destroy, while jealousy leads to the wish to imitate.

Internal response to self-esteem threats

When people experience a threat to their sense of self, they respond in a way that helps them to buoy self-esteem. This entire process may occur unconsciously. The mechanisms they use to maintain good feelings about themselves begin to develop in childhood and coalesce into fairly stable patterns by adulthood.

Responses to self-esteem threats can include inflating or deflating one's sense of self. **Grandiosity** is a massive and unwarranted overconfidence that protects people from the pain of facing their limitations. People who rely on grandiosity are often described as **narcissistic** (Kernberg, 1970). They tend to externalize their failures, become enraged and demanding, and belittle others. They are unaware that although this enables them to preserve self-esteem, it is often at the expense of their relationships with others. Think, for example, of a person who has no experience in screenwriting who says, "Most writers today are hacks. Besides, I have the name of someone in the industry—it will just take one phone call and I'll be an insider." Inflating one's self-esteem could help offset this person's insecurity, but perhaps at the cost of the good opinion of others.

In contrast, deflating one's sense of self—another response to self-esteem threats— leads to **self-deprecation** and **masochism** (Cooper, 1988). Unable to think of redeeming qualities about themselves, people who respond in this way often self-sabotage and deny their own needs. For example, a talented writer might respond to getting an "A" on a writing assignment by thinking, "The professor is just taking pity on me. I'll never make it." In the face of failure, both the grandiose and masochistic strategies often lead to depression and even the risk of suicide.

Other ways to restore self-esteem include **becoming more or less competitive**. These responses may affect a person's global ability to function and may cause difficulties and distress. The sibling of a varsity athlete might become so competitive on the tennis court that others avoid playing with them, while anxiety might make a small business owner forget deadlines and lose potential contracts. One person deals with insecurity by becoming more competitive, while the other deals with similar feelings by staying on the sidelines. The most useful responses to self-esteem threats tend to be flexible. Humor, sublimation, and altruism help people to restore good feelings about themselves without sacrificing other functions or relationships. Take, for example, a person who had to relinquish their dream of higher education in order to care for a dying parent and now feels proud of being able to help pay for their sibling to finish college. In this case, altruism is a useful way to cope with disappointment.

Use of others to help regulate self-esteem

We all desire admiration from the people we love. Nothing feels as good as hearing "great work!" for a job well done. When given in appropriate amounts, admiration is central to the development of self-esteem (see Chapter 17). Some people, however, require constant attention, praise, and validation from others to manage their self-esteem. They fish for compliments, repeatedly ask for validation, and make themselves the center of attention—often to such a degree that they deplete family and friends with their constant demands. These people require the input of others to regulate their self-esteem. They may even act as if other people exist solely to boost their self-esteem, indicating a lack of **empathy** (see Chapter 5) (MacKinnon, et al., 2006).

Others, however, have self-esteem regulation strategies that enable them to take advice, metabolize it, and make their own decisions. They take pleasure and pride in their accomplishments, and are also able to effectively rely on others to feel better about themselves.

Responses to external effects on self-esteem

Living in a society that upholds White, heteronormative, and gender-conforming norms may cause those of us who are not aligned with those values to question our place and our worth. Being the target of racism, prejudice, or daily injustices can cause us to absorb societal messages that deem our differences as less worthy, and it can be experienced as an assault on the self. (The impact of race on the self is discussed further in Chapters 16 and 20.) Some members of marginalized groups may respond to being discriminated against or oppressed by harboring hatred toward their own or other disadvantaged groups (sometimes called **lateral violence**) (Maracle, 1996). Another reaction is **mimicry** (Eng & Han, 2000; Fanon, 1952/1967), which has been described in Black and Indigenous People of Color (BIPOCs) who have implicitly adopted assigned racial roles or attempted to align with White values rather than their own. The end result can be a feeling of fraudulence that has been likened to a **false self** (Eng & Han, 2000; Winnicott, 1965). The false self is a way of relating to other people and to the world through compliance or passivity; doing so protects against having to expose a more authentic, hidden experience of oneself (the so-called **true self**). As described in Chapters 16 and 20, these responses are not necessarily pathological, and can be self-preservative when we are disadvantaged because of race, gender, religion, sexual orientation, gender expression, or disabilities.

Many authors (DuBois, 1897; Erikson, 1968; Harris, 2012; Hong, 2020; Yi, 2014) have described how those of us who are BIPOC can also respond to systemic oppression with feelings of pride and belonging. Additionally, those of us from marginalized groups can question the systems of oppression rather than ourselves, and can respond with resilience, righteous indignation, and anger.

Learning about patterns related to the self: opening questions, then stories

It's generally hard for us to talk about ourselves, particularly when we are discussing aspects of our lives that make us feel vulnerable. We can keep that in mind when we ask our patients about self-perception and self-esteem. The following suggested questions can help us to listen actively and sensitively ask about this important domain of function. Beginning with opening questions and following with requests for stories helps us to learn the most about the ways that people consciously and unconsciously think about themselves.

Learning about self-perception, including identity

Sometimes, direct questions about identity and fantasies can be helpful. For example:

> *How accurate do you think your sense of your strengths and difficulties is? What do others say about that? Do they tend to think that you can do more than you think that you can?*
>
> *Do you think that you won't be able to do things that you actually can—or is it the other way around?*
>
> *Would people describe you as someone who knows who they are?*
>
> *With what groups do you feel identified? Has that been consistent throughout your life?*

Learning about self-esteem regulation

Learning about self-esteem vulnerability

Asking direct questions about envy, jealousy, and self-esteem vulnerability can make people anxious and defensive. Instead, try asking questions about common situations to learn about this area:

> *How do you feel when you're in a group of people who seem to be wealthier/more accomplished/ more highly educated than you are?*
>
> *Tell me about a time when you didn't get something you really wanted. How did it make you feel?*
>
> *How do you feel when a friend accomplishes something that you haven't been able to do?*
>
> *All people have things that make them feel less than good about themselves. What kinds of things make you feel that way?*

Learning about internal responses to self-esteem threats

Listen for stories that reference disappointments or failures, and ask questions that will help you learn about the person's response. For example:

> *Do you tend to feel that others around you are incompetent?*
>
> *Do you generally feel like the smartest/least intelligent person in the room?*
>
> *Do you think that people would tend to describe you as competitive?*
>
> *How do you generally go about getting something you want?*

Learning about external effects on self-esteem

Ask about stories that relate to the effects of society on the person's sense of self:

> *Can you tell me about a place where you feel like you really belong? Are there places where you feel you really don't belong? How do you feel in each?*
>
> *Can you tell me about a time when others made you feel bad because of things about you that seemed beyond your control? How did you respond?*
>
> *Do you feel like you've been subject to discrimination or prejudice, and if so, in what way?*

Learning about the use of others for self-esteem regulation

Ask for stories that relate to the use of others for self-esteem regulation:

> *How do you know when you've done a good job? Can you feel this without hearing it from others? Are you able to make decisions without input from others?*

Describing self-experience

Now, let's consider Sam, and the way that we can use the variables outlined in this chapter to describe his patterns related to the self:

> *Sam is a 45-year-old man who is married, has two children, and supports his middle-class family by working in advertising. He says he loves his children and being a father. He explains that his husband "sent" him to therapy because, "I'm apparently more irritable since I didn't get that promotion." By his report, "My annual reviews don't do justice to my talents. I'm better than most of the people at my level." When asked about his ability to tolerate criticism, he says, "I'm a calm guy. Like yesterday—a guy intentionally cut me off on the highway. I don't care. Just that boss . . . but I'll get that promotion soon." He says that he has "wonderful" relationships with others: "The kids at the office all think I'm great, they look up to me . . . and I'm terrific at a dinner party."*

Here's how we might DESCRIBE his patterns related to self.

> *In his patterns related to his sense of self, Sam has prominent difficulties and some strengths. He has difficulty with **self-perception**, as evidenced by his prediction that he will be promoted despite repeated negative annual reviews. This suggests that he may have grandiose **fantasies of the self** that are not consonant with his actual abilities. He has a fairly consolidated **identity** related to his family, as he is proud of being an involved father. He has significant difficulty with **self-esteem**. Although Sam can tolerate minor **self-esteem threats**, such as being cut off by another driver on the highway, he is extremely vulnerable to more significant threats, such as being criticized by his boss at work. These threats lead him to become irritable and intolerant of others, including the members of his family (**internal response to self-esteem threat**). He frequently **uses others for self-esteem regulation**; for example, at dinner, he will often talk exclusively about himself and his accomplishments. He also tends to have friends who are younger than he is and who look up to him, and he will occasionally flirt with younger men in the office whom he is convinced see him as very attractive.*

As we can see from this example, self-experience also has a major impact on **relationships**, which is the subject of Chapter 7.

Variables for describing the SELF

Self-perception

- Identity
- Fantasies about the self

Self-esteem

- Vulnerability to self-esteem threats
- Internal responses to self-esteem threats
- Use of others to regulate self-esteem
- Responses to external effects on self-esteem

Suggested activity

Can be done by individual learners or in a classroom setting

How would you describe Dave's patterns related to the self?

Dave, a middle aged man, has had many different jobs over the years—he drifts from job to job without a real sense of direction. At one point, he decided that he wanted to be an artist and gave up his paying job, rented a nearby garage, and began painting—despite never having had any art training. He has contempt for people who "settle" for "mainstream" careers, despite the fact that he often envies their lifestyles. "They're working stiffs, but they get everything good in life," he complains. His wife and children have followed him in his meanderings—when they get frustrated, he says that they don't appreciate him.

Comment

Dave has difficulty with **self-perception** and **self-esteem regulation**. His sense of **identity** seems vague, as evidenced by his erratic career trajectory. His attempt to become a painter without training or indication of aptitude suggests that his **fantasies about himself** are not consistent with his realistic talents and limitations. He **regulates self-esteem** by becoming grandiose and contemptuous of others, and he is exquisitely **vulnerable to self-esteem threats**. His lack of empathy for the difficulties he is causing his family members suggests that he **uses others to help regulate his self-esteem**.

References

1. Auchincloss, E.L. & Samberg, E (2012) Psychoanalytic terms and concepts, Yale University Press.
2. Blos, P. (1972). The function of the ego ideal in adolescence. *The Psychoanalytic Study of the Child*, 27(1), 93–97. https://doi.org/10.1080/00797308.1972.11822711
3. Bromberg, P. (1998). *Standing in the spaces: Essays on clinical process, trauma, and dissociation.* Routledge.
4. Cooper, A. (1988). The narcissistic-masochistic character. In R. A. Glick & D. I. Meyers (Eds.), *Masochism: Current psychoanalytic perspectives* (pp. 117–138). Analytic Press. Inc.
5. DuBois, W. E. B. (1897). Strivings of the negro people. *The Atlantic Monthly*. https://www.theatlantic.com/magazine/archive/1897/08/strivings-of-the-negro-people/305446
6. Eng, D. L., & Han, S. (2000). A dialogue on racial melancholia. *Psychoanalytic Dialogues*, 10(4), 667–700. https://doi.org/10.1080/10481881009348576
7. Erikson, E. H. (1968). *Identity: youth, and crisis.* Norton.
8. Fanon, F. (1967). *Black skin, white masks.* Grove Press. (Original work published in 1952).
9. Freud, S. (1966). On narcissism. In J. Strachey (Ed.), *The standard edition of the complete psychological works of Sigmund Freud, volume XIV (1914–1916): On the history of the psycho-analytic movement, papers on metapsychology and other works* (pp. 67–102). Hogarth Press. (Original work published in 1914).
10. Harris, A. (2012). The house of difference, or white silence. *Studies in Gender and Sexuality*, 13(3), 197–216. https://doi.org/10.1080/15240657.2012.707575
11. Hong, C. (2020). *Minor feelings: An Asian American reckoning.* One World.
12. Kernberg, O. F. (1970). Factors in the psychoanalytic treatment of narcissistic personalities. *Journal of the American Psychoanalytic Association*, 18(1), 51–85. https://doi.org/10.1177/000306517001800103
13. Kohut, H. (1972). Thoughts on narcissism and narcissistic rage. *The Psychoanalytic Study of the Child*, 27(1), 360–400. https://doi.org/10.1080/00797308.1972.11822721
14. Kohut, H. (1977). *The restoration of the self.* International Universities Press, Inc.
15. Kohut, H., & Wolff, E. S. (1978). The disorders of the self and their treatment, an outline. *International Journal of Psychoanalysis*, 59, 413–414.
16. MacKinnon, R. A., Michels, R., & Buckley, P. (2006). *The psychiatric interview in clinical practice.* American Psychiatric Association Publishing.
17. Maracle, L. (1996). *I am woman: A native perspective on sociology and feminism.* Press Gang Publishers.
18. Neubauer, P. B. (1982). Rivalry, envy, and jealousy. *The Psychoanalytic Study of the Child*, 37(1), 121–142. https://doi.org/10.1080/00797308.1982.11823360
19. Reich, A. (1960). Pathologic forms of self-esteem regulation. *The Psychoanalytic Study of the Child*, 15(1), 215–232. https://doi.org/10.1080/00797308.1960.11822576
20. Sandler, J., Holder, A., & Meers, D. (1963). The ego ideal and the ideal self. *The Psychoanalytic Study of the Child*, 18(1), 139–158. https://doi.org/10.1080/00797308.1963.11822927
21. Sue, D. W., Sue, D., Neville, H. A., & Smith, L. (2019). *Counseling the culturally diverse: Theory and practice.* John Wiley & Sons, Inc.
22. Winnicott, D. W. (1965). The maturational processes and the facilitating environment: Studies in the theory of emotional development. International Universities Press.
23. Yi, K. (2014). Toward formulation of ethnic identity beyond the binary of white oppressor and racial other. *Psychoanalytic Psychology*, 31(3), 426–434. https://doi.org/10.1037/a0036649

7 Relationships

Key concepts

The capacity to have relationships is central to the way people develop and function.

We can describe a person's relationship patterns according to the following variables:

- Trust
- Sense of self and other
- Security
- Intimacy
- Mutuality

For most of us, relationships with family, friends, significant others, and colleagues provide us with some of the most rewarding experiences of our lives. Yet, relationships can also be a source of frustration, pain, and confusion. For example, consider someone who wants a relationship but is always attracted to people who are not available, or a person who continuously jeopardizes chances for promotion by alienating managers. By the time we are adults, we tend to form relationships according to certain patterns that can be more or less satisfying to us. Being able to describe these patterns is central to understanding how people function (Fairbairn, 1952; Mitchell, 1988).

Defining the area: relationships

Relationships are the interactions we have with people in our lives. Varying kinds of relationships exist, including the parent–child relationships of early childhood, the peer friendships of later childhood, and the romantic and sexual relationships of adolescence and adulthood. Relationships can be fleeting or long term, deep or superficial. Some people have numerous relationships, while others have only a few. Most people are capable of having many different types of relationships.

Psychodynamic Formulation: An Expanded Approach, First Edition. The Psychodynamic Formulation Collective.
© 2022 John Wiley & Sons Ltd. Published 2022 by John Wiley & Sons Ltd.

Variables for describing patterns related to relationships

As previously mentioned, we can describe a person's patterns of relationships with others using the following variables:

- Trust
- Sense of self and other
- Security
- Intimacy
- Mutuality

Trust

Many different types of trust exist (Smith, 2010). There is interpersonal trust of those in one's immediate environment, such as family members; trust of people in one's close community, such as friends and members of groups with which one identifies; and **generalized trust** of other members of society (Yamigishi, 2001). A person could be very trusting of those in their immediate circle but not trust people in general. This is particularly important to consider for those of us who are in nondominant groups and who face discrimination and unfair treatment from society at large. Consider this example:

> A White trans woman who identifies as gay is assigned to see a therapist who is a White cisgender man who identifies as straight. During the first few sessions, the woman asks the therapist if he has ever had a trans woman as a patient, and wonders aloud whether a straight cisgender man can understand her. She misses a session, then calls the head of the clinic to inquire as to whether she can be reassigned to a queer therapist. In supervision, the therapist notes that the patient seems not to trust him, and begins to think about whether this lack of trust could have originated in her early relationship with her primary caregiver. The therapist's supervisor helps the therapist to consider that because he is male, cisgender, and straight, he represents membership in three dominant groups. Consequently, the patient's apparent mistrust could be related to these qualities of the therapist rather than to her early relationships.

In this example, the therapist's experience of the patient's wariness about him made him consider that the patient had global difficulties with trust. In order to collaboratively understand this mistrust in the formulation, the therapist will need to explore the patient's experience of trust in her immediate and community environments, and consider her experience of people in society at large.

Trust in others develops throughout life. During the earliest years, a combination of both temperament and early relationships with caregivers (Benedek, 1959; Erikson, 1993; Winnicott, 1958) are important to the development of trust (see Chapter 10). Throughout life, one's experience of their own and their loved one's treatment at the hands of others and by society at large will affect the development of generalized trust (Smith, 2010).

The ability to trust others is essential for having meaningful, mutually satisfying relationships with a family member, lover, spouse, or colleague. Trust enables people to count on one another, to believe that they will be taken care of, and to have confidence in the consistency of their relationships. Lack of trust leads to constant fear of aggression from others, a sense of being neglected, and a perennial feeling of aloneness.

Lack of generalized trust, or a general wariness of people in general, may be adaptive for victims of violence and those who have been treated unfairly by society. It is also important to note that too much trust (e.g., trusting everyone, or trusting people who are dangerous or abusive) may lead to difficulties.

Sense of self and other

Being able to think about oneself and others in a three-dimensional way is critical to having mutually satisfying relationships (Greenberg & Mitchell, 1983; Klein, 1946). When we say three dimensional, we mean that people can think about themselves and others as having

- both bad and good qualities
- separate and unique feelings, beliefs, needs, or motivations
- generally consistent feelings about self and others from past to present

Consider two people who do not receive the bonus they hoped for from a manager at work. One vilifies the manager, saying, "I liked this guy to begin with, but now I see that he's just a jerk who only cares about his own promotion." Even when the manager explains that everyone in the department had to take a bonus cut, this person badmouths the manager, calling him "weak," and considers quitting. In contrast, the second person makes an appointment to speak with the manager about the bonus. Once the manager explains the situation, this person remains disappointed but understands that the manager is under pressure from higher management. Both workers were disappointed and frustrated with their managers. However, one could see only one side of the story and only one aspect of the manager, while the other could appreciate the complexity of the situation. The first person's way of conceptualizing others can be thought of as **splitting** (Auchincloss & Samberg, 2012)—that is, seeing people as all good or all bad. While splitting is normally found in small children, if it persists it may prevent people from being able to think about others three dimensionally and to have ongoing meaningful relationships. In the previous example, the first person also has difficulty with **mentalization**—that is, thinking about what might be going on in the manager's mind. An impaired capacity for mentalization can limit a person's sense of self and others, and consequently, their ability to have satisfying relationships (Fonagy, 1991, 2001).

Security

Security refers to the state of being safe; security in a relationship refers to feeling safe with another person (Bowlby, 1958; Mahler, 1972). This means believing that the relationship will persist even if there are

- physical separations
- disagreements
- negative feelings

In development, this is often called having a **secure attachment** (see Chapters 13 and 24) (Slade, 2000). People with more secure relationships are generally able to

- tolerate a range of ambivalent feelings about other people,
- have a variety of long-lasting relationships, and
- form relationships more slowly, taking time to get to know others (Slade, 2008)

Consider for example, two people, each of whom goes to a party with their partner. In each case, the partner spends most of the party talking animatedly to a very attractive person. After the party, the first person accuses the partner of wanting to have an affair with the person they met at the party, while the second feels a little left out but realizes that this doesn't affect the security of their relationship. We can say that the first person is less secure in their relationship than the second. The concept of the security of attachments may have different meanings for different cultures; we consider this in more depth in Chapter 24.

Intimacy

Intimacy refers to closeness and familiarity. People are intimate with one another if they share things about themselves, such as feelings, vulnerability, experiences, wishes, and disappointments. The degree of intimacy that people generally share with others is an important aspect of their relationship patterns (Stern, 1985). Depending on the relationship type, intimacy manifests in different ways. Between lovers, sexuality may be an important way of being intimate; between friends, sharing stories, hopes, and fears might forge intimacy. Without at least some intimacy, relationships are superficial. However, because intimacy involves sharing private thoughts and feelings, it makes many people feel anxious and vulnerable.

Some people tend toward extremes, sharing either too much or too little, while others are better able to modulate their degree of intimacy. For example, one person might tell a person sitting next to them on the bus the story of their life, while another might not mention to a long-term friend that a family member has a mental health problem.

Patients often use the word *intimacy* when they talk about having sex, as in, "I was intimate with my girlfriend last night." However, just because two people are having sex does not mean that they are being intimate. For example, there are people for whom sex may be best described as a casual or recreational experience. It is important to determine whether people are sharing feelings and private thoughts with their sexual partners before we can say that their relationships are intimate.

Mutuality

Consider these situations: a friendship in which one person constantly talks about themselves, while the other listens; a couple who both work full time, but one does all the housework; and a baseball-loving parent who forces their reluctant child to play little league every year. Each of these situations feels unfair, because it seems as if one person is doing all the giving, while the other does all the taking. The takers have a limited capacity for empathy (see Chapter 6), and thus do not consider the needs of others. Without this, relationships are unbalanced and lack mutuality. The givers may be more empathic, but they also are missing something about what makes a relationship balanced. Relationships are mutual when both people involved are able to give and take (Beebe & Lachman, 1988; Winnicott, 1989). It's a two-way street.

Variability in relationship patterns

A good definition of an "ideal" relationship does not exist. In clinical practice, we encounter a variety of relationships that work, even though they might not conform to what we consider as being ideal. As with all areas of function, people may have pockets of strength and difficulty. For example, a person may be able to be emotionally intimate with friends but not with romantic partners. Another person might have a very secure relationship with their partner but lack sexual intimacy. Finally, people may have strengths in some aspects of their relationships while having difficulty in others. For example, two people who live together and care for one another might have security and mutuality but lack intimacy because they don't tell each other anything private. Clarifying without judging this variability in relationship patterns is helpful for understanding this critical area of function.

Learning about relationships: opening questions, then stories

Asking patients to tell us about the people in their lives will help us learn the most about this important area of function. We can bring these people to life by asking their first names and referring to them by those names. Asking for stories about these people will reveal the most about them and about our patients relationships with them. Here are a few examples of how to facilitate this:

> *Can you tell me more about your grandmother? Tell me about a moment you really remember in your relationship with her.*

> *So, Ted is the person you rely on most in the world. Can you tell me about a time he really came through for you?*

As the treatment deepens, asking about our patients' relationship with us—the therapist—will also illuminate their patterns in this area.

Learning about trust

Interpersonal trust

To learn about interpersonal trust, you can start by asking:

> *Whom do you trust most in your life? Tell me about this person and your relationship with them.*

> *Do you think that person would help you in an emergency?*

Do you think that person really cares about you?

Do you think that I am likely to be able to help you?

Generalized trust

To learn about generalized trust, you can start by asking:

Do you generally feel that people will look out for you?

Do you generally feel that people are trustworthy?

Do you tend to feel that you will be treated fairly by others?

Learning about one's sense of self and others

To learn about one's sense of self and others, you can start by asking:

Tell me about someone who is important to you. What are they like?

If this leads to a very two-dimensional answer, follow up by asking:

Are they always like that? They sound wonderful/terrible, but do they have any flaws/good traits?

Asking about how people see themselves can be tricky; don't be satisfied with "I don't know." Questions like these can be helpful:

How do you think others see you?

Do you think others see you as basically the same person over time, or as a very changeable person?

You will also want to get a sense of a person's capacity to mentalize by asking questions such as:

Tell me about a time when a person close to you disagreed with you. Why do you think they felt that way?

Learning about security

The following questions will help you to describe your patient's patterns of security in relationships:

How do you feel when you're alone? Does it make you feel nervous or panicky?

Are you still able to feel confident about your relationships when your loved ones aren't with you?

Are you often worried that you will be left alone?

Do you have close friends? How many, and for how long?

Do you tend to stay in touch with old friends?

Do you date? If so, how long do your relationships generally last?

Do you tend to start relationships slowly or quickly?

Do you tend to worry that the people you feel close to will leave you?

Can other people soothe you when you are upset?

Learning about intimacy

To learn about emotional intimacy, you can start by asking:

How do you think your friends/partners would describe the way you are with them?

Would you describe yourself as relatively open emotionally?

Can you tell me about a time when you shared with someone an aspect of yourself about which you're less than proud?

Is there someone whom you feel you can tell almost anything?

Do you tend to push people away when they try to get close?

Are you generally more interested in sex early in a relationship? Later in a relationship?

How close do you feel to your partner during sex?

Does having sex with your partner make you feel closer or more distant from them?

Learning about mutuality in relationships

Because mutuality involves give and take, you can ask questions such as:

Do you feel your partner/friend/parent gives you what you need? If not, what is missing?

Do you think that your partner/friend/parent gets what they need from you?

Describing relationships

Now, let's consider the way that we describe relationship patterns:

Jorge, a 30-year-old man, presents saying he wants help "with women." He has difficulty begin-ning the treatment, as he misses a few appointments and is then upset when the therapist reminds him that he charges for missed sessions. Once the sessions begin, he reports that since leaving the army, he has had few relationships—both with friends and lovers. "The women I date seem amazing at first—we spend tons of time together—and then they get so needy." Looking away from the therapist, he says, "I have to tell you—I had girlfriends in high school, but I was a virgin until I had sex with a prostitute in the service." When asked about his family, he says, "My parents are amazing—they hate each other and divorced long ago—but I talk to each of them every week." Without close friends, he spends most weekends alone, playing his guitar and reading.

Here's how we might DESCRIBE Jorge's relationships:

*Jorge seems to have significant difficulty in his **relationships** with others. In particular, he has trouble achieving **intimacy**, both with friends and romantic partners. His pattern of having intense crushes and then becoming quickly annoyed with his girlfriends' "neediness" suggests he has a superficial **sense of self and other** and lacks a capacity for **mutuality**. His early suspiciousness about the therapist's fees and policy of charging for missed sessions suggests he might have difficulty with **trust**.*

Variables for describing RELATIONSHIPS

- Trust
- Sense of self and other
- Security
- Intimacy
- Mutuality

Suggested activity

How would you describe AJ's relationship patterns?

AJ is a 68-year-old trans man whose partner of 40 years recently died. He describes him as "the love of my life" and says that they took care of each other in every way, adding, "It was almost like we were the same person." They had no children and few friends. He is very lonely now. He says he doesn't know how to make friends and sometimes sees no one for many days.

Comment

Strengths: The length of AJ's relationship and the closeness he felt to his partner of 40 years indicate his deep **trust** and **security** in that relationship. He also describes the relationship as quite **mutual**.

Difficulties: The intensity of AJ's relationship with his partner, although positive, may be problematic for him. His **sense of himself and other** was merged with his partner to the degree that he feels lost without him. AJ's trouble making friends suggests that he may have difficulty with **intimacy**.

References

1. Auchincloss, E. L., & Samberg, E. (2012). *Psychoanalytic terms and concepts.* Yale University Press.
2. Beebe, B., & Lachman, F. M. (1988). The contribution of mother-infant mutual influence to the origins of self and object representation. *Psychoanalytic Psychology, 5,* 305–337.
3. Benedek, T. (1959). Parenthood as a developmental phase—A contribution to the libido theory. *Journal of the American Psychoanalytic Association, 7,* 389–417.
4. Bowlby, J. (1958). The nature of the child's tie to his mother. *International Journal of Psychoanalysis, 39,* 350–373.
5. Erikson, E. (1993). *Childhood and society.* Basic Books.
6. Fairbairn, W. R. D. (1952). *Psychoanalytic studies of the personality.* Tavistock Publications Limited.
7. Fonagy, P. (1991). Thinking about thinking: Some clinical and theoretical considerations. *International Journal of Psychoanalysis, 72,* 639–656.
8. Fonagy, P. (2001). *Attachment theory and psychoanalysis.* Other Press.
9. Greenberg, J. R., & Mitchell, S. A. (1983). *Object relations in psychoanalytic theory.* Harvard University Press.
10. Klein, M. (1946). Notes on some schizoid mechanisms. *International Journal of Psychoanalysis, 27,* 99–110.
11. Mahler, M. S. (1972). On the first three subphases of the separation-individuation process. *International Journal of Psychoanalysis, 53,* 333–338.
12. Mitchell, S. A. (1988). *Relational concepts in psychoanalysis.* Harvard University Press.
13. Slade, A. (2000). The development and organization of attachment: Implications for psychoanalysis. *Journal of the American Psychoanalytic Association, 48,* 1147–1174. https://doi.org/10.1177/00030651000480042301
14. Slade, A. (2008). Attachment theory and research: Implications for the theory and practice of individual psychotherapy with adults. In J. Cassidy & P. R. Shaver (Eds.), *Handbook of attachment: Theory, research and clinical applications* (pp. 762–782). Guilford Press.
15. Smith, S. S. (2010). Race and trust. *Annual Review of Sociology, 36,* 453–475.
16. Stern, D. N. (1985). *The interpersonal world of the infant.* Basic Books.
17. Winnicott, D. W. (1958). The capacity to be alone. *International Journal of Psychoanalysis, 39,* 411–420.
18. Winnicott, W. (1989). The mother-infant experience of mutuality. In D. W. Winnicott, C. Winnicott, R. Shepherd, et al. (Eds.), *Psychoanalytic explorations* (pp. 251–261). Harvard University Press.
19. Yamigishi, T. (2001). Trust as a form of social intelligence. In K. S. Cook (Ed.), *Trust in society* (pp. 121–147). Russell Sage Foundation.

8 Adapting

Key concepts

Every day, we must adapt to stress. Stress can be internal (e.g., guilt) or external (e.g., rejection).

The unconscious processes we use to adapt to stress are sometimes called **defense mechanisms** because they help protect us from internal and external stress.

All defense mechanisms were adaptive at one point in life.

Characteristic patterns of defense mechanisms vary according to their

- Current benefit and cost
- Emotionality
- Flexibility and range.

Trauma, discrimination, and disadvantage affect the development of defense mechanisms.

Terms such as *primitive, immature*, and *maladaptive* may not take into consideration the many ways that human beings need to adapt to stress.

Life is not constant. Every day, we face different amounts of stimulation, both from outside and inside us, that threaten our usual functioning. Some of this stimulation, such as the excitement of success, love, or joy, is welcome; while some, such as bad news, loss, or anxiety, is unwelcome. Overwhelming stimulation is sometimes called **stress** because it places strain on the way we live our lives (Koolhass et al., 2011). Thus, we all need ways to adapt to or manage both internal and external stimulation (Bellak, 1989; Bellak & Goldsmith, 1984; Bellak & Meyers, 1975; Vaillant, 1977, 1992).

Defining the area: adapting

Adapting means adjusting. Many types of internal and external stimulation exist, to which we need to adjust on a daily basis.

Psychodynamic Formulation: An Expanded Approach, First Edition. The Psychodynamic Formulation Collective.
© 2022 John Wiley & Sons Ltd. Published 2022 by John Wiley & Sons Ltd.

Internal stimulation includes

- Thoughts and fantasies
- Feelings and anxiety
- Pain and other physical sensations

External stimulation includes

- Relationships with others
- Economic and work-related pressures
- Trauma and other environmental events
- Discrimination, disadvantage, and systemic oppression

Everyone has their own threshold for tolerating stimulation. Some people can tolerate high levels of affect, anxiety, and environmental stress, while others develop difficulties at much lower levels. In the same way that all people have their own fingerprints, most adults have their unique, characteristic ways of adapting to internal and external stressors (Freud, 1894/1962; Pine, 1990; Perry et al., 2009).

When we respond to, adapt to, or manage stress, we try to keep the amount of excess stimulation at a level that enables us to continue functioning. We do this in various ways, including blocking out feelings, filtering stimuli, forgetting things, or focusing our attention elsewhere. Sometimes, we do these things purposefully and consciously, for example, when we say to ourselves, "I can't deal with this right now. I'm going to think about it later." Generally, however, we deal with stress without ever knowing we are doing it. We call unconscious ways of adapting to stress **defense mechanisms** (Gabbard, 2005; Kernberg, 1976; Vaillant, 1977). Defenses function the way our sense of balance operates when we keep ourselves upright on the deck of a boat—automatically and continuously making tiny adjustments without our awareness. Just as our balance system automatically senses the tiny movements of the boat and deploys muscles to keep us upright, our mind senses tiny changes in our anxiety and emotional tone and deploys defenses to keep us functioning on an even keel.

Adapting and early life stress

All defense mechanisms were adaptive at one point in life. However, defenses that arose early in life to respond to high-stress environments may have been adaptive at that time *and* may cause problems later in life. We are beginning to understand the neurobiology of this dichotomy. Using mouse models, early life stress (ELS) has been shown to have a variety of neurodevelopmental effects, including a reduced proliferation of neurons, enhanced dendritic turnover, decreased synaptic density, and decreased brain volume (Bath et al., 2016). Many of these effects serve to accelerate brain (i.e., neuronal) maturation. One hypothesis is that accelerated brain maturation may be adaptive in a stress-filled environment because it allows the organism to

- function independently at a younger age
- maintain a high arousal state needed to survive

However, this maturation may come at the expense of the development of important brain regions. This idea has been called the "stress acceleration hypothesis" (Callaghan & Tottenham, 2016, p. 76). These findings suggest that exposure to ELS may affect the range and flexibility of defense mechanisms, and that coping strategies found to be problematic in adulthood may have been important for survival early in life.

Modes of adapting and cultural norms

Some modes of adapting to stress may be common among people who identify with particular religious or faith practices, norms, and rituals. For example, after being fired, a devout member of a religious group may calmly say, "I can't worry about having lost my job. I'm leaving it in the Lord's hands." This mode of adapting may be commonly shared by others in their group. Thus, input from the individual's immediate and community environment should be considered when describing patterns of adapting.

Variables for describing patterns of adapting

We can describe defense mechanisms using the following variables:

- Current benefit and costs
- Emotionality
- Flexibility and range

Current benefit and cost

One way to describe defenses is to consider their current ability to help people cope with stress while preserving function. We can think about this as the current benefit of the defense. Defenses with more current benefit and less current cost preserve or enhance function, while defenses with less current benefit and more current cost hinder function (See Table 8.1) (Caligor et al., 2007; Kernberg et al., 1989; Perry & Bond, 2005). For example, if someone is angry with a friend, **rationalizing** the friend's behavior helps to maintain the relationship, while **devaluing** the friend threatens it. Defenses with less benefit decrease the awareness of a painful feeling, but incur such high cost that they impair function. Other examples of potentially high cost defenses are the use of **splitting** to handle strong opposing feelings at the expense of being able to have meaningful relationships, or **dissociating** to escape overwhelmingly bad feelings at the expense of being able to connect to reality (Herman, 1992).

Note that what has high benefit and low cost in one situation may not have the same ratio in another. For example, if survival is at stake during wartime, it may be beneficial to use **denial** to stave off panic, but denial of a medical condition may preclude attaining lifesaving care. Also, remember that people adjust to stress as well as they can in a given situation, and that even less beneficial defenses developed because they were needed at some point in the person's life. Defenses that seem problematic in adulthood likely developed as survival mechanisms early in life.

Benefit, cost, and systems of disadvantage

"For a [B]lack man," wrote psychiatrists William Grier and Price Cobbs in their book *Black Rage*,

> . . .*survival in America depends in large measure on the development of a 'healthy' cultural paranoia. He must maintain a high degree of suspicion toward the motives of every [W]hite man and at the same time never allow this suspicion to impair his grasp of reality* (Grier & Cobbs, 1968/1992, p. 161).

Grier and Cobbs suggest that for those of us disadvantaged by society's hierarchies, NOT being somewhat paranoid has a higher cost than being paranoid. Thus, when we describe the defenses people use, we should not assume they have the same cost for all people in all circumstances. Terms such as *primitive, immature,* or *maladaptive,* may be judgmental if they do not take into consideration the myriad ways human beings need to react in order to survive trauma, disadvantage, discrimination, and systemic oppression.

Emotionality

People differ in terms of the amount of emotion they experience and show. These differences may relate to cultural variation in emotionality, familial traits, and individual temperament. In fact, temperament is generally defined as "early appearing variation in emotional reactivity" (Rettew & McKee, 2005). These differences are reflected in the variable emotionality of the way people adapt to stress—that is, in their defenses.

Some defenses work by keeping stressful **feelings** out of awareness, while others work by keeping stressful **thoughts** out of awareness. For example, one person might keep the emotional pain of a divorce out of awareness, saying, "It's a good time for a divorce; property values are high" (**rationalization**), while another might experience the emotions of a divorce as headaches and stomach pains (**somatization**).

People who tend to use defenses that keep *feelings* out of awareness are sometimes said to have an **obsessive** defensive style, while others who tend to use defenses that keep *thoughts* out of awareness are sometimes said to have a **hysterical** defensive style (Shapiro, 1973).

Flexibility and range

No matter how good a strategy is for coping with stress, it does not work in every situation. Consequently, people need to be **flexible** enough to use a range of strategies. People without defensive flexibility often seem controlling, difficult, or brittle. Think of the person who always has to win an argument, or who always manages stress by making a joke—even when it's not a moment for humor. In addition, while a certain defense may work well at a particular time in life, the same strategy may become a hindrance later on.

Table 8.1 Defense Mechanisms

Defense	Definition
Acting out	Expressing unacceptable thoughts or feelings (particularly those that come up in therapy) in actions *(Eating a gallon of ice cream after a difficult therapy session)*
Altruism	Turning painful feelings into doing for others *(Finding comfort in starting a foundation to provide support for patients with cancer and their families after the death of a parent)*
Denial	Disavowing unacceptable feelings and thoughts *(Claiming to have excellent health despite having a palpable growth on one's skin)*
Displacement	Redirecting feelings or impulses to other people or activities *(Exploding in anger at one person when actually upset with another)*
Dissociation	Disconnecting unacceptable thoughts and feelings from current reality *(Having no memory of being yelled at by a boss at work)*
Excessive emotionality	Forgetting a thought while remaining aware of the associated feeling *(Being irritable while planning one's wedding because of ambivalence about whether to get married)*
Externalization	Perceiving internal conflicts or experiences as arising from external circumstances *(Blaming a coworker for one's self-esteem issues)*
Humor	Expressing uncomfortable thoughts or feelings as jokes *(Laughing while saying, "This will give me more time to read comics," after being fired)*
Idealization and devaluation	Attributing overly positive or negative feelings to others *(Telling a therapist at the first session, "You are clearly the best therapist in the city. Much better than my last therapist, who was an idiot.")*
Identification	Striving to be like another person in order to deal with jealous or competitive feelings *(Gradually beginning to dress exactly like a more popular roommate)*
Intellectualization	Replacing painful or uncomfortable feelings with excessive thinking *(Dealing with a cancer diagnosis by focusing on extensive research data about the disease)*
Isolation of affect	Forgetting a feeling while remaining conscious of the associated thought *(Having no feelings after being left by a partner)*
Projection	Perceiving unacceptable qualities or feelings as originating outside of the self *(Feeling hostility coming from a friend with whom one is actually very angry)*

(continued)

Table 8.1 *(continued)*

Defense	Definition
Projective identification	Projecting a thought or feeling into another person, then interacting with that person to make them experience the projected feeling *(Coming late to a date with a person with whom one is upset)*
Rationalization	Explaining unacceptable behavior or feelings in a logical manner *(Expressing relief at being fired because "I never liked that job.")*
Reaction formation	Reversing an unacceptable feeling by experiencing it as its opposite *(Becoming overprotective of a toddler who is difficult to soothe)*
Regression	Using coping strategies from earlier developmental periods to deal with stressful events or feelings *(Not eating well or doing laundry during exam week)*
Repression	Keeping uncomfortable thoughts, feelings, and fantasies from conscious awareness *(Forgetting a therapy appointment after an unpleasant session)*
Sexualization	Expressing uncomfortable thoughts or feelings as flirtatiousness or overly sexual behaviors *(Dressing in overly revealing clothing for a job interview)*
Somatization	Experiencing uncomfortable feelings or thoughts as physical symptoms *(Developing a headache and taking a sick day after receiving a bad review at work)*
Splitting	Keeping good and bad feelings separate in order to protect the good *(Experiencing one's mother as all good and one's sister as all bad)*
Sublimation	Converting unacceptable impulses into more useful forms *(Painting beautiful but mournful scenes when sad)*
Suppression	Consciously deciding not to focus on difficult thoughts or feelings *(Deciding to wait until after a vacation to figure out how to pay the rent)*
Turning against the self	Blaming oneself rather than experiencing unacceptable feelings toward another person *(Feeling like a bad person after being emotionally abused)*
Undoing	"Fixing" unacceptable thoughts or feelings or behavior by opposing behaviors *(Giving money to charity after cheating on one's taxes)*

Note. Adapted from Gabbard (2005).

Learning about adapting: opening questions, then stories

Here are some questions that can help us to learn about our patients' style of adapting:

How do you generally react to anxiety and strong feelings? Would family, friends, or other people in your life agree? Tell me about a time when this happened recently.

Is your sense that you react to stress in a similar way to other people in your life? Particularly those in your family/social circle/community?

Do you feel you always react in the same way, or do you feel you use different strategies depending on the circumstances?

Are you happy with the way that you respond to stress? What do you think works? What do you think could be more helpful?

Here are some questions you can ask yourself to help contextualize your patient's style of adapting:

Did this person have traumatic early life experiences? Has there been trauma in this person's later life that affected their patterns of adapting to stress?

Does this person belong to one or more disadvantaged groups? How has that aspect of their life experience affected their patterns of adapting to stress?

Does this person's defensive style seem to get in the way of their interpersonal relationships?

If you offer alternative ways of looking at things, is the person flexible or unable to shift perspective?

In talking to you, does the person use many feeling-filled words?

Does what the person says seem dry or devoid of feelings, even when they are talking about something painful or exciting?

When talking about something painful, does the person show their feelings? Do they offer an explanation/excuse for the feelings?

Do you feel caught up in the patient's dramatic storytelling? Or do you feel bored and detached from what the person is saying?

Describing adapting

Let's consider Mira as we think about how to DESCRIBE patterns of adapting:

Mira has had severe rheumatoid arthritis since childhood. Teased as a child for her need to use a cane, she now runs a foundation for children with disabilities that raises millions of dollars annually and that gives her significant satisfaction. She presents for therapy after she became very upset at a recent board meeting, saying, "I have this major job and I'm 57 years old— I should stop crying and getting so upset every time I get into a stressful situation." As she comes into her first session, she puts her cane in the umbrella stand, adding (with a wink), "OK for all kinds of sticks?"

Here's how we might DESCRIBE Mira's patterns of adapting:

*Mira's ability to cope with stress is a major strength. Chronically ill with rheumatoid arthritis since childhood, her defenses generally seem to offer her **high benefit and low cost**. For example, running a foundation for children with disabilities seems to represent **sublimation**, and her playful comment to the therapist suggests that she uses **humor** to deflect pain. In highly stressful* *situations, she can cry and become dramatic, using defenses that tend to **emphasize emotions**. Her range of coping strategies is fairly **flexible**. For example, although she may use humor with strangers, she also deals with her anger at being disadvantaged because of her physical disability with advocacy.*

Variables for describing ADAPTING

Defense mechanisms include the following:

- Current benefit and cost
- Emotionality
- Flexibility and range

Suggested activity
How would you describe Jim's patterns of adapting?

Jim, a sales executive, who is set to retire in two years at the age of 65, has just been told that he has prostate cancer. He begins complaining of headaches and toothaches, in addition to constantly shuttling back and forth to doctors and dentists. He is irritable and tells everyone he knows how frightened he is. His incessant phone calls lead his friends to begin to avoid him. In order to try to take his mind off his impending treatment, his husband tries to engage him in refinishing their dining room table, which he has wanted to do for many years, but he is unable to refocus. His husband is becoming increasingly exasperated with him, saying that this is exactly how he behaved when their son had trouble with drugs many years before.

Comment

Jim's primary defense is **somatization**. This defensive strategy, which leads him to over-use medical and dental care and threatens his relationships, seems high cost and low benefit. His inability to shift coping strategies during the current crisis, as well as the similarity between his current mechanisms and those he employed many years ago, suggest that his patterns for dealing with stress are quite **inflexible** and of **limited range**.

References

1. Bath, K. G., Manzano-Nieves, G., & Goodwill, H. (2016). Early life stress accelerates behavioral and neural maturation of the hippocampus in male mice. *Hormones and Behavior, 82*, 64–71. https://doi.org/10.1016/j.yhbeh.2016.04.010. Epub 2016 May 4.
2. Bellak, L. (1989). *Ego function assessment (EFA): A manual.* C.P.S., Inc.
3. Bellak, L., & Goldsmith, L. A. (Eds.) (1984). *The broad scope of ego function assessment.* Wiley.
4. Bellak, L., & Meyers, B. (1975). Ego function assessment and analyzability. *International Review of Psychoanalysis, 2*, 413–427. http://www.mindmeister.com/generic_files/get_file/9559058?filetype=attachment_file
5. Caligor, E., Kernberg, O. F., & Clarkin, J. F. (2007). *Handbook of dynamic psychotherapy for higher level personality pathology.* American Psychiatric Publishing, Inc.
6. Callaghan, B. L., & Tottenham, N. (2016). The stress acceleration hypothesis: Effects of early-life adversity on emotion circuits and behavior. *Current Opinion in Behavioral Sciences, 7*, 76–81. https://doi.org/10.1016/j.cobeha.2015.11.018
7. Freud, S. (1962). The neuro-psychoses of defense. In J. Strachey (Ed.), *The standard edition of the complete psychological works of Sigmund Freud, volume III (1893–1899), early psychoanalytic publications* (pp. 41–61). Hogarth Press. (Original work published 1894).
8. Gabbard, G. O. (2005). *Psychodynamic psychiatry in clinical practice* (4th ed.). American Psychiatric Publishing, Inc.
9. Grier, W. H., & Cobbs, P. M. (1992). *Black rage.* Basic Books. (Originally published in 1968).
10. Herman, J. L. (1992). *Trauma and recovery.* Basic Books.
11. Kernberg, O. F. (1976). *Object-relations theory and clinical psychoanalysis.* Aronson.
12. Kernberg, O. F., Selzer, M. A., Koenigsberg, H., Carr, A. C., & Appelbaum, A. H. (1989). *Psychodynamic psychotherapy of borderline patients.* Basic Books.
13. Koolhass, J. M., Bartolomucci, A., Buwalda, B., de Boer, S. F., Flugge, G., Korte, S. M., Meerlo, P., Murison, R., Olivier, B., Palanza, P., Richter-Levin, G., Sgoifo, A., Steimer, T., Stiedl, O., van Dijk, G., Wohr, M., & Fuchs, E. (2011). Stress revisited: A critical evaluation of the stress concept. *Neuroscience and Biobehavioral Reviews, 35*(5), 1291–1301. https://doi.org/10.1016/j.neubiorev.2011.02.003. Epub 2011 Feb 21.
14. Perry, C. J., & Bond, M. (2005). Defensive functioning. In J. Oldham, A. E. Skodol, & D. S. Bender (Eds.), *The American psychiatric publishing textbook of personality disorders* (pp. 523–540). American Psychiatric Publishing, Inc.
15. Perry, C. J., Beck, S. M., Constantinides, P., & Foley, J. E. (2009). Studying change in defensive functioning in psychotherapy using the defense mechanism rating scales: Four hypotheses, four cases. In R. A. Levy & S. J. Ablon (Eds.), *The handbook of evidence-based psychodynamic psychotherapy* (pp. 121–153). Humana Press.
16. Pine, F. (1990). *Drive, ego, object, and self: A synthesis for clinical work.* Basic Books.
17. Rettew, D. C., & McKee, L. (2005). Temperament and its role in developmental psychopathology. *Harvard Review of Psychiatry, 13*(1), 14–27. https://doi.org/10.1080/10673220590923146
18. Shapiro, D. (1973). *Neurotic styles.* Basic Books.
19. Vaillant, G. E. (1977). *Adaptation to life: How the best and the brightest came of age* (1st ed.). Little, Brown and Co.
20. Vaillant, G. E. (1992). *Ego mechanisms of Defense: A guide for clinicians and researchers* (1st ed.). American Psychiatric Publishing, Inc.

9 Cognition

Key concepts

The way people think is central to the way they function.
We can describe cognitive function using the following variables:

- Variables for describing cognition
  - Basic cognitive functions
  - Higher (executive) cognitive functions
    - Emotional expression and regulation
    - Impulse control
    - Judgment
    - Sensory stimulus regulation
    - Decision-making and problem-solving
  - Reflective (metacognitive) functions
    - Reality testing
    - Self-reflection
    - Mentalization

Defining the area: cognition

Cogito ergo sum—Descartes famously asserted that thinking is evidence of our existence (Descartes, 1637/1998). The way we think is reflected in almost everything that we do, including problem-solving, organizing thoughts, remembering things, and focusing our attention. Some people have strengths in one area of cognitive function and difficulties in another. Consider the absent-minded professor who, while being a brilliant lecturer, is disorganized and always late to appointments. Rather than placing value on one type of thinking over another, we want to describe the many ways people solve problems, make decisions and judgments, and think about their own minds and the minds of others.

Describing cognitive function is essential to the process of psychodynamic formulation for several reasons. First, the way we think is key to our functioning, and thus

Psychodynamic Formulation: An Expanded Approach, First Edition. The Psychodynamic Formulation Collective.
© 2022 John Wiley & Sons Ltd. Published 2022 by John Wiley & Sons Ltd.

we want to hypothesize about its development. Second, because cognitive functions develop and change over the course of a person's lifetime, carefully observing and describing problems in this area can provide us with clues as to when problems may have occurred for an individual during development.

Ableism and cognitive differences

Lastly, and perhaps of particular importance, the way we think can affect other aspects of our development. For example, when children have problems with attention or organization, it may affect the way they perceive themselves (self-esteem) and are viewed by others (family, community, and society at large). Children who are identified as learning disabled may be stigmatized and stereotyped in ways that can have lasting academic and emotional effects (Hehir, 2002). **Ableism** is defined as prejudicial treatment of people with disabilities and/or people who are perceived to be disabled based on underlying socially constructed assumptions that those who are disabled are inferior to those who are nondisabled (Friedman & Owen, 2017). Peers, teachers, and parents who are not sufficiently aware of their ableist assumptions about students with learning disabilities (e.g., assuming that learning to spell is "better" than using spell-check or that students with learning disabilities are less intelligent and productive in life) may reinforce dominant cultural prejudices against disability and devaluation of people with disabilities.

We do not have to be disabled to experience ableism. A child who is, by nature, quiet may be less inclined to communicate verbally but possess perfectly "normal" receptive language skills. Strict milestones about what children should be able to do by a specified age (e.g., all children should be able to read by age 7) may lead a child to be inappropriately flagged as having a language delay (Galatzer-Levy & Cohler, 1993). Individual children develop along their own trajectory and at their own pace. All of these experiences relate to the person's cognitive abilities and should be considered when formulating psychodynamically.

Variables for describing cognition

Reviewing the wide range of cognitive functions is beyond the scope of this book. However, we can think of some general clusters of cognitive functions that are essential to describe. They are

- **Basic cognitive abilities**
- **Higher (executive) functions**
  - Emotional regulation
  - Impulse control
  - Judgment
  - Sensory stimulus regulation
  - Decision-making and problem-solving
- **Reflective (metacognitive) functions**
  - Reality testing/Sense of reality
  - Self-reflection
  - Mentalization

Basic cognitive ability

How smart is he? Why does she keep forgetting things? Why can't he keep track of his homework? As therapists, we ask ourselves these questions about our patients every day, relating to our patients' **basic cognitive abilities**. These abilities are the built-in intellectual/cognitive capacities with which a person is innately equipped and include intelligence, memory, attention, perception, speech and language, and the ability to organize thought (see Table 9.1). While assessing these areas of function sometimes requires formal testing (e.g., intelligence, memory, attention) (Cournos et al., 2008), we can and should comment on general function in these areas, particularly when they represent clear strengths or difficulties. While one patient may have started winning science contests in the third grade, another could never focus on homework, and still another arrives at every session having forgotten something. The cognitive function of these individuals affects their functioning in every other area—the way they think about themselves, their relationships with others, how they adapt to stress, their values, and their work and play. This is true for all of us, but it is particularly significant when cognitive function represents a major strength or difficulty.

Table 9.1 Basic cognitive abilities

Intelligence
Memory
Attention
Speech and Language
Linear thinking
Perception

Higher (executive) functions

After an argument with a teenage child, a parent is tempted to have a stiff drink but remembers that it is likely to cause a migraine so does deep breathing exercises instead.

A student has a term paper due after the weekend but also wants to fit in a friend's birthday party, so maps out a homework schedule that allows for both.

These are examples of **higher (executive) cognitive functions** (see Table 9.2) at work. They are a set of mental processes that help people manage themselves and their basic cognitive resources to achieve desired goals. Higher cognitive functions are often called into action when a person needs to override responses that might otherwise be automatically elicited by stimuli in the environment. Higher cognitive functions include emotional regulation, impulse control, judgment, stimulus regulation, decision-making and problem-solving.

Table 9.2 Executive (Higher Cognitive) Functions

Emotional regulation
Impulse control
Judgment
Stimulus regulation
Decision-making and Problem-solving

Emotional expression and regulation

The excitement of taking one's first steps, the pride of graduating from college, the joy of watching one's child being born—without these feelings, life would be colorless. It's also important to be able to experience more painful feelings, such as sadness, loss, and disappointment. Painful feelings help us to understand ourselves and others—without them we would have trouble learning from experience, feeling empathy, and having relationships. Feelings also motivate us and give us "zest" for life. Some people are more able to experience, tolerate, and express a wide range of feelings than others, as in these examples:

> *I just love being with my grandchildren. They're so full of life! Just watching them go back and forth on the swing takes my breath away. I can't wait to see them again!"*

> *We spent the day with the grandchildren. We had lunch. My daughter has her hands full. Guess we'll see them again in a few weeks.*

Two grandparents, two different experiences. The first is full of feeling - you can almost hear the exclamation points. The second sounds flatter, less feeling filled. Noting whether the person has a range of feelings is also important—the feelings expressed can't be all good or all bad.

While it's important to be able to experience feelings, it's also important to be able to manage them. Out-of-control feelings, whether they're pleasurable or not, can be overwhelming and stressful. Every individual has a different capacity to tolerate feelings, including anxiety. For example, consider the behavior of two people after a partner texts to break up with them:

> *One person begins screaming uncontrollably, and then begins breaking plates against the wall.*

> *One person sits quietly, takes a hot bath, and cries while telling the story to a roommate over dinner.*

While they are both upset, the second person seems to be able to manage their feelings and stay reasonably calm, while the first cannot. Note, people may have difficulty managing emotions either because they have trouble handling even small amounts of feeling, or because they are overwhelmed by chronic anxiety or mood symptoms.

Culture and emotions

Emotional expressiveness can be related to many things—some people have deep feelings but don't tend to express them for personal or cultural reasons. Societal/cultural norms and expectations about controlling emotions also vary and may influence the way parents socialize their children (Tummula-Narra, 2016). Differing attitudes about autonomy, self-reliance, and individuality in western and eastern cultures influence the degree to which emotional regulation is prioritized. Cross-cultural studies have shown that in South Asian countries such as India, or in Latin American cultures such as Puerto Rico, parents teach children to control their expression of emotions in the interest of observing societal duty and preserving social harmony. In western countries, like Germany, parents usually encourage their children to express emotions so they will become self-assertive individuals who are comfortable showing their own needs (Keller et al., 2005; Trommsdorff & Cole, 2011; Trommsdorff et al., 2012).

Impulse control

Impulses come in many forms. People with difficulty controlling impulses can have trouble with the following:

- Managing appetites (e.g., substances, food, sex)
- Gambling
- Controlling aggression/violence
- Stealing

Being impulsive isn't necessarily always bad. Sometimes, being overly controlled can be problematic. The person who is unable to do anything spontaneous—from buying a new pair of shoes to agreeing to an impromptu after-work gathering—often has difficulties in relationships with others. Similarly, risk-taking, which is inversely related to impulse control, can lead to self-destructive behavior but can also be essential for large-scale career moves. For some, risk-taking activities like bungee jumping and scuba diving in caves, are pleasurable, while for others they are terrifying.

People control their impulses in many ways. They learn to slow down, delay gratification, and count to 10. Some do it on their own, but others need the support of 12-step programs or religious beliefs. Understanding and describing a person's successful strategies for self-control are as important as documenting their struggles with impulse control—again, remember to note patients' strengths as well as their difficulties.

Judgment

The capacity to consider the consequences of behavior, often called **judgment** (Cabaniss et al., 2017), is another higher cognitive function. Judgment involves not only being aware of the appropriateness and likely consequences of an intended behavior but also behaving in a way that reflects this awareness. As with other cognitive functions, judgment is not an "on or off" function; it can wax and wane in different circumstances. For example, generally responsible people who have too much to drink may forget to pick up a child after a school basketball game, or may not use a condom when having sex with a new partner. These people may "know" the right thing to do and even have a sense of the consequences of their behavior, but sometimes not act on them. Judgment can have an enormous impact on every aspect of their functioning and is thus important to describe. Chapter 10 will have more to say about the values that guide peoples' judgment.

Sensory regulation

Stimuli like noise, smells, and textures are everywhere, and we need to be able to adjust to them. As with the other types of stimuli we have discussed, people vary widely in their ability to tolerate and adapt to these sensations. Some people startle easily when they hear a telephone ring, or become nauseated if they sense a whiff of a bad odor, while others are oblivious. Some people enjoy very stimulating environments like rock concerts or Times Square on New Year's Eve; others are disturbed by the sounds of children playing in the park. Difficulty adjusting to sensory stimuli can be a major impediment to functioning. For example, a person who is very sensitive to smell might never be able to use public transportation or fly on an airplane, leading them to miss important out-of-town conferences or family gatherings.

Decision-making and problem-solving

People make decisions and solve problems in very different ways. Think about the variety of methods these people use when choosing a new car:

I always buy Buicks because that's the car my father drove.

Who has time? I just go into a dealership and buy whatever I see first.

It's all about the color!

I read 3 years' worth of Consumer Reports articles about cars, tested five models, created a rating system, and ultimately bought the car that got the most points according to my scale.

These people all have the capacity to make decisions, but they make them in different ways. Some people are very detail oriented, while others are more impressionistic; some people make decisions based on research, while others are guided by "hunches." Some people are planners, and some "take things as they come." Still others have considerable creative talents that help them not only with solving problems but also with everything from inventing new recipes to making scientific discoveries. One person may plan a party months in advance with a checklist, while another might pull it all together on a whim at the last minute. Ultimately, both parties could be great successes, but the thought process that went into planning them would have been quite different. Our job is not to judge which is better, but to describe our patients' problem-solving styles and to think about how they positively or negatively affect function.

Problem-solving requires the ability to organize thinking, plan ahead, and think creatively. As with general cognitive abilities, these capacities can have a major impact on the development of other functions as well. For example, it can be difficult to hold positions of responsibility if organization is a problem.

Reflective (metacognitive) functions

Reflective or **metacognitive functions** enable us to observe our own thoughts and feelings (**self-reflection**), understand and think about the mental states of others (**mentalizing**), and discriminate between perceptions that are real and those that are not (**reality testing**) (Dimaggio & Lysaker, 2010; Flavell, 1987; Levy, 2010; Semerari et al., 2003, 2014).

Self-reflection

An important aspect of reflective cognitive function is the capacity to examine one's own thoughts and behaviors, known as **self-reflection** (Cabaniss et al., 2017). Some people do this naturally, asking themselves questions like, "I wonder why I said/did that?", while others are more likely to say, "It is what it is," and go no further. Self-reflection is the ability to step back, sometimes just a little bit, from one's experience in order to try to understand it. **Psychological mindedness** (Cabaniss et al., 2017), which is related to self-reflection, is the ability to think about possible unconscious motivations for one's thoughts, feelings, and behavior. Being able to self-reflect helps people to learn about and improve their feelings about themselves and their relationships with others. Think of the person whose partner is disappointed to only receive a card on a birthday, then is mystified the next year when the card is once again met with tears. Unable to be self-reflective, this person does not consider the way that they might have contributed to the situation.

Reality testing and sense of reality

The capacity for reflective cognition is also related to **reality testing** (Bellak & Meyers, 1975; Cabaniss et al., 2017) and **sense of reality** (Bellak & Meyers, 1975). Reality testing refers to the ability to discriminate between perceptions that are real and those that are not (as opposed to having hallucinations, delusions, illusions, or grossly distorted perceptions of events). Needless to say, it is essential for every aspect of function, from relationships to work. Some people intermittently lose the capacity to test reality during periods of stress. Still others can test reality but sometimes doubt their conclusions (Lysaker et al., 2014). The person who is sure their boss is out to fire them because, "He found out that I have special powers and feels threatened," seems generally unable to test reality, while the person who says, "I know that my job is secure, but I sometimes worry about being fired right before a deadline," may have intermittent difficulty with this. Both types of difficulty with reality are important to note and describe.

Having a good sense of reality means that external events as well as one's own body are experienced as real and familiar. Examples of loosening in the sense of reality include feelings of derealization and depersonalization, déjà-vu experiences, dream-like states, out-of-body experiences, feelings of merger with others, and having a distorted body image (Bellak & Meyers, 1975). People with panic disorder, eating disorders, and a history of trauma may have these experiences while having intact reality testing. They may also be part of religious or spiritual experiences in the absence of psychopathology (e.g., members of certain religious groups speaking in tongues) (Keri et al., 2020).

Mentalization

Reflecting about the minds of others is called **mentalizing** (see Chapters 7 and 24). Mentalization is the capacity to understand that other people have thoughts and feelings that are different from one's own, and to make inferences about what they may be feeling or thinking (Spezzano, 2012). Consider the responses of two patients to their therapist's one-time lateness:

> *How could you do this to me? You know my driving test is tomorrow and I'm crazy with anxiety! What were you thinking?*

> *Huh, it's weird—you're never late. I hope that everything is OK. I wondered if you had an emergency. It can't be easy to be a therapist.*

The first person can't imagine that things could be going on in the mind and life of the therapist, while the second person can. Being able to describe this ability is important for understanding cognitive function.

Mentalization—truly trying to think about what is going on in the mind of another person—is different from making inferences based on cultural stereotypes and implicit biases about social groups. (Kang & Falk, 2020; Mattan et al., 2018; Reihl et al., 2015; Stoute, 2019; West & Eaton, 2019). For example, a person might say, "I know what that guy is thinking. They [all members of a particular group] hate the government." Despite the fact that the person believes that they are thinking about what goes on in the mind of another person, it is actually evidence of implicit bias and stereotyping.

Learning about cognition: opening questions, then stories

Learning about basic cognitive function

Information about basic cognitive function will come from your direct experience with people. You can notice things like

When they tell their story, is it organized in a coherent way?

Are they able to remember appointments and plan for new ones?

Do they come to appointments and pay bills on time?

Do they have a reasonable fund of knowledge?

You can also ask direct questions, such as

Are you someone who is usually on time, or are you often late?

At your job/school, are you generally able to concentrate and get your work done?

Are you generally well organized? Disorganized?

If your evaluation suggests significant problems in basic cognitive function, you may want to consider administering a brief cognitive screening test, such as the Mini-Mental Status Examination (MMSE) (Cournos et al., 2008), or referring the patient for neuropsychological testing. The presence of cognitive problems in association with other psychiatric disorders, such as depression or anxiety, should lead you to consider the potential impact of these disorders on cognition.

Learning about higher (executive) cognitive functions

Managing emotions

Particularly when asking about feelings, you'll learn the most by asking for stories:

What happens when you get angry or anxious? Can you "sit" with the feeling or do you feel driven to do something? Can you tell me about a time when you got really upset?

Would people describe you as calm and even-tempered? As volatile?

Do you ever become physically violent with others? Can you tell me about a time when that happened?

Impulse control

Many clinicians ask about substance use and eating disorders, but learning about impulse control and judgment involves much more than that. We want to be able to describe the kinds of problems people have with impulses, but we also want to describe the individual ways they try to curb their impulses. Questions like these can be helpful:

> *Would your friends describe you as a risk-taker? Can you tell me the story of a risk you've taken?*
>
> *Do you ever feel that you're too impulsive? Tell me about a time when you felt you were.*
>
> *Would someone describe you as having a quick temper?*
>
> *Do you tend to hang back or just jump into things?*
>
> *Do you find it hard to keep from doing things you think you probably shouldn't do? Has that happened recently? Can you tell me about it?*
>
> *Do you ever drink/eat to excess? If so, how much? Can you tell me about a time when that happened?*
>
> *What types of things do you do to keep yourself from being impulsive?*

Judgment

To assess judgment, consider asking questions like

> *Are you a person who tends to follow rules?*
>
> *Have there been times when you broke rules? How did you decide to do that?*
>
> *Would people who know you describe you as someone with good judgment?*

Here again, listening to stories can help. Stories about poor investments, rule bending, failure to use condoms and other methods of birth control, and driving while intoxicated can tell you a great deal about a person's judgment. If you think that a story clearly illustrates impaired judgment, find out whether the person thinks that they acted wisely. This can help you to differentiate judgment from impulse control. For example, consider this exchange:

> *Patient #1: So, I met this guy at a bar and we went back to his place and had sex.*
>
> *Therapist: Did you use a condom?*
>
> *Patient #1: No.*
>
> *Therapist: Was that what you meant to do?*
>
> *Patient #1: Yeah, it's fine. I haven't had anything bad happen yet.*

This patient clearly used questionable judgment. On the other hand, consider another patient's response to the same question:

> *Patient #2: No, are you kidding? It's so dangerous. But in the moment, I just can't stop to make sure that I'm safe—I just act.*

This patient knows how to act safely but shows poor impulse control. Judgment is still impaired, but the difference is important for the treatment.

Sensory regulation

Do you think that you're particularly sensitive to things like loud noises or smells? What bothers you most?

Do you ever experience the environment in ways that you think that others don't?

Decision-making and problem-solving

You will often learn about this from the chief complaint or from the way a person finds time to meet or decides about starting treatment. Direct questions, followed by requests for stories, will help you learn the most about people make decisions:

Do you find it easy/hard to make decisions?

Tell me about a recent decision that you made. How did you reach it?

Do you typically research options, or do you tend to "trust your gut?"

When you have many things to do, do you make a list?

Learning about reality testing and sense of reality

Hearing "yes" to any of these questions can prompt you to ask about a story with, "Tell me about a time when that happened."

Reality testing

Do you ever have trouble deciding if something really happened or if it was a dream?

Have you ever wondered if a thing happened only in your mind?

Have you ever been told by people that what you say doesn't make sense? That your ideas are way off? Can you tell me about a time when that happened?

Have you ever heard strange sounds in your ears or thought you heard a voice that you couldn't account for? Have you ever thought you saw something in the corner of your eye, and then looked around and it wasn't there? In those moments, have you known that what you are hearing (or seeing) couldn't be real even though it seemed real at the time?

Have you ever wondered if you might be hallucinating? Tell me about that time.

Do you often feel people are against you in some way? Following you? Monitoring you?

Sense of reality

Most people sometimes have the experience that things are happening that have happened before, like a déjà vu experience. Has that ever happened to you? Did you wonder if it really happened or was just your imagination?

Have you ever felt as though you were walking around in a trance? That people or things around you felt unreal or two-dimensional? Like you were living your life in a movie?

Have you ever felt you or your body were not real? Have you ever had the experience that parts of your body felt much bigger or smaller than usual? As if some part of your body is changing?

Have you ever had trouble feeling yourself to be a person separate and independent from other people? Do you frequently have the sense that you are somehow merging with other people?

Learning about reflective (metacognitive) cognitive function

Self-reflection

A good way to assess self-reflection is by gently suggesting that a thought, feeling, or behavior has a possible underlying meaning, which is sometimes called a **trial interpretation**. Consider the following exchange between a patient and a therapist:

Patient: I can't believe I slept through my sister's baby shower! I was so tired. I think my alarm clock must have malfunctioned.

Therapist: Well, last time you were talking about how hard it is for you that your sister is having a baby when your relationship with your partner has just ended. Do you think maybe you didn't want to go to the shower?

Patient: Wow, are you saying I overslept on purpose? That does kind of sound like me. I really didn't want to go. She doesn't even ask me how I'm doing.

Psychological mindedness does not mean understanding everything right away. This person does not immediately consider ambivalence but is receptive and thoughtful when the therapist asks about possible unconscious motivations. A less psychologically minded person might have replied to the therapist's comments by saying,

No way! Of course, I'm happy for her. Therapists always think there's double meaning in everything.

Mentalization

A good way to assess mentalization is to ask the patient to think about how another person thinks or feels, as in this example:

Patient: I'm so mad at my friend—she hasn't responded to my last phone call, and I'm sure it's because she's angry at me.

Therapist: When did you call her?

Patient: About 20 minutes ago.

Therapist: Do you think that there could be another reason why she hasn't called back yet?

Patient: No—if people like you, they get back to you right away.

This patient's difficulty thinking of another reason for a friend's behavior suggests problems with mentalizing. Asking people questions like . . .

How might that person be looking at things differently?

How do you imagine that I might be feeling?

. . .can help you to gauge their ability to mentalize.

Describing patterns related to cognition

We can now try to DESCRIBE patterns related to cognition Consider Monica:

> Monica came to this country for college and has lived here since she graduated 15 years ago. She has a green card and works as a university librarian. She presents for therapy requesting support after she was left by her partner of five years. So far, she arrived at all four sessions on time and has paid for the evaluation. Although English was not her first language, the therapist notes that Monica speaks flawless English with only a trace of an accent. Monica says that she is having difficulty sleeping, but that she is managing to work and has just closed on a new apartment. "Even though," she adds, "I was deciding between two places until the very last minute." She describes her childhood as "happy," then says that her mother was very depressed and abused alcohol; when the therapist notes this discrepancy, she says, "That's interesting, I didn't think about it like that." When asked about the circumstances of the break-up, Monica says, "I really don't know. Since I ended my affair, I thought things were going really well."

Here's how we might DESCRIBE Monica's patterns related to cognition:

> Monica seems to have good **basic cognitive function**. She arrived on time for her evaluation sessions, is able to manage her finances, and has excellent language skills. She is capable of **making decisions, problem-solving**, and exercising **judgment**, as evidenced by her recent ability to choose and buy her own apartment, despite her last-minute difficulties with making choices. Her ability to consider the therapist's comments suggest that she has a capacity for **self-reflection**, although her inability to imagine that her recent affair might have affected her partner suggests that she might have difficulty with **mentalization**.

Suggested activity

How would you describe the cognitive function of these patients?

> Simone, who works as a landscape architect, was doing very well at work until she was promoted to manage others. She is now alternately angry and anxious and unable to keep track of what her team members are doing. She has difficulty delegating work and ends up redoing much of what they do. She dreads the weekly meeting when she has to report to her boss—the first time she walked in with 10 lists that ended up scattered all over the floor.

> Gerry says he is "fed up" with his wife because she spends too much time at work. She has a high-profile job at a bank that pays for their lavish lifestyle, which Gerry enjoys. "Our marital problems are all due to the fact that she's a workaholic," he says, "The only way for things to get better is for her to just say NO the next time her boss tells her to stay late!"

Comment

Simone seems to have **creative talent**; however, she lacks **organizational abilities**. She also has difficulty **making decisions**, particularly relating to managing her team.

Gerry is unable to **mentalize** and lacks capacity for **self-reflection**.

References

1. Bellak, L., & Meyers, B. (1975). Ego function assessment and analysability. *International Review of Psychoanalysis, 2*, 413–427. http://www.mindmeister.com/generic_files/get_file/9559058?filetype=attachment_file

2. Cabaniss, D. L., Cherry, S., Douglas, C. J., & Schwartz, A. (2017). *Psychodynamic psychotherapy: A clinical manual* (2nd ed.). Wiley Blackwell.

3. Cournos, F., Lowenthal, D. A., & Cabaniss, D. S. (2008). Clinical evaluation and treatment: A multimodal approach. In A. Tasman, J. Kay, J. A. Lieberman, M. First, & M. Mario (Eds.), *Psychiatry* (3rd ed., pp. 525–545). Wiley Blackwell. https://doi.org/10.1002/9780470515167

4. Descartes, R. (1998). *Discourse on method and meditations on first philosophy*. (D. Cress, Trans.). Hackett Publishing Company. (Original work published in 1637).

5. Dimaggio, G., & Lysaker, P. H. (Eds.) (2010). *Metacognition and severe adult mental disorders: From basic research to treatment*. Routledge.

6. Flavell, J. H. (1987). Speculations about the nature and development of metacognition. In F. E. Weinert & R. H. Kluwe (Eds.), *Metacognition, motivation, and understanding* (pp. 21–29). Lawrence Erlbaum Associates.

7. Friedman, C., & Owen, A. L. (2017). Defining disability: Understandings of and attitudes towards ableism and disability. *Disability Studies Quarterly, 37*(1), 2–30. http://dsq-sds.org/article/view/5061/4545

8. Gabbard, G. O., Litowitz, B. E., & Williams, P. (Eds.) (2012). *Textbook of psychoanalysis* (2nd ed.). American Psychiatric Publishing, Inc.

9. Galatzer-Levy, R. M., & Cohler, B. J. (1993). *The essential other: A developmental psychology of the self*. Basic Books.

10. Hehir, T. (2002). Eliminating ableism in education. *Harvard Educational Review, 72*(1), 1–32. https://doi.org/10.17763/haer.72.1.03866528702g2105

11. Kang, Y., & Falk, E. B. (2020). Neural mechanisms of attitude change toward stigmatized individuals: Temporoparietal junction activity predicts bias reduction. *Mindfulness, 11*, 1378–1389. https://doi.org/10.1007/s12671-020-01357-y

12. Keller, H., Voelker, S., & Yovsi, R. D. (2005). Conceptions of parenting in different cultural communities: The case of West African Nso and Northern German women. *Social Development, 14*(1), 158–180. https://doi.org/10.1111/j.1467-9507.2005.00295.x

13. Keri, S., Kallai, I., & Csigo, K. (2020). Attribution of mental states in glossolalia: A direct comparison with schizophrenia. *Frontiers in Psychology, 11*, 638. Published online 2020 Apr 15. https://www.frontiersin.org/articles/10.3389/fpsyg.2020.00638

14. Levy, A. (2010). *Tools of critical thinking: Metathoughts for psychology*. Waveland Press, Inc.

15. Lysaker, P. H., DiMaggio, G., & Brüne, M. (2014). *Social cognition and metacognition in Schizophrenia: Psychopathology and treatment approaches* (1st ed.). Elsevier Inc. Academic Press.

16. Mattan, B. D., Wei, K. Y., Cloutier, J., & Kubota, J. T. (2018). The social neuroscience of race-based and status-based prejudice. *Current Opinion in Psychology, 24*, 27–34. https://doi.org/10.1016/j.copsyc.2018.04.010

17. Reihl, K. M., Hurley, R. A., & Taber, K. H. (2015). Neurobiology of implicit and explicit bias: Implications for clinicians. *The Journal of Neuropsychiatry and Clinical Neurosciences, 27*(4), 248–253. https://doi.org/10.1176/appi.neuropsych.15080212

18. Semerari, A., Carcione, A., Dimaggio, G., Maurizio, F., Nicolo, G., Procacci, M., & Alleva, G. (2003). How to evaluate metacognitive function in psychotherapy? The metacognition assessment scale and its applications. *Clinical Psychology & Psychotherapy, 10*, 238–261. https://doi.org/10.1002/cpp.362

19. Semerari, A., Colle, L., Pellecchia, G., Buccioni, I., Carcione, A., Dimaggio, G., Nicolo, G., Procacci, M., & Pedone, R. (2014). Metacognitive dysfunctions in personality disorders: Correlations with disorder severity and personality styles. *Journal of Personality Disorders*, *28*(6), 1–16. https://doi.org/10.1521/pedi_2014_28_137

20. Spezzano, C. (2012). Intersubjectivity. In G. O. Gabbard, B. E. Litowitz, & P. Williams (Eds.), *Textbook of psychoanalysis* (2nd ed.). American Psychiatric Publishing, Inc.

21. Stoute, B. J. (2019). Racial socialization and thwarted mentalization: Psychoanalytic reflections from the lived experience of James Baldwin's America. *Journal of the American Academy of Child and Adolescent Psychiatry*, *57*(10), S117. https://doi.org/10.1016/J.JAAC.2018.09.015

22. Trommsdorff, G., & Cole, P. M. (2011). Emotion, self-regulation, and social behavior in cultural contexts. In X. Chen & K. H. Rubin (Eds.), *Socioemotional development in cultural context* (pp. 131–163). Guilford Press.

23. Trommsdorff, G., Cole, P., & Heikamp, T. (2012). Cultural variations in mothers' intuitive theories: A preliminary report on interviewing mothers from five nations about their socialization of children's emotions. *Global Studies of Childhood*, *2*, 158–169. https://dx.doi.org/10.2304/gsch.2012.2.2.158

24. Tummula-Narra, P. (2016). *Psychoanalytic theory and cultural competence in psychotherapy* (pp. 125–132). American Psychological Association.

25. West, K., & Eaton, A. A. (2019). Prejudiced and unaware of it: Evidence for the dunning-Kruger model in the domains of racism and sexism. *Personality and Individual Differences*, *146*, 111–119. https://doi.org/10.1016/j.paid.2019.03.047

10 Values

As part of a study, a three-year-old child is told the following story:

> *A mother tells a child and his younger sibling not to touch the bathroom shelf where the Band-Aids are kept. After the mother leaves, the children play and the younger sibling cuts himself and asks the child for a Band-Aid.*

Then the child is asked, "Show me and tell me what happens next" (Oppenheim et al., 1997, p. 947). The researchers who devised this scenario found that even at this young age, many children could acknowledge and even resolve the dilemma. Thus, they were beginning to have and use a sense of right and wrong. Developing before the child's ability to consciously delineate rules, this set of values is out of their awareness, or unconscious. Although we are consciously aware of some of our values, many aspects of our value system are unconscious and implicit. Understanding the way that a person's values affect their thoughts, feelings, and behaviors is an essential part of the psychodynamic formulation.

Psychodynamic Formulation: An Expanded Approach, First Edition. The Psychodynamic Formulation Collective.
© 2022 John Wiley & Sons Ltd. Published 2022 by John Wiley & Sons Ltd.

Defining the area: values

Pinocchio called it "Jiminy Cricket", and Freud called it the **super-ego** (Freud, 1923/1971). Whatever you call it, our system of values is a major part of who we are. Our values guide the way we think about ourselves and our actions, how we behave, and how we judge others and our culture. Values are called by many names—morals, ethics, super-ego function, conscience, and prosocial behavior (Hoffman, 2008), and they continue to develop throughout our lives (Emde et al., 1991). These terms mean different things to different people in different fields. Rather than choosing definitions that suit us, we will consider the fundamental aspects of this important domain of function.

Variables for describing values

We can think about three aspects of a person's values:

- Sense of right and wrong
- Right/wrong behavior
- Personal values

While these overlap, they are different, and thus it's important to describe them all in the following text.

Sense of right and wrong

Our internal "shoulds" and "shouldn'ts" begin to develop during our very first years of life. They ultimately form our **sense of right and wrong**. Their development is influenced by temperament, our earliest caregivers, our peers, our belief systems, and the culture in which we live (Emde et al., 1991). They guide how we think about ourselves, others, and society in general. Although we may be consciously aware of them, they are, in large part, automatic and unconscious. Consider, for example, a healthcare professional who uses their "for emergencies only" tag to park in a tow-away zone so they can pick up medication for a family member. They might think, "this is justified," but then feel irritable and have a restless night of sleep. While they consciously justified their choice, it is likely that unconscious internal values affected their mood and sleep. As psychodynamic psychotherapists, we must have a sense of our patients' unconscious values as they can affect many aspects of their lives and can even cause symptoms.

A person's sense of right and wrong can be described using the following variables, each of which is along a continuum.

Right/wrong system

What is someone's **system of right and wrong**, and how does it work? Or, because people may have different right/wrong systems in different situations (Jensen 2015), what are their systems of right and wrong? People base their systems of right and wrong on various things. Some abide by civic codes and laws, others by religious codes, and some by cultural standards. Most of us use a combination. Rather than suggesting that a person does or doesn't have a sense of right and wrong, it's more important to understand how someone's right/wrong systems function. Some may have very consistent systems of right and wrong, others may vary their systems depending on the situation (Jensen, 2015), and still others may have times when their systems seem to dissolve.

Harshness

Do someone's values lead them to excessively judge themselves or others? Traditionally, this was known as having a harsh super-ego. **Harshness** or leniency relates to whether the amount and quality of value judgment seems to match the perceived infraction. What's important here is understanding what harshness means to the person. We hear harshness in the person who, raised in poverty, saves all their money and deprives themself of any luxuries, thinking, "Why should I have luxuries when my parents had none?" As therapists, our job isn't to judge the harshness and whether it is justified, but rather to try to understand what the harshness means and to reflect upon the accuracy of a harsh assessment.

Flexibility

For some, values are values, while for others situations may affect the way they see right and wrong (Jensen, 2015). For example, in Toni Morrison's novel *Beloved*, a mother kills her child (Morrison, 2012). While the values of most people would condemn this act, the consideration that the mother was a fugitive slave pursued by slave catchers may allow many people to flexibly judge this act. This kind of **flexibility** may foster empathy and forgiveness.

Right/wrong behavior

How we think, feel, and judge others is one thing—how we act is another (Gibbs, 2019, p. 8). We can call the behavior that is guided by our values **right/wrong behavior**. This behavior is a major dimension of who we are and how we are perceived by others. We can usefully separate it from internal values because, while these two dimensions of our value system may overlap and intersect, they are not necessarily identical. We can describe our right/wrong behavior using the following variables.

Consistency with one's sense of right and wrong

Think of the person who says, "I know it's wrong but I'm going to do it anyway" versus the person whose behavior more consistently matches their internal sense of right and wrong. A classic question in the mental status exam is, "What would you do with a $100 bill you found on the street?" Some people say, "It belongs to someone else—I'd take it to the police," while others might say, "Yeah, I know you shouldn't take things, but who would know?" Knowing that something is wrong but using the measure of how likely one is to be caught to guide behavior is quite different from choosing one's actions in the absence of that consideration.

Consistency with one's family or culture

Is the individual's right/wrong behavior similar to or different from that of the people around them? This can be very important to describe. For example, consider an 18-year-old adult who refuses to go to parties or date, saying that it's "sinful." If this person lived in a culture in which all 18-year-old adults shared this belief, we might view that behavior one way while if they lived in an environment in which 18-year-old adults generally socialized, we might think about their behavior in another way. Contextualizing a person's behavior helps us to understand it, rather than judge it.

Prosocial behavior

The opposite of antisocial behavior, **prosocial behavior**, is defined as "social action intended to benefit others . . . without anticipation of personal reward" (Gibbs, 2019, p. 157). This particular kind of value-driven behavior is important to describe in its presence or absence (again, along a continuum). Consider two people who don't litter: one who is driven by the wish to have a beautiful city, and the other who is driven by the wish to leave the Earth greener for the next generation. We would say that the second person's behavior is more prosocial.

Personal values

What motivates us? What gives our lives meaning? What is important to us? These are what we can call our **personal values**. Personal values vary from person to person, guiding everything from the choice of a partner to the choice of a career. They can include motivators such as money, status, religion and family, as well as more abstract concepts such as integrity, hard work, inclusion, justice, honesty, and spirituality. For example, consider four women, each of whom has chosen to work while raising their children. One might work because she wants her family to have more money, the second might work because she finds it personally fulfilling, the third might work because she feels that it's important for women to be treated equally in society, and the fourth might work in order to survive. They're four women with similar behaviors, each guided by different personal values. As therapists, it's important for us to understand our own personal values in order to describe and explore the values of our patients without judgment.

Values and cultural context

Although early theories of moral development favored the concept of universal values (Kohlberg, 1981), current research suggests that the way we think about right and wrong is shaped by the culture (or cultures) in which we live (Pandya & Bhangaonkar, 2015).

For example, in one study, investigators found that adults were more inclined to choose to help others when it was suggested to them that "God was watching" (Shariff & Norenzayan, 2007). Others have found that school-age children in the United States raised in conservative religious households had different ideas about values compared to those raised in more progressive households (Jensen, 2015). In his book *The Making of a Racist*, historian Charles Dew, who was raised in a conservative Southern family, writes about how his experiences as a student at Williams College (in Massachusetts) helped to transform his views on race and racism (Dew, 2016). Our lived experiences and the cultures in which they occur affect the development of our values through life.

Learning about values: opening questions, then stories

When learning about someone's values, we enable ourselves to be guided by the individual's life experience and situation. People come to therapy because they are under stress—they may be in some type of trouble, be traumatized, have regrets, feel guilty, or simply be confused about an upcoming decision. We must learn how their values are intertwined with the specifics of their stories. For all of the following, it will also be useful to ask whether the person shares these values with members of their immediate and community environments.

Learning about a person's sense of right and wrong

The best way to learn about values is to work with the individual's personal experience. For example, we can ask a patient who feels guilty or who is self-punishing about the thoughts that guide those feelings. We can also learn about internal values through the transference. For example, the way that patients handle time and money may shed light on conscious or unconscious values. Confronting inconsistencies can help us to learn about harshness—for example, asking a person who says that they don't deserve therapy why they feel that way. Here are some other sample questions that you can adapt and modify:

> *When (you or another person) did that, did you think that was right?*
>
> *What do you think about that decision? Do you wish you'd made another choice?*
>
> *You say that you feel guilty—what do you think you did wrong?*
>
> *Who taught you about right and wrong?*
>
> *Has your sense of what's right and wrong changed over your lifetime? Why do you think that happened?*
>
> *Is your sense of right and wrong linked to your personal belief system or your cultural background? Do you think it's different from your family's sense of right and wrong, or that of your cultural background?*

Learning about right/wrong behavior

Learning about right/wrong behavior also begins with the stories people tell. Are they talking about a fight with a loved one? Are they in some kind of trouble? Have they just done something they regret? Getting people to talk about these stories can tell us a great deal about their right/wrong behavior. Talking about their feelings about us (the **transference**) can help as well. Here are a few ideas:

If you could do that again, would you do it the same way?

You've talked a lot about how much you regret how you treated your sister. What do you think you did wrong?

You seem angry with me about the way that I handled the session you missed. What do you think I did wrong?

Learning about personal values

What feels most important to you in life? Why?

What values motivate you?

What are you looking for out of life?

If you could ask for one thing in the world, what would it be? How would that improve your life?

Who are your role models? Why?

Describing VALUES

Let's consider Carlos as we think about DESCRIBING values:

Carlos presents at the suggestion of his pastor, who became concerned about Carlos after a recent conversation in which Carlos said he was "guilt ridden" about not being able to attend church services during the pandemic. "I've had a lot of lapses," Carlos tells the therapist. "I drank a lot as a young man. If my God-fearing father had known, he would have thrown me out of the house—and with good reason." Carlos says he spends all of his spare time working as a deacon in his church, and that he is dedicated to raising his children to "love God" and to do service for others.

Here's how we might DESCRIBE Carlos' patterns related to values:

*Raised in a religious household, Carlos has a clear **sense of right and wrong** that can sometimes be quite **harsh and inflexible**—particularly toward himself. Examples of this are guilt about not attending church during the pandemic (when this was impossible for most people), and his internal preoccupation with what he calls "lapses" in his **right-wrong behavior**. Now, he holds himself to rigid behavioral guidelines that are **consistent with his internal values and those of his community**, abstaining from alcohol altogether and spending all his free time working as a deacon in his church. His **primary values** relate to raising children who share his beliefs and behaviors.*

Variables for describing VALUES

Sense of right/wrong includes:

- Right/wrong system
- Harshness
- Flexibility

Right/wrong behavior includes:

- Consistency with sense of right/wrong
- Consistent with one's family/culture
- Prosocial behavior

Personal values includes:

- Types (e.g., education, family, money)
- Consistent with/divergent from those around them

Suggested activity
Can be done by individual learners or in a classroom setting

Think of a patient with whom you are working in any clinical setting. Can you list that person's personal values? How did you learn about them? What questions were useful in eliciting this information? Share your ideas if you are in a learning group.

References

1. Dew, C. B. (2016). *The making of a racist: A southerner reflects on family, history and the slave trade*. University of Virginia Press.
2. Emde, R. N., Biringen, Z., Clyman, R. B., & Oppenheim, D. (1991). The moral self of infancy: Affect core and procedural knowledge. *Developmental Review, 11*, 252–270.
3. Freud, S. (1971). The ego and the id. In J. Strachey (Ed.), *The standard edition of the complete psychological works of Sigmund Freud, Volume XIX (1923–1925): The ego and the id and other works* (pp. 1–66). Hogarth Press. (Original work published in 1923).
4. Gibbs, J. C. (2019). *Moral development and reality* (4th ed.). Oxford University Press.
5. Hoffman, M. L. (2008). Empathy and prosocial behavior. In M. Lewis, J. M. Haviland-Jones, & L. F. Barrett (Eds.), *Handbook of eemotions* (pp. 440–455). The Guilford Press.
6. Jensen, L. A. (Ed.) (2015). *Moral development in a global world*. Cambridge University Press.
7. Kohlberg, L. (1981). *Essays on moral development (volume I): The philosophy of moral development*. Harper & Row.
8. Morrison, T. (2012). *Beloved*. Alfred A. Knopf Inc.
9. Oppenheim, D., Emde, R. N., Hasson, M., & Warren, S. (1997). Preschoolers face moral dilemmas: A longitudinal study of acknowledging and resolving internal conflict. *The International Journal of Psycho-Analysis, 78*, 943–957.
10. Pandya, N., & Bhangaonkar, R. (2015). Divinity in children's moral development: An Indian perspective. In L. A. Jensen (Ed.), *Moral development in a global world*. Cambridge University Press.
11. Shariff, A. F., & Norenzayan, A. (2007). God is watching you: Priming God concepts increases prosocial behavior in an anonymous economic game. *Psychological Science, 18*(9). https://doi.org/10.1111/j.1467-9280.2007.01983.x

11 Work and Play

Key concepts

We spend most of our lives engaged in some type of work or play. Thus, it is an important area of function to understand when we create psychodynamic formulations.
We can describe people's work and play using the following variables:

- Consistency with developmental level/talents/limitations
- Comfortable/satisfying/pleasurable/restful
- Adequate for care of self and dependents
- Culturally sanctioned
- Limited because of restricted access

We spend our time doing myriad things. We work and study, relax and socialize. As mental health professionals, we are less interested in what people *should* do in life, and more interested in understanding what they *choose* to do and how it *serves* them. In order to do this, we must be able to describe how people spend their time. Freud is reputed to have said that people need to be able to *love and work* (Masson, 1985), and to this many have added *play* (Benveniste, 1998; Brown, 2009). Having discussed *love* in Chapter 7, let's now think about work and play.

Defining the area: work and play

Work

Webster's Dictionary defines **work** as "physical or mental effort exerted to do or make something; purposeful activity" (Webster's, 1970, p. 1638). Most people in the world engage in some type of work. Although we generally think about work as something that someone does to earn money, work can be any of the following:

- **Paid or unpaid**—A second grader's work is going to school, and a stay-at-home parent's work is taking care of children. When cleaning, cooking, child-rearing,

Psychodynamic Formulation: An Expanded Approach, First Edition. The Psychodynamic Formulation Collective.
© 2022 John Wiley & Sons Ltd. Published 2022 by John Wiley & Sons Ltd.

and elder care are conducted within a family, they are generally unpaid forms of work. Volunteering is also considered unpaid work.

- **Consistent or sporadic**—Two adolescents might both work as babysitters, but if one works every weekend and the other one only works now and then, their work patterns are very different.
- **Skilled or unskilled**—Some work can be done with very little instruction, while other work requires extensive training. Note, that training can take many forms, including education via technical schools, graduate schools, and apprenticeships.

Play

Relaxing on a beach, watching TV, reading fiction, socializing, throwing a football, traveling, cooking—everyone has a different way of playing. People who know how to play may have healthier emotional lives and may age more successfully (Terr, 1999; Vaillant, 2002). As mental health professionals, we often forget to ask about what people do to relax, but patterns of play are central to a person's functioning. When thinking about play, consider

- **How much time it occupies in the person's life**—Two people might say that they enjoy reading, but if one reads a few magazines a month and the other goes to two book clubs per week, they have different patterns of play.
- **Alone or with others**—Some people enjoy solitary forms of relaxation, such as building models in the basement, while others enjoy going to huge rock concerts or throwing weekly dinner parties.
- **Depth and breadth of involvement**—Some people are very involved in only one form of play, while others try many forms. For example, one person might cite walking as their only leisure activity while doing it intensely; in contrast, another person might cite numerous pastimes while engaging in them superficially.
- **Sex as play**—Sex can be an important aspect of the way people relax and enjoy themselves. Sexual activity has also been shown to be important for an adult's mental and emotional health (DeLamater, 2012). It is important to ask about this part of our patients' lives, including whether they regularly engage in sexual activity, whether it is satisfying, with whom they are sexually active, whether their sexual activity is recreational, and whether it is in the context of a loving relationship.
- **Play and rest**—Some forms of play can be as stressful as work. It's important to find out whether people have ways to rest and decompress from life's stressors.
- **No play**—If people do not mention any leisure activity, be sure to ask about it. It's crucial to find out whether there's something the person enjoys doing—even if it's watching TV or reading the newspaper. Some people, however, have no leisure activities, which could indicate that they have difficulty relaxing and enjoying themselves.

Variables for describing work and play

Along with describing *what* a person does for work and play, we also want to think about how well these patterns serve them and those around them. To do this, we must consider whether the person's work and play patterns are

- Consistent with developmental level/talents/limitations
- Comfortable/satisfying/pleasurable/restful
- Adequate for care of self and dependents
- Culturally sanctioned
- Limited because of restricted access

Are work and play consistent with the person's developmental level, training, talents, and limitations?

A 16 year old who works in a fast-food restaurant to make extra money during high school may be highly motivated, but a 45-year-old chemist with a PhD in the same job may be underemployed. A 12 year old who plays video games on weekends with friends may be having developmentally appropriate fun, but a 55 year old who plays video games all day at work may be jeopardizing their job. When thinking about work and play, we not only have to think about what the person is doing, but also whether it matches the person's developmental phase, training, talents, and limitations.

Are work and play comfortable and pleasurable?

Fun is not just for kids—everyone needs to do things they enjoy. Some people love their work, while for others it is simply something they do to put food on the table. Work can also be satisfying but not necessarily enjoyable. Interestingly, some people do not find their leisure activities pleasurable. Sometimes, this is because of the "play preferences" of partners or family members. Consider the person who hates camping but is constantly dragged into the woods by their partner, or a child who hates basketball but feels compelled to play with their parent every weekend. For others, play becomes compulsive and ceases to be enjoyable. Think of the person who feels compelled to run 20 miles a day despite numerous injuries and daily post-run nausea. Hearing about these leisure choices will likely help us to understand the person.

Are work and play adequate for care of self and dependents?

People may love their work, but it may not pay the bills. Consider the writer who enjoys creating a novel but can't pay for health insurance. For some people, making a lot of money is not a high priority, but they still must have enough money to provide food, shelter, and health care for themselves and their dependents. Sometimes, a person is supported by a spouse or other family members. In this situation, it's important to assess whether this is a mutually agreed-upon situation, and if it is satisfactory to the individual. The couple who mutually decides that one partner will stay home to raise children may be very happy with this arrangement, while the family who continues to support an adult child who seems to be avoiding work may be less satisfied.

Play is also important with regard to self-care, because regular physical exercise is essential for physical and mental health (Paluska & Schwenk, 2000). If a person is unable to exercise, for example, because they have to work three jobs to feed their family, then their pattern of play is inadequate for self-care.

Are work and play health-promoting and culturally sanctioned?

In order to fully understand a person's work and play patterns, it's important to know *how* they fit into the world in which the person lives and whether they are health-promoting patterns. For example, if people make their living through illegal activities, or if their leisure involves harming others or substance misuse, then it's hard to say that their work and play patterns are health promoting or well suited to life in their environment.

Aside from work and leisure activities involving substance misuse and illegal activities, thinking about whether work and play patterns are culturally sanctioned can be tricky, particularly in cross-cultural situations. For example, a person who recently immigrated from another country may look askance at their office's weekly happy hour, while a therapist treating someone from another culture might question that person's wish to take all their vacations with their extended family. Once again, understanding these leisure patterns requires sensitivity to cultural background.

Are work and play limited because of restricted access?

An individual's work and play may be limited because of access. Consider the following:

A person who trained as a physician in their country of origin but works in a laundromat after immigrating because they lack the language skills to take the qualifying exam

A person who grew up playing tennis and continues to enjoy it but cannot play now because the only courts in the area are part of a club which denied them admission

A person who would like a more challenging job but has to work for minimum wage because their family was not able to pay for higher education

Through no fault of their own, these people do not have access to work and play that would serve them.

Learning about work and play: opening questions, then stories

Here are some sample questions you can adapt to learn about various aspects of work and play

Learning about whether work and play are consistent with developmental level, talents, and limitations

For people who are working:

> *How long have you been doing the work you do?*
>
> *Have you been at the same job since you started working, or have you moved from workplace to workplace?*
>
> *Did this work require training? If so, what kind?*
>
> *Is this what you would ideally like to be doing? If not, what is keeping you from doing what you prefer to do?*
>
> *Tell me about something you are currently doing at work.*

For students:

> *How did you choose what and where you are studying?*
>
> *Does this course of study seem like a good fit?*
>
> *Are you working toward something, such as a career?*

For play:

> *When did you begin this leisure activity?*
>
> *Do you do this activity with people your age?*
>
> *How much time does it take up in your life?*
>
> *How does it fit in with other things you do in your life?*

Learning about whether work and play are comfortable and pleasurable

> *How do you like your work? Is it hard to go to work in the morning?*
>
> *Do you find your work satisfying? Are there things about it that you find more or less enjoyable than others?*
>
> *Are there things that you look forward to doing? Do you have fun? Tell me about something that you are looking forward to.*
>
> *How do you decompress? Are your leisure activities restful?*

Learning about whether work and play are adequate for care of self and dependents

> *Are you able to make ends meet? For yourself? For your family?*
>
> *Are you satisfied with the way in which you support yourself financially?*

Do you receive financial help from someone else (including the government)? How do you feel about this? Are you in debt?

Are you able to get regular physical exercise? If not, why?

Learning about whether work and play patterns are culturally sanctioned and/or healthy

Have you ever been in trouble with the law? For what type of activity?

Do your leisure activities ever involve illegal substances?

Are you ever concerned that something you are doing might not be legal?

Learning about whether work and play are limited because of restricted access

Is there something that you'd rather be doing but are unable to because of discrimination?

Do you feel that your choices in life have been restricted because of who you are or where you are from? Can you tell me about a time when that happened?

Describing work and play patterns

Using the variables that we outlined earlier in the chapter, let's consider Kimberly:

Kimberly presents with irritability after a recent orthopedic surgery. "I was a Division I athlete in college. I need physical activity to stay sane, and now I'm really sidelined. How am I going to wind down without tennis?" Kimberly, who was trained as a chemist, has worked in the home, caring for her two daughters since she had her first child 18 years ago. "I wanted to really be a mom, and my wife really wanted to go back to work. We have plenty of money with her salary and have been happy with this all these years." Kimberly loves being what she calls a "perennial class parent" and is a bit anxious about losing this when her children attend college.

Here's how we might DESCRIBE Kimberly's patterns of work and play:

*Kimberly has considerable strengths in her patterns of **work and play**. Although her work is **not consistent with her level of training**, it is a mutually agreed upon arrangement with her wife with which she is **comfortable** and from which she derives great **pleasure**. Her patterns of play— most of which involve athletics—have brought her great **enjoyment** but might be too limited now that she has been injured. Similarly, she is concerned that she will not be able to do the things she enjoys once her children leave home.*

Variables for describing WORK AND PLAY

- Consistent with developmental level/talents/limitations
- Comfortable/satisfying/pleasurable
- Adequate for care of self and dependents
- Culturally sanctioned
- Limited because of restricted access

Suggested activity

Can be done by individual learners or in a classroom setting

How would you describe the work/play of the following people?

Alvin has been married for 30 years, has two grown sons, and has worked as a sanitation engineer since he was 22 years old. He's proud of the fact that, although he did not graduate from high school, he owns his own home, which he says is the "hub" where his family gathers for dinners on Sundays, Thanksgiving, and Christmas. He and his wife enjoy watching TV, which they do for approximately two to three hours each night after dinner. An avid fisherman, he enjoys going to his fishing cabin at least once a month, joined by his best friend and his brother.

Katy is in the 10th year of her PhD program at a prestigious university. She finished her class-work and oral exams six years ago and has been writing her thesis ever since. Most of her classmates have graduated, and some even have faculty positions. She is an excellent teacher who has received teaching awards as a graduate student. She is still supported by her elderly parents, who are themselves having difficulty making ends meet. She is unhappy with her academic progress and is unable to move forward with her writing.

Xavier has been married for eight years and has two small children. He works in his father's business, where he struggles to keep up with his peers. He lives beyond his means and constantly feels stressed about money. He was a mediocre student in college but matriculated at a prestigious business school with the help of his father's friends. Unbeknownst to his wife, he has been using prescription opioids to relax.

Comment

Alvin has steady work that allows him to care for himself and his family, with which he is comfortable. He takes great enjoyment from being with his family and fishing.

While Katy's work is consistent with her level of training, she is not comfortable with her work, and it is not adequate for self-care.

It is likely that Xavier's work is not consistent with his level of ability because he is performing at a level that, if not for his family connections, he might not have attained. Although his work enables him to care for himself and his family, his anxiety suggests that his work is not comfortable for him. His method of relaxing is neither culturally sanctioned nor health promoting.

References

1. Benveniste, D. (1998). The importance of play in adulthood: A dialogue with Joan Erikson. *The Psychoanalytic Study of the Child*, *53*, 51–64.
2. Brown, S. (2009). *Play: How It shapes the brain, opens the imagination, and invigorates the soul.* Penguin Books.
3. DeLamater, J. (2012). Sexual expression in later life: A review and synthesis. *Journal of Sex Research*, *49*(2–3), 125–141. https://doi.org/10.1080/00224499.2011.603168
4. Masson, J. M. (Ed.) (1985). *The complete letters of Sigmund Freud and Wilhelm Fliess 1887–1904.* Belknap Press.
5. Paluska, S. A., & Schwenk, T. L. (2000). Physical activity and mental health: Current concepts. *Sports Medicine*, *29*(3), 167–180. https://doi.org/10.2165/00007256-200029030-00003
6. Terr, L. (1999). *Beyond love and work: Why adults need to play.* Touchstone.
7. Vaillant, G. E. (2002). *Aging well: Surprising guideposts to a happier life.* Little, Brown and Co.
8. Websters. (1970). *In Webster's new world dictionary of the American language* (2nd college ed.) (pp. 1638). Merriam-Webster.

Putting It Together—DESCRIBE Problems and Patterns

In this first "Putting It Together" section, we'll illustrate how to DESCRIBE the six areas of function we reviewed in Part Two. "Putting It Together" sections can be also be found at the ends of Parts Three and Four. As we move throughout the book, we'll continue to build the formulation. Note that each of these sections will highlight different patients. We'll always begin with the presentation, since that's what we hear first.

DESCRIBING a person's problems and patterns is the first step toward creating a formulation. The six areas that we have outlined—**self, relationships, adapting, cognition, values,** and **work/play**—give us the scaffolding necessary to describe the way a person functions in life.

Let's look at Jonathan to see how we might **describe his patterns** in the six areas of function:

Presentation

Jonathan is a White, 64-year-old cisgender gay man who presents for an evaluation after the death of his mother four months ago. Jonathan's mother was 90 years old and had dementia. Several years before her death, she had moved to a nursing home in Jonathan's hometown to be near him. In the past few years, Jonathan visited her nearly every day. Since his mother's death, Jonathan feels "aimless" and "like I'm just drifting." Jonathan says, "I know she had a long, good life, and I have someone in my life now. I think I should be dealing with this better."

Jonathan has been with his husband, Charles, for 15 years. Jonathan and Charles love each other and are fully devoted to one another, but live somewhat separate lives. Jonathan works mostly from home working as a computer consultant, while Charles has a busy life as a bank manager. Together, they support their middle-class lifestyle. Charles, who is 10 years younger than Jonathan, often comes home from work quite late after long meetings or work-related dinners. Charles also travels for work, sometimes for up to 2 weeks at a time. Jonathan says that this arrangement has mostly served them well, because he prefers to have time alone and Charles is more social and enjoys the activity. When laws changed allowing them to marry, Jonathan and Charles were quick to hold a wedding, to which they invited about 50 family members and friends. Jonathan says that although people were very supportive of them, the guests were mostly Charles' friends, and that he felt somewhat marginal at the event. Nevertheless, Jonathan enjoyed himself and was able to manage these feelings. Jonathan's mother was present at the wedding. Although Jonathan's father, who died 20 years ago, did not approve of his gay life, his mother was more accepting and had become very fond of Charles.

Since the wedding, Jonathan says he has started to feel more lonely. He says his work is slowing down, while Charles' work seems only to be getting busier. In addition, Jonathan says he's started feeling jealous of the time Charles spends with colleagues and even occasionally feels fearful about Charles' commitment to him. Jonathan says, "Charles always reassures me . . . but I don't know why he thinks I'm so great. He's smarter, more successful, and everyone loves him. Sometimes, I think that I just bring him down. I'm lucky that he has wanted to be with me all this time." Jonathan says that he is looking forward to retiring, but that he's not sure what he'll do with "all that time," adding, "I've never had many outside interests."

DESCRIBE

Problem

Jonathan is having trouble adjusting to his mother's death. He feels lonely, aimless, and has some sense that he should be "getting over" the loss more quickly.

Patterns

Self

*Jonathan's **identity** is not fully consolidated. Jonathan identifies as a good caretaker (of his mother and Charles) and as a gay man, and he has been reasonably successful in the computer consulting business. However, in the face of retirement, Jonathan feels lost and cannot identify any interests outside of work. Jonathan seems somewhat vulnerable to **self-esteem threats**, particularly in his relationship with Charles, who he fears could be cheating on him, although Jonathan has no concrete reason to suspect it. Jonathan's self-deprecating stance toward Charles suggests that he may have **difficulty with his internal response to self-esteem threats**.*

Relationships

*Jonathan has both strengths and challenges in this area. His committed 15-year relationship with Charles is a strength. Lately, however, Jonathan has had some difficulty with **trust**, and struggles with feelings that Charles could leave their relationship. While Jonathan must have a good enough **sense of self and other** to have maintained this meaningful relationship, some difficulties have risen in this area. Jonathan idealizes Charles, which has the effect of not allowing Jonathan to see either of them in more complex ways. Jonathan feels less **secure** in this relationship with Charles than may be warranted, given the strength and longevity of their commitment to each other. His lack of close friendships confirms that Jonathan has challenges in this area. Yet, Jonathan is able to tolerate some degree of **intimacy** in that he has stayed with Charles, and that he had a very close relationship with his mother. In the area of **mutuality**, Jonathan seems to give much more than he takes (in caring for his mother and in his stance towards Charles).*

Adapting

*In general, Jonathan adapts to stress quite well. He uses a **range of defenses**, some of which are of more benefit to him than others. For example, Jonathan rationalizes that Charles' business trips suit his own need for time for himself. When stressed, Jonathan **idealizes** and **projects**, as illustrated by worry that Charles will leave him. Jonathan's use of **altruism** (caring for his mother) indicates that while he is a caring person, he has difficulty receiving care and affection from others. Jonathan is a fairly **emotional** person who can adapt reasonably well when there are fewer stressors; however, in the face of his mother's death and upcoming retirement, Jonathan has become **less flexible** in the use of defenses.*

Cognition

*Cognition is mostly an area of strength for Jonathan. The ability to run a successful business suggests that Jonathan has relatively strong **general cognitive functions**, is reasonably intelligent, and has the skills and abilities to manage his work and business finances. Jonathan **manages emotions**, has good **impulse control**, and does not report difficulty with **stimulus regulation**. Jonathan's thoughts are well organized, and his memory appears intact. Jonathan's capacity for **self-reflection** is only fair: while Jonathan understands that he is likely reacting to his mother's death, he is less able to question his jealous feelings about Charles. This may also indicate some difficulty with **mentalization**, as it is unclear whether Jonathan can fully imagine Charles' perspective (it must be frustrating for Charles to feel that Jonathan can not fully take in his love). There is no evidence that Jonathan has difficulty with judgment.*

Values

*Jonathan seems to have a **sense of right and wrong** and demonstrates **prosocial behavior** (caring for his mother). Jonathan's values seem to revolve around **family and relationships**.*

Work and play

*Jonathan has more strengths in work life than in play. His work is **consonant with his talents and training** and provides **satisfaction** and **support**. His worry about retirement suggests that Jonathan is not able to enjoy activities outside of work—in this regard, his capacity for play and relaxation seems limited. Work may serve a defensive function for him, but nevertheless the way Jonathan works and plays seems to be **culturally sanctioned**.*

Suggested activity

Can be done by individual learners or in a classroom setting

Now that you've learned about DESCRIBING, try writing a DESCRIBE section for one of your patients. If you're an independent learner, consider sharing it with a supervisor or a peer. If you're a supervisor or a teacher, consider assigning this as a class exercise. It can be instructive to have all of the learners in a class read each other's papers to see how this looks for different patients. You don't have to write about a patient in psychodynamic psychotherapy; this is an important thing to do with all patients so that you can begin to construct psychodynamic formulations across many different clinical situations. Include both problems and patterns. For patterns, use the six headers we've reviewed—self, relationships, adapting, cognition, values, and work and play—and consider each of the variables in each area. The writing needn't be long—certainly no more than a page. Remember—don't repeat the history, rather consolidate your thoughts about the problems and patterns.

PART THREE: Review

Introduction

Key concepts

When we formulate psychodynamically, we create hypotheses about how people develop their characteristic ways of thinking, feeling, and behaving.

Thus, once we have a good sense of a person's problems and patterns, the next step in creating a psychodynamic formulation is to **review their life story.** A life story includes everything that happens during peoples' lives which helps to shape their dominant patterns of functioning; that is, it includes how they think about themselves, have relationships with others, adapt to stress, think, conceptualize right and wrong, and work and play.

When we learn about a person's life story, we are guided by these principles:

- Include nature *and* nurture
- Relationships are key
- Society and culture affect development
- Trauma is critical
- Chronology is relevant
- Development is lifelong

Our understanding of our patients' lived experience deepens throughout our work together.

Learning about the life story

Once we have described a person's major problems and patterns, our next step in creating a psychodynamic formulation is to think about when those problems and patterns might have developed. We do this by **reviewing their life story** to get a sense of what happened to the person during each phase of their life. This review differs from taking other types of histories. For example, when we review the **history of present illness**, we focus on the recent history of the person's most pressing **problems**, and when we review the **past psychiatric history**, we review the lifetime history of the person's psychiatric symptoms and disorders. On the contrary, a life story focuses on everything that helps shape the **person**—that is, their dominant patterns of functioning.

Guiding principles for learning about the life story

When we listen to a life story, we are guided by the following principles.

Include nature *and* nurture

As we reviewed in Chapter 1, people are shaped both by what they bring into the world—their endowment—and by their interactions with their environment. Sometimes when we're thinking about psychodynamics, we think only about the impact of the individual's relationships with others. This is a mistake. An old joke says that psychoanalysts don't consider the role of genetics in development until they have their second child. This speaks to the different ways in which two siblings might interact with the same parents—presumably because of their unique endowments. Thus, as we learn about a life story, we must ask questions to help us understand the way the person's endowment, sometimes referred to as *temperament*, affects their development (see Chapter 12).

Relationships are key

Beyond endowment, we are largely shaped by our relationships and interactions with others. As we discussed in Chapter 7, throughout our lives we have relationships with all kinds of people—family members, friends, colleagues, and acquaintances—and each of these relationships is different. Particularly early in our lives, the way we think, feel, and behave largely depends on how we respond to others and how they respond to us. Although this effect is very powerful in our earliest years, it continues throughout our lives, and thus our later relationships can profoundly influence our patterns as well. Learning about someone's relationships means more than just finding out the names of the key players—it means learning about what those people are/were like and really trying to understand the nature of their relationships with the patient.

Society and culture affect development

Every person exists in a sociocultural environment that shapes the opportunities available to them; their experiences throughout development; and ultimately how they make sense of themselves, their problems, and the world around them. Understanding an individual's presenting challenge requires some knowledge of the broader sociocultural context that informs their experiences. For example, how does a Muslim-American boy living in a majority White and Christian suburb after 9/11 navigate Islamophobia? How does this affect and inform his interactions with his peers and his sense of self if he experiences his faith and identity as devalued in his own neighborhood?

The field of **ecology** has helped us to understand that a plant or animal doesn't exist in a vacuum; to understand it, we must study it in the context of its environment and the organisms located around it. The field of **human ecology** takes a similar approach to thinking about people, suggesting that there are several human environments which influence and affect people throughout their lives (Bronfenbrenner, 1977). The **Ecological systems model** conceptualizes these as the immediate environment, the community environment, and the broader society.

The immediate environment (microsystem) includes the person's primary caregivers, and close relatives. Examples of contributions from the immediate environment include:

- A secure attachment to a primary caregiver
- Loss of a parent at an early age
- Trauma or abuse at the hands of the primary caregivers
- Good enough parenting from the primary caregivers

The community environment (mesosystem) includes groups to which someone belongs, such as schools, religious organizations, or neighborhoods. Examples of contributions from the community environment include:

- The mentorship of a caring teacher
- The feeling of belonging to a neighborhood
- The hostility of a community toward a family of immigrants
- The support of a local religious community

The broader society (macrosystem) includes the influence of laws, public policies, economic structures, and broad cultural values. Examples of contributions from the broader society (macrosystem) include:

- The chronic stress of belonging to a minority group
- Chronic fear of bodily harm
- Lifelong disadvantage of being a Black person living under Jim Crow laws
- Expectations of success when in a majority group

All of these environments affect the development of the individual's conscious and unconscious mind. The immediate, community, and broader environments should all be considered when creating the psychodynamic formulations of all patients—not just those who are disadvantaged by social hierarchies. Society at large powerfully affects everyone's implicit mental processes. We will revisit the ecological systems model again in Chapter 20, focusing there on how this model helps us to link life stories to problems and patterns.

Trauma is critical

Compared with the general population, patients who see mental health professionals tend to have a higher rate of adverse early life events, such as physical/sexual abuse and neglect (Floen & Elklit, 2007). These events may predispose people to difficulties in adulthood, such as depression, anxiety, substance use disorder, eating disorders, and borderline personality (Clemmons et al., 2007; Cohen et al., 2001; Edwards et al., 2003; Green et al., 2010; Kessler et al., 1997; Lansford et al., 2002; Van der Kolk et al., 1994). Thus, trauma can have a major impact on development. However, for a variety of reasons, when we talk to patients, we sometimes shy away from asking about a history of trauma. It can be profoundly distressing and overwhelming to hear about the terrible things our patients have endured. We may be afraid of upsetting or retraumatizing them by inquiring, and sometimes, we don't know how to respond. Nevertheless, it is essential not only to ask whether trauma has occurred at any point in development but also to try to understand the meaning of that trauma to that particular person. The following are examples of the kinds of questions we might ask to elicit this information:

Can you tell me the story of what happened to you?

What did you feel when it was happening?

How did you try to understand what was going on at that time? How do you understand it now?

Did you talk to anyone about it when it happened or any time after?

Do you see that experience (the trauma) as having lasting effects on you? If so, what are they?

Do you think that the experience shaped who you are today? If so, how?

Has the experience shaped how you think about other people and how you think about life in general?

When we listen to our patients' histories of trauma, we must be careful to differentiate between *our* feelings and *theirs* about what happened. Exclaiming, "Oh my goodness!" in response to a story of trauma might alarm someone who is disconnected from their own feelings. On the other hand, making gently empathic remarks such as, "That must have been difficult," can help the patient to recognize you were listening and trying to understand.

We also need to make our patients feel as safe as possible when they tell us their stories, and to let them know we don't have preconceptions about what they're telling us. For example, listening in an interested, empathic but nonjudgmental way to a woman telling her experience of being raped may help her more easily tell the story. Letting patients know that many people have difficulty talking about these things can also be helpful.

Chronology is relevant

In development, *when* things happen is often as important as *what* happened. If the same event happened early in life, it can have a very different effect than if it happened later. Generally, earlier disturbances are more likely to cause pervasive problems than later ones. For example, a separation of several months from a primary caregiver at age 1 is likely to cause more global difficulties than a separation of the same length at age 7. We say a problem is **global** if it affects many aspects of a person's functioning, and we say that it is **circumscribed** if it affects fewer functions. If a person cannot form any intimate relationships, for example, their difficulty is more global than that of a person who has many close friends but cannot form an intimate romantic relationship.

Once you have a sense of the person's problems and patterns, you will have some idea about how global their issues are. This can help guide you as you explore their life story. Because the timing of events is so important, we recommend chronologically conceptualizing their life story. We will discuss the phases of development chronologically in Chapters 12–17.

Development is lifelong

To many people, "taking a developmental history" means learning about the history of early childhood milestones. While these milestones are clearly relevant, it is important to remember that development continues throughout life, and thus the full life story must include everything from before birth through the person's entire lived experience. People grow and change in numerous ways in their adult years. They have successes, losses, trauma, discrimination, disadvantage, illnesses, later relationships, and psychotherapeutic experiences—all which affect the way they think, feel, and behave.

The evolving history

When we first meet a patient, we try to get a sense of the major aspects of their life story, including basic information about prenatal exposures, developmental milestones, relationships with primary caregivers, major traumas, patterns of relationships later in life, access to resources, and the patient's education and work history. This helps us to create an initial formulation of the patient that will guide the treatment. However, we cannot learn everything about them at the beginning. Not only does it take a very long time to learn everything, but patients gradually reveal new aspects of their life stories as the treatment unfolds. The bottom line is that we need not ask about every aspect of development in our first meetings with patients, AND that we need to remember to continue building our understanding of a patient's life story throughout our work together.

How extensive should the life story be?

Chapters 12–17 are chock-full of detailed information about the life story—ranging from genetics to issues related to aging. We have included all of this

- to give you a sense of the range of information that we can learn about our patients
- because mental health professionals learn different amounts about development during their training

- to offer you a review of this material
- to highlight the aspects of the life story that affect the development of conscious and unconscious thoughts and feelings

There is so much information here, however, that we cannot possibly learn all of it about every patient. In some clinical situations like psychopharmacologic treatments and acute care settings (see Part Five), we may have very little time to get any of this information at all. Whether you are an individual learner or an educator, please use these chapters as a reference. As you read, try to highlight the major points of each life phase. Then, when you hear about a difficult period, you can refer back to the related chapter to help you to gain more details. The "Putting it together" example at the end of Part Three illustrates the type of life story that a clinician could write after getting to know a patient in greater detail. On the other hand, you will find many brief life stories in Parts Four and Five. The type of life story review we do in a given clinical situation depends on the amount of time we have with the patient, as well as the goals of the treatment. Regardless of the clinical situation, we need some sense of the person's life journey to formulate psychodynamically.

Now, let's move on to Chapter 12 and the beginning of the life story.

References

1. Bronfenbrenner, U. (1977). Toward an experimental ecology of human development. *American Psychologist, 32*(7), 513–531. https://doi.org/10.1037/0003-066x.32.7.513

2. Clemmons, J. C., Walsh, K., DiLillo, D., et al. (2007). Unique and combined contributions of multiple child abuse types and abuse severity to adult trauma symptomatology. *Child Maltreatment, 12*(2), 172–181.

3. Cohen, P., Brown, J., & Smaile, E. (2001). Child abuse and neglect and the development of mental disorders in the general population. *Development and Psychopathology, 13*(4), 981–999.

4. Edwards, V. J., Holden, G. W., Felitti, V. J., et al. (2003). Relationship between multiple forms of childhood maltreatment and adult mental health in community respondents: Results from the adverse childhood experiences study. *American Journal of Psychiatry, 160*(8), 1453–1460.

5. Floen, S. K., & Elklit, A. (2007). Psychiatric diagnoses, trauma, and suicidiality. *Annals of General Psychiatry, 6*(1)). https://doi.org/10.1186/1744-859x-6-12

6. Green, J. G., McLaughlin, K. A., Berglund, P. A., et al. (2010). Childhood adversities and adult psychopathology in the National Comorbidity Survey Replication (NCS-R) I: Associations with first onset of DSM-IV disorders. *Archives of General Psychiatry, 67*(2), 113–125.

7. Kessler, R. C., Davis, C. G., & Kendler, K. S. (1997). Childhood adversity and adult psychiatric disorder in the US National Comorbidity Survey. *Psychological Medicine, 27*(5), 1101–1119.

8. Lansford, J. E., Dodge, K. A., Pettit, G. S., et al. (2002). A 12-year prospective study of the long-term effects of early child physical maltreatment on psychological, behavioral, and academic problems in adolescence. *Archives of Pediatric Adolescent Medicine, 156*(8), 824–830.

9. Van der Kolk, B. A., Hostetler, A., Herron, N., et al. (1994). Trauma and the development of borderline personality disorder. *Psychiatric Clinics of North America, 17*(4), 715–730.

12 What We're Born With

Key concepts

The life story begins before birth. What we're born with is affected by

- Heredity (genetic and epigenetic)
- Prenatal development, exposures and events
- Peripartum events
- Transgenerational transmission of trauma

Adult problems and patterns that suggest origins in prenatal development include

- Psychiatric disorders, particularly when associated with a family history
- Stable temperamental traits beginning in childhood
- Cognitive and emotional difficulties associated with a history of prenatal exposures

Learning about development that occurred during this period involves asking patients about

- Family history of psychiatric disorders, temperamental traits, and trauma
- Adverse events and exposures during pregnancy or birth
- Maternal health and habits during pregnancy

When we think about a psychodynamic formulation, we generally think about how a person's relationships and life story have affected the development of their unique problems and patterns. However, more and more, we're learning that people are born with a **unique endowment** that influences the way their relationships and environment affects them. Thus, we must consider the impact of this endowment when we think about the psychodynamic formulation. We can think of this endowment as everything we bring into the world at birth. It includes contributions from

- Genetics and heredity
- Prenatal development, including the mother's physical and emotional health during pregnancy

---

Psychodynamic Formulation: An Expanded Approach, First Edition. The Psychodynamic Formulation Collective.
© 2022 John Wiley & Sons Ltd. Published 2022 by John Wiley & Sons Ltd.

- Peripartum events
- Transgenerational transmission of trauma

This chapter reviews some of the ways the prenatal and peripartum periods contribute to adult development so that you can consider ideas about this period in your psychodynamic formulation.

Heredity: genetics, and epigenetics

We know we can inherit physical traits like height and eye color, but can we also inherit the way we think, feel, and behave? This is a complicated question that we have yet to fully understand, but research increasingly suggests that many aspects of our adult problems and patterns have significant hereditary components. To better understand this, let's define two types of types of heredity:

- **Genetic inheritance** refers to the collection of genes (**genotype**) that a person inherits from their parents. Changes in our genetic inheritance come about through changes to the genes themselves (i.e., changes to our DNA sequence).
- **Epigenetic inheritance** refers to inherited information about whether our genes are active or inactive (**gene expression**). Changes in our epigenetic inheritance come about in ways *other* than changes to the DNA sequence (Deans & Maggert, 2015), such as how the DNA is wrapped around proteins called **histones**, making it more or less likely that certain genes will be expressed.

The concept of epigenetics helps us to understand the way in which parents' behavior and life experiences may be passed on to their children, as there is evidence that a parent's life experiences may lead to heritable epigenetic changes (Meaney & Szyf, 2005). These epigenetic changes, which can lead to an under- or overexpression of genes, have been shown to play a role in causing various adult psychiatric, autistic, and neurodegenerative disorders (Jirtle & Skinner, 2007).

Epidemiological studies have also provided evidence that prenatal and early postnatal environmental factors influence the adult risk of developing various behavioral disorders. For example, adults exposed to famine conditions prenatally have been reported to have a significantly higher incidence of schizophrenia (St Clair et al., 2005). Both the environment and individual lifestyle can interact with the genome, not just in the womb but throughout life, and cause epigenetic change (Heijmans et al., 2008).

Psychiatric disorders

Twin, adoption, and family studies have long supported a role for heredity in many psychiatric disorders, including mood and anxiety disorders, psychotic illnesses, attention-deficit/hyperactivity disorder (ADHD), and autism (Hyman, 2000; Plomin et al., 1994). Molecular genetics now provides compelling corroborating evidence for this (Byrne et al., 2020; Ferreira et al., 2008; Kang et al., 2011; Lee et al., 2021; Ripke et al., 2011; Sklar et al., 2011; Sullivan, 2010). Although the child of an affected parent will not necessarily develop the parent's disorder, hearing about psychopathology in a parent should alert the clinician to a possible genetic contribution. For example, if a person presents with depression in the context of a current life stressor and says that there is depression in the family, it could suggest a genetic predisposition.

Temperament

"I've always been a shy person," says a patient. "My parents say I hid behind my mother from the time I could walk." Hearing about personal characteristics that people report they have had for as long as they—or their family members—can remember should make us wonder whether they are describing traits related to **temperament**. We can define temperament as the heritable, biologically based patterns of responding and behaving that are

- Present from earliest infancy
- Consistent across situations
- Relatively stable over time (Bratko et al., 2017; Rothbart, 2011)

Scientists say that 20–60 percent of temperament variations may be determined by genetic factors (Bouchard et al., 1990; Bratko et al., 2017; Power & Pluess, 2015; Rothbart, 2011). Epigenetic changes may also contribute. Several temperamental styles have been shown to be remarkably consistent throughout development. For example, Kagan (2010) found that the four-month-old infants he described as having **inhibited temperament**, based on their upset reactions to unfamiliar stimuli, were significantly more likely to develop anxiety symptoms by age seven than infants with **uninhibited temperament** who had responded calmly (Kagan et al., 2007). These temperamental distinctions have been found to predict behavior in adolescence, as well as MRI findings related to the amygdala in early adulthood (Schwartz et al., 2003).

In other studies, Thomas et al. (1963) found that **easy, difficult,** and **slow-to-warm up temperaments** were remarkably stable over the first 7–8 years of life. **Sensation seeking and avoidance** are other temperamental traits that seem to be heritable and linked to biological markers (Zald et al., 2008; Zuckerman, 1991, 2007). Finally, neurobiological studies have demonstrated that **impulsive aggressivity** may be rooted in heritable mechanisms for regulating emotions (Coccaro & Siever, 2007; Frankle et al., 2005; Hoermann et al., 2011; Siever, 2008). These studies suggest that many traits, which have been considered "maladaptive defenses," may be genetically based, disordered brain functioning that makes it hard for people to act in ways that benefit them most (Hoermann et al., 2011).

A person who seeks therapy after receiving three speeding tickets in one year says their preferred leisure activities are bungee jumping and solo rock climbing. They report having been told that they climbed out of the crib at age 10 months, which suggests they may have a sensation-seeking temperament. But do these early ways of reacting to the world predict our adult personality? Not necessarily. Although some temperamental types are quite stable over time, environmental factors, including early interactions with caregivers as well as other life experiences, can bring about significant changes in temperament. For example, if caregivers gradually expose an infant with inhibited temperament to new situations and challenges, they can change the child's propensity to avoid the unfamiliar (Cicchetti et al., 1991, pp. 15–48; Partridge, 2003). Again, although these early ways of reacting to the world do not necessarily predict adult behavior, when a patient describes characteristic patterns of behavior that have been fairly stable since infancy, it's worth considering whether these are temperamental traits.

Prosocial traits

Children differ markedly in the degree to which they exhibit attitudes and behaviors that focus on the benefit of others. Called **prosocial traits** (see Chapter 10), these include sharing, social concern, kindness, helping, and empathic concern for others. Recent research suggests that both genetic and environmental factors contribute to this variability (Eisenberg et al., 2015; Knafo-Noam et al., 2015). For example, some evidence exists that variations in the oxytocin receptor gene may lead to an initial genetic predisposition for empathy and may indirectly predict a tendency for prosocial behavior across development (Christ et al., 2016; Shang et al., 2017).

Prenatal development

Genes aren't the only things that contribute to our endowment. There are nine long months during which the fetus' brain is affected by a number of other factors, including everything the mother eats, drinks, and, perhaps, feels. The following are among the most common influences on fetal brain development:

Maternal habits

Intrauterine exposure to alcohol or cigarette smoke has long been recognized as a risk factor for various cognitive and emotional difficulties in later life (Huizink & Mulder, 2006; Milberger et al., 1996; Nichols & Chen, 1981; Zammit et al., 2009). Children born to women who **smoke** during pregnancy have been found to have two- to fourfold increased risk of ADHD (Huizink & Mulder, 2006; Lindblad & Hjern, 2010; Obel et al., 2011), as well as suspected or definite psychotic symptoms (Zammit et al., 2009).

Prenatal **alcohol** exposure, which is the most common known cause of intellectual disability, may cause more subtle but still significant cognitive and learning problems, and, when associated with fetal alcohol syndrome, may cause various psychiatric disorders (Famy et al., 1998; Fryer et al., 2007; Steinhausen & Spohr, 1998; Streissguth et al., 2004). This etiology should be considered as a possible contributing factor in patients presenting with problems such as learning difficulties and ADHD when there is a history of maternal alcohol misuse.

Maternal physical and emotional health

Increasingly, researchers are finding that the physical health of a woman during pregnancy may affect her child's later problems and patterns. Viral and parasitic illnesses, as well as malnutrition in the pregnant mother, have been linked to the later development of various cognitive and emotional difficulties in adulthood (Blaser et al., 2001; Brown et al., 2001, 2004, 2005; Brown & Susser, 2008; Chess et al., 1971; Kodesh et al., 2021; Libbey et al., 2005; Lim et al., 1995; Mednick et al., 1988; Moreno et al., 2011; Yamashita et al., 2003). Though it is likely that autism is caused by multiple factors, congenital viral infections may play a role (Libbey et al., 2005; Yamashita et al., 2003). High rates of anxiety disorders, ADHD, conduct disorder, and oppositional defiant disorder have been described in children and adolescents with prenatally acquired HIV (Mellins et al., 2009).

We are used to thinking about the way the emotional health of a person's parents affects their development, but we're learning that we must include the mother's distress *during* pregnancy as well—specifically, perceived stress, life events, depression, and anxiety (Monk et al., 2019). Recent studies suggest that the offspring of mothers with high levels of anxiety and stress during pregnancy have an elevated risk of a variety of psychiatric conditions, including ADHD, anxiety, depression, autism, and schizophrenia (Halligan et al., 2007; Hunter et al., 2012; Karg et al., 2011; Khashan et al., 2011; Rice et al., 2007, 2010; Van den Bergh et al., 2008; Welberg & Seckl, 2001).

Prematurity and peripartum brain injury

Finally, we must remember that the events of a person's birth can also affect their development. Prematurity and low birth weight increase the risk for difficulties ranging from cerebral palsy, autism, and intellectual disability to ADHD, tic disorder, and obsessive-compulsive disorder (OCD) (Botting et al., 1997; Bhutta et al., 2002; Lindström et al., 2011; Pasamanick et al., 1956; Pinto-Martin et al., 2011; Vanderbilt & Gleason, 2010; Whitaker et al., 1997, 2001). Brain trauma resulting from hypoxia at the time of birth, the mechanical trauma of the birth process itself, or obstetric complications may also play a role in the development of later psychopathology (Beauchaine et al., 2008; Dalman, 2001; Geddes & Lawrie, 1995; Mittal et al., 2008; Rosso & Cannon, 2003).

Nature and nurture—a two-way street

Although the exact origins of our later cognitive and emotional difficulties are not known, research suggests that they are caused by some combination of "nature" and "nurture"—complex, mutually influencing interactions between variations in multiple genes and the environment. These are often called **gene by environment interactions** (Duncan & Keller, 2011). It has long been recognized that our endowment can influence the quality of our early experiences with caregivers and may, in turn, be modified by these relationships and other environmental factors. For example, a baby who startles easily, cries often, and is difficult to soothe may overwhelm the already limited reserves of an insecure and depressed mother who then withdraws from the child, further exacerbating the baby's distress. The quality of early parental care can even modify the expression of genes that regulate the developing infant's behavioral and neuroendocrine responses to stress (Bagot & Meaney, 2010; McGowan et al., 2009).

Transgenerational transmission of trauma

Interest is growing in the theory that the effects of trauma such as slavery, war, famine and genocide may reverberate across generations through epigenetic mechanisms. Although studies have not yet demonstrated this in humans (Yehuda & Lehrner, 2018), findings in animal models have implicated epigenetic mechanisms in the transmission of maternal and paternal trauma, not only postnatally, but also *in utero* and even through preconception effects on the germ cell line (Jawaid et al., 2018; Yehuda & Lehrner, 2018). Several studies in humans have suggested that parental post-traumatic stress disorder (PTSD) is a strong correlate for the development of PTSD in offspring and is associated with transmission of biological alterations of the hypothalamic-pituitary-adrenal (HPA) axis (Bowers & Yehuda, 2016; Curry, 2019; Perroud et al., 2014).

From a broader sociocultural perspective, collective trauma, such as slavery, colonialism, or genocide, are not simply factors in the past that may have some residual influence but ongoing oppressive forces that shape physical and psychological well-being and social opportunity (Syed & Fish, 2018). Brave Heart et al. (2011) referred to historical trauma as the "cumulative emotional and psychological wounding across generations, including the lifespan, which emanates from massive group trauma (p. 283)." Historical trauma shapes the broader societal beliefs and identity development for individuals within a given culture over generations. For some in Black communities, the impact of centuries of unaddressed trauma related to enslavement and White racism is still evident, and may well prove to be related to epigenetic mechanisms as well as ongoing social injustice (DeGruy, 2017; Jackson et al., 2018).

Resilience

It's not only our susceptibility to later difficulties that may be related to genetics and prenatal development; researchers are now finding that our capacity for **resilience** may also be hereditary (Horn et al., 2016; Jackson et al., 2018). Differences in the gene that codes for a protein which regulates serotonin movement in synapses (the serotonin transporter, the target of many antidepressants), may explain why only certain people develop serious depression after stressful life experiences (Caspi et al., 2003, 2010; Wankerl et al., 2010), while differences in genes that regulate the metabolism of neurotransmitters may explain why some teenagers who use cannabis develop psychotic illnesses when adults and others do not (Caspi et al., 2005). Genetic differences of this nature may also affect an individual's response to early childhood maltreatment and trauma (Belsky et al., 2009; Caspi et al., 2002; Kim-Cohen et al., 2006; Kloke et al., 2011; Reif et al., 2007; Taylor et al., 2006). A recent genome-wide association study on resilience revealed several genome-wide significant polymorphisms (Maul et al., 2020; Stein et al., 2019).

Adult problems and patterns that suggest a prenatal origin

Several types of adult problems and patterns suggest a prenatal origin:

- Psychiatric disorders, particularly if they begin in childhood and/or are associated with a family history
- Stable temperamental traits, such as inhibition, sensation seeking or avoidance, and impulsive aggression, also beginning in childhood
- Cognitive and/or behavioral problems with a history of prenatal exposure

Psychiatric disorders, particularly if they begin in early childhood and/or associated with a family history

Hank is a divorced computer programmer who seeks help with what he calls "social isolation." He reports that he drove his ex-wife crazy with his constant lectures on esoteric topics of interest only to him, and that had few friends outside of work. As a boy, he was considered exceptionally smart but "quirky," couldn't connect with most of his classmates, and was teased mercilessly on the playground when he approached other kids and said, "Seven times seven is equal to 49." He adds, "My mother is like me. We even have the same balanced translocation on chromosome 16."

Hank's lifetime lack of social skills, trouble with social communication, rigid preoccupation with certain topics, and family history of similar difficulties in his mother suggest that his social isolation may be related to a genetically based autism spectrum disorder.

Stable temperamental traits

Iris is a recent college graduate who seeks help with "interview phobia." She was recently turned down for a number of positions for which she felt "way overqualified" because she "froze up" at the interviews. Iris remembers that she was always timid and quiet. Her mother told her that as an infant she cried if she was placed on the rug in an unfamiliar place, and that as a two-year-old baby she sobbed whenever someone she didn't know came to the door.

Iris' "interview phobia" may be one manifestation of a lifelong pattern of temperamental inhibition.

Cognitive and/or behavioral problems with a history of prenatal exposure

Now in his 20s, Josh presents because he is having difficulty at work. "I sort of faked it through school, but now that it's about my job I just can't make all these careless mistakes anymore." He says that he has had significant academic and behavioral problems since kindergarten, and that at one point he was diagnosed as having ADHD. During the interview, he pulls out a pack of cigarettes and asks, "Do you mind? I know . . . it's a horrible habit, but I've been smoking two packs a day since high school. I was raised in a cloud of smoke—my mother was completely addicted. She died last year of lung cancer."

Josh's history of ADHD may be related to other risk factors, but his likely prenatal exposure to cigarette smoke may have been a contributor.

Learning about the life story of the prenatal period

How do you learn about the time before a person was born? In the treatment of a child, parents come in to give the history, but in the treatment of adults, we generally have to rely on what they know and tell us.

Family history of psychiatric disorders and temperamental traits

Note that this should include asking about the extended family - patients generally only tell us about their nuclear family.

Does anyone in the family have a history of mood, anxiety, or psychotic disorder?

Was anyone in the extended family ever hospitalized for a psychiatric problem?

Did anyone in the extended family ever commit or attempt suicide?

Does/did anyone in the family ever use substances?

If the person seems to have a particular temperament, such as an inhibited or sensation-seeking temperament, you can ask the following:

Does anyone else in the family have those traits?

Do your family members think that you remind them of another family member?

Prematurity and birth

Were you born prematurely? If so, at how many weeks? Were you in an incubator? For how long?

Do you know if your mother had any illnesses during her pregnancy with you?

Did you have any surgeries immediately following birth? Do you know what they were for? Do you have any medical problems that you've had since you were born?

Do any genetic disorders run in your family?

Maternal habits and health

Even if your adult patients do not know if they had any toxic exposures while they were *in utero*, asking about maternal habits can give you a sense of whether this might have been a possibility.

Did your mother smoke, drink alcohol, or use drugs when you were little? What about now?

Is there a possibility that your mother was not eating well, or that she was ill when she was pregnant with you?

Have you ever heard that your mother might have been depressed or under a lot of stress when she was pregnant with you? What were the circumstances?

Learning about the life story from adults who do not know their biological parents

In the era of assisted reproduction, more and more patients likely will not know their biological parents. This has generally been true of adoptees, but now sperm and egg donation are increasingly common, as is the use of a surrogate to carry a pregnancy.

Some people may have some information about a donor's genetic background, or the conditions of the surrogate's pregnancy, yet many will not. Some may have information about one parent but not the other. Nevertheless, it is always important to find out the conditions of the patient's birth. Questions like the following can help:

Did your biological parents raise you?

If not, can you tell me more about how that came about?

In Chapter 13, we move from nature to nurture as we consider the person's earliest years, focusing on the way in which relationships shape subsequent development and adult relationships.

Suggested activity

Can be done by individual learners or in a classroom setting

As you read the following example, think about the possible contribution of prenatal factors to Nel's presenting problems and patterns:

Nel is 22 years old when she presents after having her first panic attack. She tells you that she was the product of a surrogate pregnancy using a donor egg and her father's sperm. Her parents, who were wealthy and in their 40s when they met, spent years trying to conceive, to no avail. They told her that the surrogate they chose did not smoke or drink during pregnancy, and that she had maintained excellent nutrition throughout. According to Nel's mother, there were no problems during the surrogate pregnancy, labor, and delivery. However, her mother said, "Your father was a wreck throughout the whole thing! He couldn't believe that we were going to trust the pregnancy to someone else. He was sure that something would go wrong. He didn't sleep for months." There is no known history of psychiatric illness in her father's family.

Comment

There is no known family history of psychiatric illness in Nel's paternal relatives, and no known problems in prenatal development or delivery that might have increased Nel's risk for developing an anxiety disorder in adulthood. However, Nel's father may have symptoms of anxiety, and thus it is possible that Nel's susceptibility to an anxiety disorder may have been inherited. It is also possible that emotional difficulties were not adequately screened for in the egg donor—this is very difficult to rule out in this situation.

References

1. Bagot, R. C., & Meaney, M. J. (2010). Epigenetics and the biological basis of gene x environment interactions. *Journal of the American Academy of Child and Adolescent Psychiatry, 49*(8), 752–771. https://doi.org/10.1016/j.jaac.2010.06.001

2. Beauchaine, T. P., Hinshaw, S. P., & Gatzke-Kopp, L. (2008). Genetic and environmental influences on behavior. In T. P. Beauchaine & S. P. Hinshaw (Eds.), *Child and adolescent psychopathology* (pp. 58–92). Wiley.

3. Belsky, J., Jonassaint, C., Pluess, M., Stanton, M., Brummett, B., & Williams, R. (2009). Vulnerability genes or plasticity genes? *Molecular Psychiatry, 14*, 746–754. https://doi.org/10.1038/mp.2009.44

4. Bhutta, A. T., Cleves, M. A., Casey, P. H., Cradock, M. M., & Anand, K. J. S. (2002). Cognitive and behavioral outcomes of school-aged children who were born preterm. *Journal of the American Medical Association, 288*(6), 728–737. https://doi.org/10.1001/jama.288.6.728

5. Blaser, S., Venita, J., Becker, L., Ford-Jones, E.L. (2001). Neonatal brain infection. In M. Rutherford (Ed.), *MRI of the neonatal brain* (4th ed., pp. 201–224). W.B. Saunders Ltd.

6. Botting, N., Powls, A., Cooke, R., & Marlow, N. (1997). Attention deficit hyperactivity disorders and other psychiatric outcomes in very low birth weight children at 12 years. *Journal of Child Psychology and Psychiatry, 38*(8), 931–941. https://doi.org/10.1111/j.1469-7610.1997.tb01612.x

7. Bouchard, T. J., Lykken, D. T., McGue, M., Segal, N. L., & Tellegen, A. (1990). Sources of human psychological differences: The Minnesota study of twins reared apart. *Science, 250*(4978), 223–228. https://doi.org/10.1126/science.2218526

8. Bowers, M. E., & Yehuda, R. (2016). Intergenerational transmission of stress in humans. *Neuropsychopharmacology, 41*, 232–244. https://doi.org/10.1038/npp.2015.247

9. Bratko, D., Butkovic, A., & Vukasovic, T. (2017). Heritability of personality. *Psychological Topics, 26*(1), 1–24. https://doi.org/10.1037/bul0000017

10. Brave Heart, M. Y. H., Chase, J., Elkins, J., & Altschul, D. B. (2011). Historical trauma among indigenous peoples of the Americas: Concepts, research, and clinical considerations. *Journal of Psychoactive Drugs, 43*(4), 282–290. https://doi.org/10.1080/02791072.2011.628913

11. Brown, A. S., Begg, M. D., Gravenstein, S., Schaeffer, C. A., Wyatt, R. J., Bresnahan, M., Babulas, V. P., & Susser, E. S. (2004). Serologic evidence of prenatal influenza in the etiology of schizophrenia. *Archives of General Psychiatry, 61*(8), 774–780. https://doi.org/10.1001/archpsyc.61.8.774

12. Brown, A. S., Cohen, P., Harkavy-Friedman, J., & Babulas, V. P. (2001). Prenatal rubella, premorbid abnormalities, and adult schizophrenia. *Biological Psychiatry, 49*(6), 473–486. https://doi.org/10.1016/S0006-3223(01)01068-X

13. Brown, A. S., Schaefer, C., Quesenberry, C., Liu, L., Bubalas, V. P., & Susser, E. S. (2005). Maternal exposure to toxoplasmosis and risk of schizophrenia in adult offspring. *American Journal of Psychiatry, 162*, 767–773. https://doi.org/10.1176/appi.ajp.162.4.767

14. Brown, A. S., & Susser, E. S. (2008). Prenatal nutritional deficiency and risk of adult schizophrenia. *Schizophrenia Bulletin, 34*(6), 1054. https://doi.org/10.1093/schbul/sbn096

15. Byrne, E. M., Zhu, Z., Wray, N. R., Skene, N. G., Bryois, J., Pardinas, A., Stahl, E., Smoller, J. W., Rietschel, M., Bipolar Working Group of the Psychiatric Genomics Consortium, Major Depressive Disorder Working Group of the Psychiatric Genomics Consortium, Owen, M. J., Walters, J. T. R., O'Donovan, M. C., McGrath, J. G., Hjerling-Leffler, J., Sullivan, P. F., Goddard, M. E., Visscher, P. M., . . . Wray, N. R. (2020). Conditional GWAS analysis to identify disorder-specific SNPs for psychiatric disorders. *Molecular Psychiatry, 26*, 2070–2081. https://doi.org/10.1038/s41380-020-0705-9

16. Caspi, A., Hariri, A. R., Holmes, A., Uher, R., & Moffitt, T. E. (2010). Genetic sensitivity to the environment: The case of the serotonin transporter gene and its implications for

studying complex diseases and traits. *American Journal of Psychiatry, 167*(5), 509–527. https://doi.org/10.1176/appi.ajp.2010.09101452

17. Caspi A., McClay, J. Moffit, T.E., Mill, J., Martin, J., Craig, I.W., Taylor, A., Poulton, R. (2002). Role of genotype in the cycle of violence in maltreated children. *Science, 297*(5582), 851–854. https://doi.org/10.1126/science.1072290

18. Caspi, A., Moffitt, T. E., Cannon, M., McClay, J., Murray, R., Harrington, H., Taylor, A., Arseneault, L., Williams, B., Braithwaite, A., Poulton, R., & Craig, I. W. (2005). Moderation of the effect of adolescent-onset cannabis use on adult psychosis by a functional polymorphism in the catechol-O-methyltransferase gene: Longitudinal evidence of a gene X environment interaction. *Biological Psychiatry, 57*(10), 1117–1127. https://doi.org/10.1016/j.biopsych.2005.01.026

19. Caspi, A., Sugden, K., Moffitt, T. E., Taylor, A., Craig, I. W., Harrington, H., McClay, J., Mill, J., Martin, J., Braithwaite, J., & Poulton, R. (2003). Influence of life stress on depression: Moderation by a polymorphism in the 5-HTT gene. *Science, 301*(5631), 386–389. https://doi.org/10.1126/science.1083968

20. Chess, S., Korn, S., & Fernandez, P. (1971). *Psychiatric disorders of children with congenital Rubella.* Brunner/Mazel Publishers.

21. Christ, C., Carlo, G., & Stoltenberg, S. (2016). Oxytocin receptor (OXTR) single nucleotide polymorphisms indirectly predict prosocial behavior through perspective taking and empathic concern. *Journal of Personality, 84*(2), 204–213. https://doi.org/10.1111/jopy.12152

22. Cicchetti, D., Ganiban, J., & Barnett, D. (1991). Contributions from the study of high-risk populations to understanding the development of emotion regulation. In J. Garber & K. A. Dodge (Eds.), *The development of emotion regulation and dysregulation* (pp. 15–48). Cambridge University Press.

23. Coccaro, E. F., & Siever, L. J. (2007). Neurobiology. In J. M. Oldham, A. E. Skodol, & D. S. Bender (Eds.), *The american psychiatric publishing textbook of personality disorders* (pp. 155–171). American Psychiatric Publishing, Inc.

24. Curry A. A painful legacy. Science. 2019 Jul 19;365(6450):212-215. doi: 10.1126/science. 365.6450.212. PMID: 31320518.

25. Dalman, C. (2001). Signs of asphyxia at birth and risk of schizophrenia: Population-based case-control study. *The British Journal of Psychiatry, 179*(5), 403–408. https://doi.org/10.1192/bjp.179.5.403

26. Deans, C., & Maggert, K. A. (2015). What do you mean, "epigenetic"? *Genetics, 199*(4), 887–896. https://doi.org/10.1534/genetics.114.173492

27. DeGruy, J. (2017). *Post traumatic slave syndrome: America's legacy of enduringiinjury and healing* (Rev. ed.). Joy Degruy Publications, Inc.

28. Duncan, L. E., & Keller, M. C. (2011). A critical review of the first 10 years of candidate gene-by-environment interaction research in psychiatry. *American Journal of Psychiatry, 168*(10), 1041–1049. https://doi.org/10.1176/appi.ajp.2011.11020191

29. Eisenberg, N., Spinrad, T. L., & Knafo-Noam, A. (2015). Prosocial development. In M. E. Lamb & R. M. Lerner (Eds.), *Handbook of child psychology and developmental science. Vol. 3. Socioemotional processes.* Wiley. https://doi.org/10.1002/9781118963418.childpsy315

30. Famy, C., Streissguth, A., & Unis, A. (1998). Mental illness in adults with fetal alcohol syndrome or fetal alcohol effects. *American Journal of Psychiatry, 155,* 552–555.

31. Ferreira, M. A. R., O'Donovan, M. C., & Meng, Y. A. (2008). Collaborative genome-wide association analysis supports a role for ANK3 and CACNA1C in bipolar disorder. *Nature Genetics, 40*(9), 1056–1058. https://doi.org/10.1038/ng.209

32. Frankle, W. G., Lombardo, I., New, A. S., Goodman, N., Talbot, P. S., Huang, Y., Hwang, D., Slifstein, M., Curry, S., Abi-Dargham, A., Laruelle, M., & Siever, L. J. (2005). Brain serotonin transporter distribution in subjects with impulsive aggressivity: A positron emission study with [11C]McN5652. *American Journal of Psychiatry, 162*(5), 915–923. https://doi.org/10.1176/appi.ajp.162.5.915

33. Fryer, S., McGee, C., Matt, G., Riley, E. P., & Mattson, S. N. (2007). Evaluations of psycho-pathological conditions in children with heavy prenatal alcohol exposure. *Pediatrics, 119*(3), e733–e741. https://doi.org/10.1542/peds.2006-1606

34. Geddes, J. R., & Lawrie, S. M. (1995). Obstetric complications and schizophrenia: A meta-analysis. *The British Journal of Psychiatry, 167*(6), 786–793.

35. Halligan, S. L., Murray, L., Martins, C., & Cooper, P. J. (2007). Maternal depression and psychiatric outcomes in adolescent offspring: A 13-year longitudinal study. *Journal of Affective Disorders, 97*, 145–154. https://doi.org/10.1016/j.jad.2006.06.010

36. Heijmans, B. T., Tobi, E. W., Stein, A. D., Putter, H., Blauw, G. J., Susser, E. S., Slagboom, P. E., & Lumey, L. H. (2008). Persistent epigenetic differences associated with prenatal exposure to famine in humans. *Proceedings of the National Academy of Sciences, 105*(44), 17046–17049. https://doi.org/10.1073/pnas.0806560105

37. Hoermann, S., Zupanick, C. E., & Dombeck, M. Biological factors related to the development of personality disorders (Nature). Retrieved October 28, 2011, from https://www.gracepointwellness.org/8-personality-disorders/article/41557-biological-factors-related-to-the-development-of-personality-disorders-nature

38. Horn, S. R., Charney, D. S., & Feder, A. (2016). Understanding resilience: New approaches for preventing and treating PTSD. *Experimental Neurology, 284*, 119–132. https://doi.org/10.1016/j.expneurol.2016.07.002

39. Huizink, A., & Mulder, E. (2006). Maternal smoking, drinking or cannabis use during pregnancy and neurobehavioral and cognitive functioning in human offspring. *Neuroscience and Biobehavioral Reviews, 30*(1), 24–41. https://doi.org/10.1016/j.neubiorev.2005.04.005

40. Hunter, S. K., Mendoza, J. H., D'Anna, K., Zerbe, G. O., McCarthy, L., Hoffman, C., Freedman, R., & Ross, R. G. (2012). Antidepressants may mitigate the effects of prenatal maternal anxiety on infant auditory sensory gating. *American Journal of Psychiatry, 169*(6), 616–624. https://doi.org/10.1176/appi.ajp.2012.11091365

41. Hyman, S. (2000). The genetics of mental illness: Implications for clinical practice. *Bulletin of the World Health Organization, 78*(4), 455–463.

42. Jackson, F., Jackson, L., & Jackson, Z. E. (2018). Developmental stage epigenetic modifications and clinical symptoms associated with disease susceptibility. *Nature Reviews Genetics, 8*, 253–262. http://hdl.handle.net/20.500.11990/1821

43. Jawaid, A., Roszkowski, M., & Mansuy, I. M. (2018). Chapter 12—Transgenerational epigenetics of traumatic stress. *Progress in Molecular Biology and Translational Science, 158*, 273–298. https://doi.org/10.1016/bs.pmbts.2018.03.003

44. Jirtle, R. L., & Skinner, M. K. (2007). Environmental epigenomics and disease susceptibility. *Nature Reviews of Genetics, 8*(4), 253–262. https://doi.org/10.1038/nrg2045

45. Kagan, J. (2010). *The temperamental thread: How genes, culture, time, and luck make us who we are.* Dana Press.

46. Kagan, J., Snidman, N., Kahn, V., & Towsley, S. (2007). The preservation of two infant temperaments into adolescence. *Monographs of the Society for Research in Child Development, 72*(2), 95. https://doi.org/10.1111/j.1540-5834.2007.00436.x

47. Kang, H. J., Kawasawa, Y. I., Cheng, F., Zhu, Y., Xu, X., Li, M., Sousa, A. M. M., Pletikos, M., Meyer, K. A., Sedmak, G., Guennel, T., Shin, Y., Johnson, M. B., Krsnik, Z., Mayer, S., Fertuzinhos, S., Umlauf, S., Lisgo, S. N., Vortmeyer, A., & Sestan, N. (2011). Spatio-temporal transcriptome of the human brain. *Nature, 478*(7370), 483–489. https://doi.org/10.1038/nature10523

48. Karg, K., Burmeister, M., Shedden, K., & Sen, S. (2011). The serotonin transporter promoter variant (5-HTTLPR), stress and depression meta-analysis revisited: Evidence of genetic moderation. *Archives of General Psychiatry, 68*(5), 444–454. https://doi.org/10.1001/archgenpsychiatry.2010.189

49. Khashan, A. S., McNamee, R., Henriksen, T. B., Pedersen, M. G., Kenny, L. C., Abel, K. M., & Mortensen, P. B. (2011). Risk of affective disorders following prenatal exposure to severe life events: A Danish population-based cohort study. *Journal of Psychiatric Research, 45*, 879–885. https://doi.org/10.1016/j.jpsychires.2010.12.005

50. Kim-Cohen, J., Caspi, A., Taylor, A., Williams, B., Newcombe, R., Craig, W., & Moffitt, T. E. (2006). MAOA, maltreatment, and gene-environment interaction predicting children's mental health: New evidence and a meta-analysis. *Molecular Psychiatry, 11*(10), 903–913. https://doi.org/10.1038/sj.mp.4001851

51. Kloke, V., Jansen, F., Heiming, R. S., Palme, R., Lesch, K., & Sachser, N. (2011). The winner and loser effect, serotonin transporter genotype, and the display of offensive aggression. *Physiology & Behavior, 103*, 565–574. https://doi.org/10.1016/j.physbeh.2011.04.021

52. Knafo-Noam, A., Uzefovsky, F., Israel, S., Davidov, M., & Zahn-Waxler, C. (2015). The prosocial personality and its facets: Genetic and environmental architecture of mother-reported behavior of 7-year-old twins. *Frontiers in Psychology, 6*, 112. https://doi.org/10.3389/fpsyg.2015.00112

53. Kodesh A, Levine SZ, Khachadourian V, Rahman R, Schlessinger A, O'Reilly PF, Grove J, Schendel D, Buxbaum JD, Croen L, Reichenberg A, Sandin S, Janecka M. Maternal health around pregnancy and autism risk: a diagnosis-wide, population-based study. Psychol Med.2021 Mar 26:1-9. doi: 10.1017/S0033291721001021. Epub ahead of print. PMID: 33766168; PMCID: PMC8464612.

54. Lee, P. H., Feng, Y. A., & Smoller, J. W. (2021). Pleiotropy and cross-disorder genetics among psychiatric disorders. *Biological Psychiatry, 89*(1), 20–31. https://doi.org/10.1016/j.biopsych.2020.09.026

55. Libbey, J., Sweeten, T., & McMahon, W. (2005). Autistic disorders and viral infections. *Journal of Neurovirology, 11*, 1–10. https://doi.org/10.1080/13550280590900553

56. Lim, K. O., Beal, D. M., & Harvey, R. L. (1995). Brain dysmorphology in adults with congenital rubella plus schizophrenia-like symptoms. *Biological Psychiatry, 37*(11), 764–776. https://doi.org/10.1016/0006-3223(94)00219-S

57. Lindblad, F., & Hjern, A. (2010). ADHD after fetal exposure to maternal smoking. *Nicotine & Tobacco Research: Official Journal of the Society for Research on Nicotine and Tobacco, 12*(4), 408–415. https://doi.org/10.1093/ntr/ntq017

58. Lindström, K., Lindblad, F., & Hjern, A. (2011). Preterm birth and attention-deficit/hyperactivity disorder in schoolchildren. *Pediatrics, 127*(5), 858–865. https://doi.org/10.1542/peds.2010-1279

59. Maul, S., Giegling, I., Fabbri, C., Corponi, F., Serretti, A., & Rujescu, D. (2020). Genetics of resilience: Implications from genome-wide association studies and candidate genes of the stress-response system in post-traumatic stress disorder and depression. *American Journal Medical Genetics, Part B: Neuropsychiatric Genetics, 183*(2), 77–94. https://doi.org/10.1002/ajmg.b.32763

60. McGowan, P. O., Sasaki, A., D'Alessio, A. C., Dymov, S., Labonte, B., Szyf, M., Turecki, G., & Meaney, M. J. (2009). Epigenetic regulation of the glucocorticoid receptor in human brain associates with childhood abuse. *Nature Neuroscience, 12*(3), 342–348. https://doi.org/10.1038/nn.2270

61. Meaney, M. J., & Szyf, M. (2005). Environmental programming of stress responses through DNA methylation: Life at the interface between a dynamic environment and a fixed genome. *Dialogues in Clinical Neuroscience, 7*, 103–123. https://doi.org/10.31887/DCNS.2005.7.2/mmeaney

62. Mednick, S. A., Machon, R. A., Huttunen, M. O., & Bonett, D. (1988). Adult schizophrenia following prenatal exposure to an influenza epidemic. *Archives of General Psychiatry, 45*(2), 189–192. https://doi.org/10.1001/archpsyc.1988.01800260109013

63. Mellins, C. A., Brackis-Cott, E., Leu, C. S., Elkington, K. S., Dolezal, C., Wiznia, A., McKay, M., Bamji, M., & Abrams, E. J. (2009). Rates and types of psychiatric disorders in perinatally human immunodeficiency virus-infected youth and seroverters. *Journal of Child Psychology and Psychiatry and Allied Disciplines, 50*(9), 1131–1138. https://doi.org/10.1111/j.1469-7610.2009.02069.x

64. Milberger, S., Biederman, J., Faranone, S., Chen, L., & Jones, J. (1996). Is maternal smoking a risk factor for attention deficit hyperactivity disorder in children? *American Journal of Psychiatry, 153*, 1138–1143. https://doi.org/10.1176/ajp.153.9.1138

65. Mittal, V. A., Ellman, L. M., & Cannon, T. D. (2008). Gene-environment interaction and covariation in schizophrenia: The role of obstetric complications. *Schizophrenia Bulletin, 34*(6), 1083–1094.

66. Monk, C., Lugo-Candelas, C., & Trumpff, C. (2019). Prenatal developmental origins of future psychopathology: Mechanisms and pathways. *Annual Review of Clinical Psychology, 15*, 317–344. https://doi.org/10.1146/annurev-clinpsy-050718-095539

67. Moreno, J. L., Kurita, M., Holloway, T., Lopez, J., Cardagan, R., Martinez-Sobrido, L., Garcia-Sastre, A., & Gonzales-Maeso, A. (2011). Maternal influenza viral infection causes schizophrenia-like alternations of 5-HT2A and mGlu2 receptors in the adult offspring. *The Journal of Neuroscience: The Official Journal of the Society for Neuroscience, 31*(5), 1863–1872. https://doi.org/10.1523/JNEUROSCI.4230-10.2011

68. Nichols, P., & Chen, T. (1981). *Minimal brain dysfunction: A prospective study*. Lawrence Erlbaum.

69. Obel, C., Olsen, J., Henriksen, T. B., Rodriguez, A., Jarvelin, M., Moilanen, M., Parner, E., Linnet, K. M., Taanila, A., Ebeling, H., Heiervang, E., & Gissler, M. (2011). Is maternal smoking during pregnancy a risk factor for hyperkinetic disorder? Findings from a sibling design. *International Journal of Epidemiology, 40*(2), 338–345. https://doi.org/10.1093/ije/dyq185

70. Partridge, T. (2003). Biological and caregiver correlates of behavioral inhibition. *Infant and Child Development, 12*, 71–87. https://doi.org/10.1002/icd.266

71. Pasamanick, B., Rogers, M. E., & Lilienfield, A. M. (1956). Pregnancy experience and the development of behavior disorders in children. *American Journal of Psychiatry, 112*(8), 613–618.

72. Perroud, N., Rutembesa, E., Paoloni-Giacobino, A., Mutabaruka, J., Mutesa, L., Stenz, L., Malafosse, A., & Karege, F. (2014). The Tutsi genocide and transgenerational transmission of maternal stress: Epigenetics and biology of the HPA axis. *The World Journal of Biological Psychiatry, 15*, 334–345. https://doi.org/10.3109/15622975.2013.866693

73. Pinto-Martin, J. A., Levy, S. E., Feldman, J. F., Lorenz, J. M., Paneth, M., & Whitaker, A. H. (2011). Prevalence of autism spectrum disorder in adolescents born weighing <2000 grams. *Pediatrics, 128*(5), 883–891. https://doi.org/10.1542/peds.2010-2846

74. Plomin, R., Owen, M. J., & McGuffin, P. (1994). The genetic basis of complex human behaviors. *Science, 1264*, 1733–1739.

75. Power, R. A., & Pluess, M. (2015). Heritability estimates of the big five personality traits based on common genetic variants. *Translational Psychiatry, 5*, e604. https://doi.org/10.1038/tp.2015.96; published online 14 July 2015

76. Reif, A., Rösler, M., Freitag, C. M., Schneider, M., Eujen, A., Kissling, C., Wenzler, D., Jacob, C. P., Retz-Junginger, P., Thome, J., Lesch, K., & Retz, W. (2007). Nature and nurture predispose to violent behavior: Serotonergic genes and adverse childhood environment. *Neuropsychopharmacology: Official Publication of the American College of Neuropsychopharmacology, 32*(11), 2375–2383. https://doi.org/10.1038/sj.npp.1301359

77. Rice, F., Harold, G. T., Bolvin, J., van den Bree, M., Hay, D. F., & Thapar, A. (2010). The links between prenatal stress and offspring development and psychopathology: Disentangling environmental and inherited influences. *Psychological Medicine, 40*(2), 335–345. https://doi.org/10/1017/S0033291709005911

78. Rice, F., Jones, I., & Thapar, A. (2007). The impact of gestational and prenatal growth on emotional problems in the offspring: A review. *Acta Psychiatrica Scandinavica, 115*, 171–183. https://doi.org/10.1111/j.1600-0447.2006.00895.x

79. Ripke, S., Sanders, A. R., Kendler, K. S., Levinson, D. F., Sklar, P., Holmans, P. A., Lin, D., Duan, J., Ophoff, R. A., Andreassen, O. A., Scolnick, E., Cichon, S., St. Clair, D., Corvin, A.,

Gurling, H., Werge, T., Rujescu, D., Blackwood, D. H. R., Pato, C. N., & Gejman, P. V. (2011). Genome-wide association study identifies five new schizophrenia loci. *Nature Genetics*, *43*(10), 969–976. https://doi.org/10.1038/ng.940

80. Rosso, I. M., & Cannon, T. D. (2003). Obstetric complications and neurodevelopmental mechanisms in schizophrenia. In D. C. Cicchetti & E. F. Walker (Eds.), *Neurodevelopmental mechanisms in psychopathology* (pp. 111–137). Cambridge University Press.

81. Rothbart, M. (2011). *Becoming who we are: Temperament and personality in development*. Guilford Press.

82. Schwartz, C. E., Wright, C. I., Shin, L. M., Kagan, J., & Rauch, S. L. (2003). Inhibited and uninhibited infants "grown up": Adult amygdalar response to novelty. *Science*, *300*, 1952–1953. https://doi.org/10.1126/science.1083703

83. Shang, S., Wu, N., & Su, Y. (2017). How oxytocin receptor (OXTR) single nucleotide polymorphisms act on prosociality: The mediation role of moral evaluation. *Frontiers in Psychology*, *8*, 396. https://doi.org/10.3389/fpsyg.2017.00396

84. Siever, L. J. (2008). Neurobiology of aggression and violence. *American Journal of Psychiatry*, *165*(4), 449–442.

85. Sklar, P., Ripke, S., & Scott, L. J. (2011). Large-scale genome-wide association analysis of bipolar disorder identifies a new susceptibility locus near ODZ4. *Nature Genetics*, *43*(10), 977–983. https://doi.org/10.1038/ng.943

86. St Clair, D., Xu, M., Wang, P., Yaqin, Y., Fang, Y., Zhang, F., Zheng, X., Gu, N., Feng, G., Sham, P., & He, L. (2005). Rates of adult schizophrenia following exposure to the Chinese famine of 1959–1961. *JAMA*, *294*(5), 557–562. https://doi.org/10.1001/jama.294.5.557

87. Stein, M. B., Choi, K. W., Jain, S., Campbell-Sills, L., Chen, C., Gelernter, J., He, F., Heeringa, S. G., Maihofer, A. X., Nievergelt, C., Nock, M. K., Ripke, S., Xiaoying, S., Kessler, R. C., Smoller, J. W., & Ursano, R. J. (2019). Genome-wide analysis of psychological resilience in U.S. Army Soldiers. *American Journal of Medical Genetics. Part B, Neuropsychiatric Genetics: The Official Publication of the International Society of Psychiatric Genetics*, *180*(5), 310–319. https://doi.org/10.1002/ajmg.b.32730

88. Steinhausen, H., & Spohr, H. (1998). Long-term outcome of children with fetal alcohol syndrome: Psychopathology, behavior, and intelligence. *Alcoholism Clinical and Experimental Research*, *22*, 334–338.

89. Streissguth, A., Bookstein, F., Barr, H., Sampson, P. D., O'Malley, K., & Young, J. K. (2004). Risk factors for adverse life outcomes in fetal alcohol syndrome and fetal alcohol effects. *Journal of Developmental and Behavioral Pediatrics*, *25*(4), 228–238. https://doi.org/10.1097/00004703-200408000-00002

90. Sullivan, P. F. (2010). The psychiatric GWAS consortium: Big science comes to psychiatry. *Neuron*, *68*(2), 182–186. https://doi.org/10.1016/j.neuron.2010.10.003

91. Syed, M., & Fish, J. (2018). Revisiting Erik Erikson's legacy on culture, race, and ethnicity. *Identity: An International Journal of Theory and Research*, *18*(4), 274–283. https://doi.org/10.1080/15283488.2018.1523729

92. Taylor, S. E., Way, B. M., Welch, W. T., Hilmert, C. J., Lehman, B. J., & Eisenberger, N. I. (2006). Early family environment, current adversity, the serotonin transporter polymorphism, and depressive symptomatology. *Biological Psychiatry*, *60*, 671–676. https://doi.org/10.1016/j.biopsych.2006.04.019

93. Thomas, A., Chess, S., & Birch, H. G. (1963). *Temperament and behavior disorders in children*. New York University Press.

94. Van den Bergh BR, Van Calster B, Smits T, Van Huffel S, Lagae L. Antenatal maternal anxiety is related to HPA-axis dysregulation and self-reported depressive symptoms in adolescence: a prospective study on the fetal origins of depressed mood. Neuropsychopharmacology. 2008 Feb;33(3):536-45. doi: 10.1038/sj.npp.1301450. Epub 2007 May 16. Erratum in: Neuropsychopharmacology. 2008 Aug;33(9):2301. PMID: 17507916.

95. Vanderbilt, D., & Gleason, M. M. (2010). Mental health concerns of the premature infant through the lifespan. *Child and Adolescent Psychiatric Clinics of North America, 19*(2), 211–228, vii–viii. https://doi.org/10.1016/j.chc.2010.02.003

96. Wankerl, M., Wüst, S., & Otte, C. (2010). Current developments and controversies: Does the serotonin transporter gene-linked polymorphic region (5-HTTLPR) modulate the association between stress and depression? *Current Opinion in Psychiatry, 23*(6), 582–587. https://doi.org/10.1097/YCO.0b013e32833f0e3a

97. Welberg, L. A., & Seckl, J. R. (2001). Prenatal stress, glucocorticoids, and the programming of the brain. *Journal of Neuroendocrinology, 13*, 113–128.

98. Whitaker, A. H., Feldman, J. F., Lorenz, J. M., McNicholas, F., Fisher, P. W., Shen, S., Pinto-Martin, J., Shaffer, D., & Paneth, N. (2001). Neonatal head ultrasound abnormalities in preterm infants and adolescent psychiatric disorders. *Archives of General Psychiatry, 68*(7), 742–752. https://doi.org/10.1001/archgenpsychiatry.2011.62

99. Whitaker, A. H., Van Rossem, R., & Feldman, J. F. (1997). Psychiatric outcomes in low-birth-weight children at age 6 years: Relation to neonatal cranial ultrasound abnormalities. *Archives of General Psychiatry, 54*(9), 847–856. https://doi.org/10.1001/archpsyc.1997.01830210091012

100. Yamashita, Y., Fujimoto, C., Nakajima, E., Isagai, T., & Matsuishi, T. (2003). Possible association between congenital cytomegalovirus infection and autism disorder. *Journal of Autism and Developmental Disorders, 33*(4), 455–459. https://doi.org/10.1023/A:1025023131029

101. Yehuda, R., & Lehrner, A. (2018). Intergenerational transmission of trauma effects: Putative role of epigenetic mechanisms. *World Psychiatry, 17*, 243–257. https://doi.org/10.1002/wps.20568

102. Zald, D. H., Cowan, R. L., Riccardi, P., Baldwin, R. M., Sib Ansari, M., Shelby, E. S., Smith, C. E., McHugo, M., & Kessler, R. M. (2008). Midbrain dopamine receptor availability is inversely associated with novelty-seeking traits in humans. *Journal of Neuroscience, 28*(53), 14372. https://doi.org/10.1523/JNEUROSCI.2423-08.2008

103. Zammit, S., Thomas, K., Thompson, A., Horwood, J., Menezes, P., Gunnell, D., Hollis, C., Wolke, D., Lewis, G., & Harrison, G. (2009). Maternal tobacco, cannabis and alcohol use during pregnancy and risk of adolescent psychotic symptoms in offspring. *The British Journal of Psychiatry, 195*(4), 294–300.

104. Zuckerman, M. (1991). *Psychobiology of personality*. Cambridge University Press.

105. Zuckerman, M. (2007). *Sensation seeking and risky behavior*. American Psychological Association.

13 The Earliest Years

When you build a house, the first thing you must do is to lay down a good foundation. It needs to be strong, but it also needs to be flexible enough to withstand future blows. The same is true for a developing person, and the years between birth to about 3 years are the time to lay down this internal **foundation**. These are the **earliest years**—the time when children are learning to trust and form secure attachments, establishing a stable sense of themselves and others, developing the capacity to know and regulate their own feelings and internal states, and gaining essential cognitive abilities.

Psychodynamic Formulation: An Expanded Approach, First Edition. The Psychodynamic Formulation Collective.
© 2022 John Wiley & Sons Ltd. Published 2022 by John Wiley & Sons Ltd.

Connecting to the primary caregiver

All of this development happens in the context of the child's earliest relationships. Many investigators have speculated that infants are preprogrammed to form relationships, because their survival—both physical and emotional—depends on it (Bowlby, 1958; Harlow & Zimmerman, 1958). For babies, simply being held can be literally a matter of life and death (Ainsworth et al., 1978; Bowlby, 1969; Fries et al., 2005, 2008; Jones & Mize, 2008). A lack of early tactile stimulation and physical proximity to the primary caregiver has been found to cause multiple problems, including delays in physical growth and neurobehavioral development (Johnson et al., 1992; Smyke et al., 2007), depressed levels of stress hormones (Feng et al., 2011; Fox & Hane, 2008; Fries et al., 2005, 2008), weakened immune function, (Feng et al., 2011; Suomi, 1995), and even death (Albers et al., 1997; Harmon, 2010). Lack of touch in infancy has also been linked to behavioral problems later in life, including aggressiveness, violent behavior, substance misuse, and depression (Bos et al., 2011; Goldfarb, 1947; Pederson, 2004; Prescott, 1979, 1980; Winnicott, 1987).

During the first several years of life, babies have the challenge of forming at least one reliable, consistent, nurturing relationship in which they feel unconditionally loved and completely cared for. This relationship can be with the mother, but it can also be with another person—for the purposes of this discussion, let's call that person the **primary caregiver**. Because this is a one-on-one relationship, it is often called a **dyadic relationship**.

Children who establish a solid dyadic relationship are fortunate indeed—they now have an internal foundation that will serve them well for the rest of their lives. There is a good chance that they will feel worthy of being loved, cared for, understood, and able to be angry with loved ones without feeling that they will destroy them. Conversely, children who do not establish a solid dyadic relationship are more likely to have global difficulties in one or more of these areas.

"Good Enough" parenting

The dyadic relationship does not have to be perfect—it must be what Winnicott (1987) called "good enough." Good enough parenting ensures that children are generally cared for and loved without abuse or neglect. With good enough parenting, children have a good chance of developing at least a nascent capacity for all the things that we will discuss in this chapter (Winnicott, 1987). Of course, the good enough primary caretaker does not necessarily have to be a woman.

What develops during the earliest years?

Trusting other people

Once there is a connection, children can begin to develop **trust**. Trust is vital for forming relationships (see Chapter 6). Without trust, people generally experience themselves as alone and unable to rely on others. Mutuality and intimacy, which are predicated on the capacity for dependency, are also very difficult without trust (see Chapter 7). The ability to trust others has important roots in the primary dyadic relationship of the earliest years. When an infant's primary caretaker is reliably available and appropriately responsive to the baby's needs, the growing child is mostly likely to develop **basic trust**—the core positive expectation that one's physical and emotional needs will be met and that other people can be depended on to provide comfort and safety (Erikson, 1950, 1968). Conversely, if a child's early experience is one in which physical and emotional needs are supplied inconsistently or if the child is constantly frustrated, they are more likely to develop a deep-seated conviction that the world is not a safe place and that they cannot rely on other people. Consider the person who seeks therapy for difficulty committing to a loving, adult relationship and who spent the first four years of life in an orphanage before being adopted. Even if the person had good parenting after age 4, it is possible that lack of a solid dyadic relationship during the earliest years has affected their ability to trust others. When adults have global problems with trusting others, it is important to consider that they may have had difficulties during this phase of development.

Forming secure attachments

The capacity to form **secure attachments** also has its origins in the primary dyadic relationship. **Attachment** is the deep and enduring emotional bond that connects one person to a special other across time and space (see Chapter 24) (Bowlby, 1969). Based on the work done by psychologist Mary Ainsworth, it is generally believed that children develop a particular **attachment style** around age 1. Ainsworth created an experiment called the **strange situation** in which she observed the way in which 1-year-old children reacted to being briefly left by, and then reunited with, their mothers. After observing hundreds of American children in this experimental situation, Ainsworth outlined four distinct styles of attachment (Ainsworth et al., 1978):

1. **Secure**—In this style, shown by about 50 percent of American children studied, the child cries and protests initially when the mother leaves the room, then quickly settles down. When she returns, the child greets her with pleasure, is easily consoled if still upset, and then goes back to playing.
2. **Anxious-Avoidant**—In this style, shown by about 25 percent of American children, the child seems not to notice and does not protest when the mother leaves the room. When she returns, the child may ignore her and not approach her at all. Though it may appear that the child does not react to the mother leaving and returning, the child's increased heart rate and cortisol levels demonstrate that the event is a biological stressor for the child.
3. **Anxious-Ambivalent**—The child reacts with exaggerated crying and protests to the mother's departure and remains in distress while she is gone, but on her return, the child arches away from her if held, seems angry, and is not easily comforted. About 10–15 percent of American children show this pattern of attachment.
4. **Disorganized**—About 10–15 percent of American infants protest when their mothers leave, but behave oddly when they return. For example, they may freeze in the middle of approaching the mother, walk backwards, sit, rock, or stare into space.

The caregivers of infants who have a secure attachment style tend to respond consistently and sensitively to their baby's crying and feeding signals (Ainsworth et al., 1974; Andrea & Kirkland, 1996; De Wolff & van Ijzendoorn, 1997; Schaffer & Emerson, 1964). In contrast, caregivers of children with anxious-avoidant, anxious-ambivalent, and disorganized styles tend to be inconsistent, unresponsive, or rejecting, and seem far less able to conceive of and respond sensitively to their infant's mental state. Not surprisingly, these caregivers tend to be under greater social stress (less help at home, more children, financial problems, or a disruptive partner), have more mental illness, and describe more adverse attachment experiences in their own childhood (Crockenberg, 1981; De Wolff & van Ijzendoorn, 1997; Main et al., 1985; Murray, 1992). While these environmental influences are key in shaping attachments, it is also important to recognize that inherited genetic factors may also play a role (Gillath et al., 2008), as may the influence of society, such as privilege and disadvantage (Sherry et al., 2013).

Failure to form secure attachments can have significant effects on subsequent development and adult relationships. For example, children previously classified as anxious-avoidant are likely to be less independent than securely attached children at age 4, and those who were classified as disorganized are likely to have aggressive, dissociative tendencies in later childhood and chaotic, tumultuous relationships in adulthood (Fonagy et al., 2000; Main et al., 1985; Ooi et al., 2006) (see Chapter 24 for more on attachment).

Effects of adversity and inequity later in life on the securely attached child

John Bowlby (1979), an early investigator of attachment, is famous for having asserted that early attachment experiences influence later social functioning. However, it is also true that a person's attachment pattern can change after early childhood—for the better as well as for the worse. For example, social stressors or adverse life events in later childhood, such as illness, death of a parent, or divorce, can lead children to lose the security of their attachment style (Steele et al., 1996). And despite the importance of early experience and the relative stability of attachment security (Waters et al., 2000), later life events, external circumstances, inequity, and relationships—including relationships between therapists and patients—can also affect adult attachment patterns (Coutinho et al., 2009). Still, in the balance, research suggests that early interpersonal experiences at least set the stage for adult relationship patterns (Gallo et al., 2003; Grossmann & Grossmann, 2009), and greater attachment security in infancy does seem to lead to better social functioning in adulthood (Gallo et al., 2003: Priel & Shamai, 1995).

Cross-cultural differences in attachment

Child-rearing values regarding attachment are a reflection of our culture (Mamarosh, 2015; Rothbaum et al., 2000; van Ijzendoorn & Sagi-Schwartz, 2008; Wang & Mallinckrodt, 2006). Research has revealed different ways of responding to the universal need for attachment security in infants. For example, many African communities discourage the maternal exclusivity that many attachment-based Western parenting models advocate and believe optimal care is provided by multiple caregivers (Keller et al., 2005; Otto, 2008). Among the Aka, a Congo Basin tropical forest foraging community, about 20 caregivers interact and care for children on a daily basis (Keller et al., 2005; Mechan et al., 2017). Higher maternal death rates in certain communities increase the importance of having many caregivers look after children. (Carr, 2019; Otto, 2008). Conversely, Kagan and colleagues found that indigenous Guatemalan children who spent most of their first year of life in dark huts with minimal stimulation were not adversely affected (Kagan et al., 1978). We'll return to this topic in Chapter 24.

Developing a sense of others

Infants also use their experiences with their primary caregivers to develop their feelings and fantasies about other people. With basically caring and consistent parenting—along with the maturation of the prefrontal cortex—children begin to create internal images of the primary caregiver that help them to realize that when caregivers are out of sight, it's because they have a separate permanent existence. This capacity is called **object permanence** (Piaget, 1954).

But even when children know that their primary caregivers won't disappear, they still have rudimentary ideas about other people. For example, they still do not necessarily know that someone can have both good *and* bad qualities. This is true of both themselves and others. If the child feels good, the caregiver is good; if the child feels bad, the caregiver is bad. By about age 2 or 3, however, the image of the primary caregiver becomes stable and enduring and can be maintained even when the child's needs are not being met. This enables children to understand that people can have both good and bad qualities (Akhtar 1994). This capacity, referred to as **object constancy** (Mahler, 1965), generally only develops if the experience of the primary caregiver is predominantly positive. If it isn't, for example, in the case of abuse or neglect, children may continue to separate bad from good, a process called **splitting**, in order to protect positive feelings about their caregivers (Burland 1994). This may interrupt the child's capacity to develop a more nuanced and three-dimensional view of both themself and others.

During this time, infants also develop the ability to **mentalize**—to appreciate that other people can have beliefs, feelings, desires, and motivations that are different from their own, and to make inferences about what those thoughts and feelings might be (Aschersleben et al., 2008; Fonagy & Target, 1997; Meins, 1997, 1998; Sharp et al., 2006). Sensitive caregivers help this developmental process by observing their child's internal states closely and treating the child as having a separate mind—even before the child understands this themself (Sharp et al., 2006). Doing so helps the child to appreciate their own internal experience, and, in later childhood, helps them to understand that other people have their own thoughts and feelings. Thus, caregivers who do not do this can hinder the development of their children's capacity for **empathy**.

Developing a sense of self

Along with being a time to learn about others, this period of childhood is also critical for developing a consistent sense of self as well as the capacity to regulate self-esteem. When infants have consistent, trust-inspiring experiences with early caregivers, they are likely to develop the confidence that they can safely explore the world and face life's challenges. However, if early childhood experiences with caregivers are marked by unpredictability and inconsistency—especially by trauma, neglect, or emotional withdrawal—children are more likely to lack a core sense of themselves as being safe, effective, and valued in their interactions with the world.

During these years, children also begin to have a nascent sense of their talents and limitations, which can help them to begin to regulate self-esteem. Parents who appropriately **mirror** their children are excited by what the children are able to do, without overinflating or downplaying it (Stern, 1974, 1985a, 1985b). Children who are repeatedly disappointed by their caregivers' lack of empathic feedback or sensitive support often have more extreme problems regulating self-esteem later in life. As adults, they may rely excessively on the opinions of others to keep their self-esteem afloat, and they tend to swing back and forth between overly inflated views of their own abilities and deep-seated feelings of inferiority (Kohut, 1972; Ornstein, 2006). We will return to this topic in Chapter 23.

Thinking and regulating emotions

Thinking

Numerous investigators have shown that the quality of the early dyadic relationship affects various aspects of the growing child's cognitive development during the earliest years. While general cognitive ability does not appear to be affected, language acquisition and the capacity for abstraction are influenced by the security of attachment to caregivers in infancy (Meins, 1997). At 20 months, securely attached children tend to be faster language learners and have larger vocabularies than insecurely attached children (Meins, 1997, 1998).

Learning to regulate emotions

Although infants experience feelings from birth, they do not know what those feelings are or how to regulate them (Fonagy et al., 2002; Stern, 1985b, 1990). Through their interactions with their primary caregivers, they learn both. When infants nonverbally communicate their needs for soothing, feeding, or sleep, this usually evokes a series of unconsciously coordinated and attuned responses from the primary caregivers (Gergely et al., 2002; Stern, 1974, 1985b). This has been referred to as the caregiver's **empathic responsiveness** or **affective attunement**. Imitation of the baby's actions alone is not sufficient. Caregivers must be able to "read" their infants' feeling states from the baby's behavior, and then perform some coordinated behavior that "matches" it. For example, if the baby cries, the caregiver might make a gently frowning face. In turn, infants must be able to "read" the caregiver's response as having something to do with their own original feeling experience (Stern, 1985b). This nonverbal communication helps children get to know, organize, and regulate their own internal states without being overwhelmed and is essential for the development of anxiety and affect tolerance (Beebe & Sloate, 1982; Beebe & Stern, 1977; Gergely et al., 2002).

Development of values

Just as they go through various stages of physical, emotional, and cognitive growth, children also develop values as they mature. With the help of their caregivers, by age 3 most children have started to appreciate the difference between what's "okay" and what's "not okay." For example, they might understand that, "We don't take other kids' toys because we wouldn't want them to take ours." Contemporary research suggests that some children of this age can even struggle with a situation in which they are aware of two competing sides to a conflict and reach the choice that is most likely to benefit others (sometimes called a **prosocial** solution) (Oppenheim et al., 1997). As suggested in Chapter 12, genetic factors as well as environmental influences may help explain variations in prosociality among children (Christ et al., 2016; Shang et al., 2017).

Adult problems and patterns that suggest origins in the earliest years

Anything that disrupts development during the critical period from birth to age 3, including insensitive parenting, abuse, neglect, social stress, and negative life events, tends to have pervasive effects on multiple domains of function, and may lead to global problems in adulthood. In particular, these include:

- Difficulties with self-esteem management and maintaining a stable sense of self
- Difficulties trusting others and maintaining stable relationships
- Difficulties with self-regulation

The following sections provide examples of each.

Difficulty with self-esteem management and maintaining a stable sense of self

Yuri, a 32-year-old gay man who was born in Eastern Europe, comes for therapy saying, "I just don't feel good about myself." Having obtained a business degree from a community college, Yuri works as a bookkeeper at a small auto parts company. "I doodle all the time," he says. "I love illustrating and wish I could do that for work, but I was never trained in art." Every criticism from his boss, he explains, sends him into a tailspin for days. "I just feel like I'll never amount to anything," he states. He is also having trouble with dating because, as he explains, "if a man doesn't seem totally into me right away, I just start avoiding his texts. I suffer when I am rejected." When you ask about his life story, he says that he was abandoned by his single mother when he was eight months old, and that he lived in an orphanage for four years before being adopted by his American family. "They saved my life, of course," he says, "but they don't get me. They are all about numbers and always told me to put my 'scribbles' away. I'm not even out to them."

Abandoned as an infant and sent to live in an orphanage, it is likely that Yuri missed the mirroring he needed to establish a stronger sense of self. This lack of mirroring seems to have continued with his adoptive family. Now, as an adult, he is having difficulty maintaining his sense of self in the face of criticism, or even perceived criticism, from others.

Difficulty trusting others and maintaining stable relationships

Born to wealthy parents, Malcolm has worked for the family business throughout life. Now 50 years old, he has no close friends, has never been married, has no children, and has generally had short-lived relationships. "The women I date always want to get married. I don't tell them that

I come from money, but they probably get it based on my home and my car. If it didn't work out, I'd be fleeced in a divorce." Although Malcolm insists that his parents were "the most loving," he has few happy memories of childhood and cannot recall being hugged by anyone. He was always afraid of "doing the wrong thing" and displeasing his parents. "They had strong opinions about everything and everyone," he says. "I wasn't even allowed to play with other kids. Nobody was ever good enough for us—not even other relatives."

Beginning in his earliest years, Malcolm's parents instilled in him the sense that the world was a very dangerous place, and that people are not who they seem to be. Although he claims that they were loving, his parents may not have been able to help him form secure attachments. This has likely interfered with his ability to forge meaningful adult relationships.

Difficulty with self-regulation

Yasmin seeks help because she "goes to pieces" every time her boyfriend leaves town on a business trip. She feels utterly abandoned, becomes frantic, and then angrily demands that her elderly father drive two hours from the town where he lives to stay with her. Despite the fact that she is physically healthy and able to support herself financially, she has never slept alone—"not for a single night, ever." Yasmin's mother died in childbirth, and she later learned that her father went through several years of intense grief, financial insecurity, depression, and heavy drinking during her infancy, leaving the responsibility for her care to his half-sister who had three children of her own and who resented the imposition.

Yasmin's history of early parental loss and neglect in her earliest years has likely left her unable to tolerate separations and vulnerable to anxiety when actual or perceived abandonment looms. In the absence of a reliable, loving early caregiver, she seems never to have developed the capacity to evoke a soothing presence to calm herself, and she makes frantic efforts to avoid being alone (Akhtar, 1994).

Learning about the life story of the earliest years

People don't know and will never be able to tell you what transpired in their first three years of life. It is simply the nature of memory. Areas in the brain that mediate language and autobiographical memory are not "online" and fully functioning until 18–36 months of age (Wallin, 2007). After age 3, people have what has been called **declarative** or **explicit memory** for the events they experienced—they can probably remember and tell the story of their first day in kindergarten. But to make informed guesses about events during those first few "missing" years of life, we have only the patient's **procedural** or **implicit memory** to guide us—emotional responses, patterns of behavior, and skills that are nonverbal and are unconscious in the sense that they can't be retrieved for conscious reflection. Instead of *telling* us about these events, patients *act them out* every day in their interactions with the world and in their relationships with other people, including therapists. This unconscious or procedural memory about "being in relationships" has been called **implicit relational knowing** (Lyons-Ruth, 1998).

As clinicians, how can we put together reasonable hypotheses about our patient's earliest relationships? It turns out great consistency exists between the nonverbal interactions that take place between an infant and a caregiver during the earliest years, and the observable behavior of adults in interactions with others, including therapists (Beebe & Lachman, 2005; Stern et al., 1998; Wallin, 2007). We gain valuable clues about the nature of our patients' earliest formative relationships by paying close attention to how they habitually interact with us and make us feel, in addition to listening to how they describe current relationships (Beebe & Lachman, 2005; Wallin, 2007).

The following sections cover some additional guidelines for learning about the life story of the earliest years.

Early environment

Where did you live after you were born? In what type of dwelling? How did you come to live there? With whom did you live?

What were the financial circumstances of the people with whom you lived? What major stressors did they face?

Did you grow up with your biological parents? If not, what were the circumstances (e.g., adoption, surrogacy, living in an orphanage, or extended family living situation)?

Were you adopted? If so, at what age? What were the circumstances of the adoption?

Do you think your parents wanted to have a child when you were born?

Where are you in the birth order of your family? How do you think this affected your early years? Can you tell me about your earliest memory?

Qualities of the primary caregivers

Most adults will have stories about their caregivers that they have heard from others or from the caregivers themselves. These questions can serve as prompts for those stories:

Who were your primary caregivers?

What were your primary caregivers like? Do you have memories of them during your earliest years?

Were your primary caregivers generally happy with their lives? What stressors did they face before and after you came into their lives?

Were your primary caregivers emotionally or physically ill during your early childhood? Do you know if they were drinking or using drugs?

Do you know what your primary caregivers' relationships with their parents were like?

Quality of the early relationships with the primary caregivers

Do you think that you were loved and well cared for during this period of your life? Do you remember being held and kissed? Being called pet names? Having your scribbles tacked onto the refrigerator?

Are there pictures/videos of your early family? What do they show?

Do you feel that your primary caregivers were happy to have a child?

Do you have memories of being soothed when upset? Who usually calmed you?

History of separations and/or trauma during this time

Do you have any memories of especially difficult or upsetting experiences during this time?

Were you physically ill or hospitalized as a very young child? If so, was your primary caregiver with you?

Was your primary caregiver absent or inconsistently present during this time of your life?

Do you have any memory of physical or emotional trauma or sexual abuse (either your own or that was perpetrated on people in your household) during this time? Were the perpetrators people in your household?

Note that when asking about abuse, particularly during the earliest years, you may learn more if you ask in this way:

Did you have any physical or sexual experiences that made you uncomfortable during this time?

In Chapter 14, we will follow what happens as toddlers begin to explore the wider world and broaden their social sphere.

Suggested activity

Can be done by individual learners or in a classroom setting

Consider the following example and think about what difficulties Ainsley might have had during her earliest years:

> *Ainsley presents at age 25 because she has been cutting herself at night when she is alone. "I used to do this as a kid but stopped," she says, "but it comes back late at night when I'm not with people." Raised below the poverty level, Ainsley says she lived with her single mother and never knew her father. "Mom was in and out of drug rehabs," she reports. "And I was in and out of foster care. Some placements were better than others." Ainsley says that her last family was very stable. "When I was with them, I was fine—no cutting. But now that I'm on my own, it's tough." She says that it's hard to "settle down" after work. "I don't even know what I'm feeling," she says, "It's just a jumble."*

Comment

Raised in foster care, with one parent only intermittently available, it is likely that Ainsley developed a ***disorganized attachment pattern***. This has likely impaired her ability to achieve ***object constancy***, and to ***regulate her own anxiety and affect***. This is evident in her persistent need to be with people, her inability to understand her own feelings, and her use of self-harm to regulate her affect.

References

1. Ainsworth, M. D. S., Bell, S. M., & Stayton, D. J. (1974). Infant-mother attachment and social development: Socialization as a product of reciprocal responsiveness to signals. In M. Richards (Ed.), *The integration of the child into a social world* (pp. 9–135). Cambridge University Press.

2. Ainsworth, M. D. S., Blehar, M. C., Waters, E., & Wall, S. (1978). *Patterns of attachment: A psychological study of the strange situation.* Lawrence Erlbaum.

3. Akhtar, S. (1994). Object constancy and adult psychopathology. *International Journal of Psychoanalysis, 75*, 441–455.

4. Albers, L. H., Johnson, D. E., Hostetter, M. K., Iverson, S., & Miller, S. C. (1997). Health of children adopted from the Soviet Union and Eastern Europe: Comparison with pre-adoptive medical records. *Journal of the American Medical Association, 278*, 922–924.

5. Andrea, N., & Kirkland, J. (1996). Maternal sensitivity: A review of attachment literature definitions. *Early Child Development and Care, 120*, 55–65.

6. Aschersleben, G., Hofer, T., & Jovanovic, B. (2008). The link between infant attention to goal-directed action and later theory of mind abilities. *Developmental Science, 11*(6), 862–868. https://doi.org/10.1111/j.1467-7687.2008.00736.x

7. Beebe, B., & Lachman, F. (2005). *Infant research and adult treatment: Co-constructing interactions.* Analytic Press.

8. Beebe, B., & Sloate, P. (1982). Assessment and treatment of difficulties in mother-infant attunement in the first three years of life: A case history. *Psychoanalytic Inquiry, 1*(4), 601–623. https://doi.org/10.1080/07351698209533422

9. Beebe, B., & Stern, D. N. (1977). Engagement-disengagement and early object experiences. In M. Freedman & S. Grand (Eds.), *Communicative structures and psychic structures* (pp. 35–55). Plenum Press.

10. Bos, K., Zeanah, C. H., Fox, N. A., Drury, S. S., McLaughlin, K. A., & Nelson, C. A. (2011). Psychiatric outcomes in young children with a history of institutionalization. *Harvard Review of Psychiatry, 19*(1), 15–24. https://doi.org/10.3109/10673229.2011.549773

11. Bowlby, J. (1958). The nature of the child's tie to his mother. *International Journal of Psychoanalysis, 39*, 350–371.

12. Bowlby, J. (1969). *Attachment and loss: Volume 1: Attachment.* Basic Books.

13. Bowlby, J. (1979). *The making and breaking of affectional bonds.* Tavistock.

14. Burland, J. A. (1994). Splitting as a consequence of severe abuse in childhood. *Psychiatric Clinics of North America, 17*(4), 731–734.

15. Carr, S. (2019). Parenting practices around the world are diverse and not all about attachment. *The Conversation.* Accessed November 13, 2021. Available at https://theconversation.com/parenting-practices-around-the-world-are-diverse-and-not-all-about-attachment-111281

16. Christ, C., Carlo, G., & Stoltenberg, S. (2016). Oxytocin receptor (OXTR) single nucleotide polymorphisms indirectly predict prosocial behavior through perspective taking and empathic concern. *Journal of Personality, 84*(2), 204–213. https://doi.org/10.1111/jopy.12152

17. Coutinho, J., Ribeiro, E., & Safran, J. (2009). Resolution of ruptures in therapeutic alliance: Its role on change processes according to a relational approach. *Analise. Psicológica, 4*(XXVII), 479–491.

18. Crockenberg, S. B. (1981). Infant irritability, mother responsiveness, and social support influences on the security of infant-mother attachment. *Child Development, 52*(3), 857–886.

19. De Wolff, M., & van Ijzendoorn, M. H. (1997). Sensitivity and attachment: A meta-analysis on parental antecedents of infant attachments. *Child Development, 68*, 571–591. https://doi.org/10.2307/1132107

20. Erikson, E. H. (1950). *Childhood and society.* W.W. Norton & Co.

21. Erikson, E. H. (1968). *Identity: Youth and crisis*. W.W. Norton & Co.
22. Feng, X., Wang, L., Yang, S., Qin, D., Wang, J., Li, C., Lv, L., Ma, Y., & Hu, X. (2011). Maternal separation produces lasting changes in cortisol and behavior in rhesus monkeys. *Proceedings of the National Academy of Sciences of the United States of America, 108*(34), 14312–14317. https://doi.org/10.1073/pnas.1010943108
23. Fonagy, P., & Target, M. (1997). Attachment and reflective function. *Development and Psychopathology, 9*, 679–700. https://discovery.ucl.ac.uk/id/eprint/168571/1/download8.pdf
24. Fonagy, P., Target, M., & Gergely, G. (2000). Attachment and borderline personality disorder. A theory and some evidence. *Psychiatric Clinics of North America, 23*(1), 103–122. vii– viii. https://doi.org/10.1016/S0193-953X(05)70146-5
25. Fonagy, P., Gergely, G., Jurist, E., & Target, M. (2002). *Affect regulation, nentalization, and the development of the self*. Other Press.
26. Fox, N. A., & Hane, A. A. (2008). Studying the biology of human attachment. In J. Cassidy & P. R. Shaver (Eds.), *Handbook of attachment: Theory, research, and clinical applications* (2nd ed., pp. 217–240). Guilford Press.
27. Fries, A. B. W., Ziegler, T. E., Kurian, J. R., Jacoris, S., & Pollak, S. D. (2005). Early experience in humans is associated with changes in neuropeptides critical for regulating social behavior. *Proceedings of the National Academy of Sciences of the United States of America, 102*(47), 17237–17240. https://doi.org/10.1073/pnas.0504767102
28. Fries, A. B. W., Shirtcliff, E. A., & Pollak, S. D. (2008). Neuroendocrine dysregulation following early social deprivation in children. *Developmental Psychobiology, 50*(6), 588–599. https://doi.org/10.1002/dev.20319
29. Gallo, L. C., Smith, T. W., & Ruiz, J. M. (2003). An interpersonal analysis of adult attachment style: Circumplex descriptions, recalled developmental experiences, self-representations, and interpersonal functioning in adulthood. *Journal of Personality, 71*(2), 141–181. https://doi.org/10.1111/1467-6494.7102003
30. Gergely, G., Fonagy, P., & Target, M. (2002). Attachment, mentalization, and the etiology of borderline personality disorder. *Self Psychology, 7*(1), 61–72.
31. Gillath, O., Shaver, P. R., Baek, J. M., & Chun, D. S. (2008). Genetic correlates of adult attachment style. *Personality and Social Psychology Bulletin, 34*(10), 1396–1405. https://doi.org/10.1177/0146167208321484
32. Goldfarb, W. (1947). Variations in adolescent adjustment of institutionally reared children. *American Journal of Orthopsychiatry, 17*, 449–457.
33. Grossmann, K., & Grossmann, K. E. (2009). The impact of attachment to mother and father at an early age on children's psychosocial development through young adulthood. In R. E. Tremblay, R. G. Barr, R. D. V. Peters, et al. (Eds.), *Encyclopedia on early child development* (pp. 1–8). Centre of Excellence for Early Child Development. https://citeseerx.ist.psu.edu/viewdoc/download?doi=10.1.1.485.4485&rep=rep1&type=pdf
34. Harlow, H. F., & Zimmerman, R. R. (1958). The development of affective responsiveness in infant monkeys. *Proceedings of the American Philosophical Society, 102*, 501–509. https://www.jstor.org/stable/985597
35. Harmon, K. (2010). How important is physical contact with your infant? *Scientific American*. Accessed September 11, 2011, http://www.scientificamerican.com/article.cfm?id=infant-touch
36. Johnson, D. E., Miller, L. C., Iverson, S., Thomas, W., Franchino, B., Dole, K., Kiernan, M. T., Georgieff, M. K., & Hostetter, M. K. (1992). The health of children adopted from Romania. *Journal of the American Medical Association, 268*(24), 3446–3451. https://doi.org/10.1001/jama.1992.03490240054036
37. Jones, N. A., & Mize, K. D. (2008). Touch interventions positively affect development. In L. L'Abate (Ed.), *Low-cost approaches to promote physical and mental health: Theory, research and practice* (pp. 353–370). Springer Verlag.
38. Kagan, J., Kearsley, R. B., & Zelazo, P. R. (1978). *Infancy: Its place in human development*. Harvard University Press.

39. Keller, H., Voelker, S., & Yovsi, R. D. (2005). Conceptions of parenting in different cultural communities: The case of West African Nso and Northern German women. *Social Development, 14*(1), 158–180. https://doi.org/10.1111/j.1467-9507.2005.00295.x

40. Kohut, H. (1972). Thoughts on narcissism and narcissistic rage. In P. H. Ornstein (Ed.), *The search for the self* (Vol. II, pp. 615–658). International Universities Press, Inc.

41. Lyons-Ruth, K. (1998). Implicit relational knowing: Its role in development and psychoanalytic treatment. *Infant Mental Health Journal, 19*(3), 282–289.

42. Mahler, M. S. (1965). On the significance of the normal separation-individuation phase: With reference to research in symbiotic child psychosis. In M. Schur (Ed.), *Drives, affects and behavior* (Vol. II, pp. 161–169). International Universities Press, Inc.

43. Main, M., Kaplan, N., & Cassidy, J. (1985). Security in infancy, childhood, and adulthood: A move to the level of representation. *Monographs of the Society for Research in Child Development, 50*(1–2), 66–104. https://doi.org/10.2307/3333827

44. Mamarosh, C. (2015). Emphasizing the complexity of the relationship: The next decade of attachment-based psychotherapy research. *Psychotherapy, 52*(1), 12–18.

45. Mechan, C. L., Hagen, E. H., & Hewlett, B. S. (2017). Persistence in infant care patterns among Aka foragers. In V. R. Garcia & P. Aili (Eds.), *Hunter-gatherers in a changing world* (pp. 213–232). Springer International Publishing.

46. Meins, E. (1997). *Security of attachment and the social development of cognition.* Psychology Press/Erlbaum.

47. Meins, E. (1998). The effects of security of attachment and maternal attribution of meaning on children's linguistic acquisitional style. *Infant Behavior & Development, 21*(2), 237–252. https://doi.org/10.1016/S0163-6383(98)90004-2

48. Murray, L. (1992). The impact of postnatal depression on infant development. *Journal of Child Psychology, Psychiatry and Allied Disciplines, 33,* 543–561. https://doi.org/10.1111/j.1469-7610.1992.tb00890.x

49. Ooi, Y. P., Ang, R. P., Fung, D. S. S., Wang, G., & Cai, Y. (2006). The impact of parent-child attachment on aggression, social stress and self-esteem. *School Psychology International, 27*(5), 552–566. https://citeseerx.ist.psu.edu/viewdoc/download?doi=10.1.1.925.672&rep=rep1&type=pdf

50. Oppenheim, D., Emde, R. N., Hasson, M., & Warren, S. (1997). Preschoolers face moral dilemmas: A longitudinal study of acknowledging and resolving internal conflict. *The International Journal of Psychoanalysis, 78*(5), 943–957.

51. Ornstein, P. H. (2006). Chronic rage from underground: Reflections on its structure and treatment. In A. M. Cooper (Ed.), *Contemporary psychoanalysis in America: Leading analysts present their work* (pp. 449–463). American Psychiatric Publishing, Inc.

52. Otto, H. (2008). *Culture-specific attachment strategies in the Cameroonian Nso: Cultural solutions to a universal developmental task.* Ph.D. Dissertation, Osnabruck: Faculty of Human Sciences, Department of Culture & Psychology, University of Osnabruck, Germany. Available at https://repositorium.ub.uni-osnabrueck.de/bitstream/urn:nbn:de:gbv:700-2009050119/2/E-Diss881_thesis.pdf

53. Pederson, C. A. (2004). Biological aspects of social bonding and the roots of human violence. *Annals of the New York Academy of Sciences, 1036,* 106–127. https://doi.org/10.1196/annals.1330.006

54. Piaget, J. (1954). *The construction of reality in the child.* Basic Books.

55. Prescott, J. W. (1979). Deprivation of physical affection as a primary process in the development of physical violence. In D. G. Gil (Ed.), *Child abuse and violence* (pp. 66–137). AMS Press.

56. Prescott, J. W. (1980). Somatosensory affectional deprivation (SAD) theory of drug and alcohol use. In D. J. Lettieri, M. Sayers, & H. W. Pearson (Eds.), *Theories on drug abuse: Selected contemporary perspectives* (pp. 286–296). National Institute on Drug Abuse, Department of Health and Human Services.

57. Priel, B., & Shamai, D. (1995). Attachment style and perceived social support: Effects on affect regulation. *Personality and Individual Differences, 19*(2), 235–241. https://doi.org/10.1016/0191-8869(95)91936-T

58. Rothbaum, F., Weisz, J., Pott, M., Miyake, K., & Morelli, G. (2000). Attachment and culture: Security in the United States and Japan. *American Psychologist, 55,* 1093–1104. https://doi.org/10.1037/0003-066X.55.10.1093

59. Schaffer, H. R., & Emerson, P. E. (1964). The development of social attachments in infancy. *Monographs of the Society for Research in Child Development, 29*(3), 5–75. https://doi.org/10.2307/1165727

60. Shang, S., Wu, N., & Su, Y. (2017). How oxytocin receptor (OXTR) single nucleotide polymorphisms act on prosociality: The mediation role of moral evaluation. *Frontiers in Psychology, 8,* 396. https://doi.org/10.3389/fpsyg.2017.00396

61. Sharp, C., Fonagy, P., & Goodyear, I. M. (2006). Imagining your child's mind: Psychosocial adjustment and mothers' ability to predict their children's attributional response styles. *British Journal of Developmental Psychology, 26,* 197–214. http://m2s-conf.uh.edu/class/psychology/clinical-psych/_docs/SharpFonagyGoodyer.pdf

62. Sherry, A., Adelman, A., Farwell, L., & Linton, B. (2013). The impact of social class on parenting and attachment. In W. Ming Liu (Ed.), *The Oxford handbook of social class in counseling* (pp. 275–291). Oxford University Press. https://doi.org/10.1093/oxfordhb/9780195398250.013.0017

63. Smyke, A. T., Koga, S. F., Johnson, D. E., Fox, N. A., Marshall, P. J., Nelson, C. A., Zeanah, C. H., & BEIP Core Group. (2007). The caregiving context in institution-reared and family-reared infants and toddlers in Romania. *Journal of Child Psychology and Psychiatry, and Allied Disciplines, 48*(2), 210–218. https://doi.org/10.1111/j.1469-7610.2006.01694.x

64. Steele, H., Steele, M., & Fonagy, P. (1996). Associations among attachment classifications of mothers, fathers, and their infants. *Child Development, 67*(2), 541–555. https://doi.org/10.2307/1131831

65. Stern, D. N. (1974). Mother and infant at play: The dyadic interaction involving facial, vocal and gaze behaviors. In M. Lewis & L. A. Rosenblum (Eds.), *The effect of the infant on its caregiver.* John Wiley & Sons. http://psycnet.apa.org/record/1974-22730-010

66. Stern, D. N. (1985a). *The interpersonal world of the infant: A view from psychoanalysis and developmental psychology.* Basic Books.

67. Stern, D. N. (1985b). Affect attunement. In J. D. Call, E. Galenson, & R. L. Tyson (Eds.), *Frontiers of infant psychiatry* (Vol. II, pp. 3–14). Basic Books.

68. Stern, D. N. (1990). *Diary of a baby: What your child sees, feels, and experiences.* Basic Books.

69. Stern, D. N., Sander, L. W., Nahum, J. P., Harrison, A. M., Lyons-Ruth, K., Morgan, A. C., Bruschweiler-Stern, N., & Tronick, E. Z. (1998). Non-interpretive mechanisms in psychoanalytic psychotherapy: The "something more" than interpretation. *International Journal of Psychoanalysis, 79,* 903–921.

70. Suomi, S. (1995). Touch and the immune system in rhesus monkeys. In T. Field (Ed.), *Touch in early development* (pp. 53–65). Lawrence Erlbaum.

71. van Ijzendoorn, M. H., & Sagi-Schwartz, A. (2008). Cross-cultural patterns of attachment: Universal and contextual dimensions. In J. Cassidy & P. R. Shaver (Eds.), *Handbook of attachment: Theory, research, and clinical applications* (pp. 880–905). Guilford Publications, Inc.

72. Wallin, D. J. (2007). *Attachment in psychotherapy.* Guilford Press.

73. Wang, C. D., & Mallinckrodt, B. (2006). Differences between Taiwanese and U.S. cultural beliefs about ideal adult attachment. *Journal of Consulting Psychology, 53*(2), 192–204.

74. Waters, E., Weinfeld, N., & Hamilton, C. (2000). The stability of attachment security from infancy to adolescence and early adulthood: General discussion. *Child Development, 7*(3), 703–706.

75. Winnicott, D. W. (1987). *The child, the family, and the outside world.* Perseus Publishing.

14 Middle Childhood

Key concepts

Between the ages of 3 and 6, children become more aware of relationships among people in their environment. In this context, they continue to develop their sense of self, particularly related to their bodies, gender, race, and relationships with others.

Adult problems and patterns that suggest origins in middle childhood include

- Difficulty committing to relationships
- Sexual inhibitions
- Fear of competition and inhibited ambition

Learning about a life story of middle childhood involves asking about the child's relationships with their primary caregivers and siblings, with particular regard to

- The way the caregivers responded to the child's burgeoning sexuality
- Jealousy or rivalry among the family members

What develops during middle childhood?

As children increase their awareness of themselves and their world during middle childhood, they develop a more sophisticated sense of who they are and how they relate to others. If things have gone well in their earliest years, they are likely to enter this period with a nascent sense of self and the capacity to have relationships with others based on secure attachments. During middle childhood, their growing bodies and minds enable them to develop these capacities in new ways.

Psychodynamic Formulation: An Expanded Approach, First Edition. The Psychodynamic Formulation Collective.
© 2022 John Wiley & Sons Ltd. Published 2022 by John Wiley & Sons Ltd.

Self-perception and self-esteem regulation

During middle childhood, children continue to develop their sense of self, which is fueled by many factors. Some of this development comes from new thoughts and feelings about their bodies. Most children consolidate control of their bowel and bladder function during these years, giving them newfound mastery over their bodies and a growing sense of independence.

Awareness of gender

Awareness of gender comes to the fore as children become curious about each other's bodies as well as their own (Lewis & Volkmar, 1990). By age 2, children can recognize their own genitals when shown anatomically correct dolls, although it takes until ages 6 or 7 for them to understand genitals as the basis of gender categorization, and the idea that gender, for most people, is constant and stable (Drescher & Byne, 2017).

Awareness of race and ethnicity

By the ages of 4 or 5, children show many of the same racial attitudes as adults in their culture and have learned to associate some groups with higher status than others (Dunham et al., 2008; Kinzler, 2016; Sullivan et al., 2020). By age 7, children can define group preferences and affiliation and come to appreciate that ethnic affiliation is constant (Derman-Sparks, 1980; Piaget, 1951; Stoute, 2019). Children whose caregivers encourage them to identify positively with regards to their racial and ethnic identity will have an important base from which to explore as they develop and encounter the wider, but not always encouraging, world.

Relationships with others

In middle childhood, children develop the capacity to think about people as having relationships with each other as well as relationships with them. This enables them to feel like part of a family, and even a community (e.g., a day care center or nursery school). While this can enrich their sense of security, it can also lead to jealousies and rivalries as they struggle between wanting someone all for themselves and being able to share that person with others. Learning to tolerate jealousy and competition is an important developmental goal of this phase.

Changing relationships with primary caregivers

As children grow, their feelings toward the people in their lives become more complex (Lewis & Volkmar, 1990). Beyond attachment, children now wish for love, intimacy, and physical closeness. For some children, their awareness that the central people in their lives have feelings of love for each other changes the one-on-one closeness they felt in the two-person dyadic relationships of their earliest years. For these children, their nascent feeling of being excluded increases their need for love, as there is now a rival for their affection. These childhood longings, although different from adult experiences, often include physical feelings that are the precursors to later sexual feelings (Lewis & Volkmar, 1990). Because the child is generally still solidly focused on the nuclear family (usually, but not always, composed of parents and siblings), these feelings tend to land on the caregivers. Freud (1905/1968) believed that the three-person (**triadic**) relationship of middle childhood, consisting of the child and two primary caregivers, was central to development. He named his theory after Oedipus, the fictional Theban king who married his mother and killed his father, calling it the Oedipus complex (Freud, 1894/1962). Although family members, particularly primary caregivers, are generally central to the lives of children in this period, the triadic relationships of this period can involve any constellation of primary caregivers including grandparents, single parents, two same sex parents, or nonfamily members.

Conflicts in three-person relationships

Although Freud believed in the universality of the Oedipus complex, this is probably not the case. For those children who do begin to think about relationships in groups of three, however, we can think of these three-person relationships as having three basic roles:

- A child
- A desired caregiver
- A rival caregiver

Although children may naturally alternate in their choice of a "desired caregiver," predictable patterns exist, depending on the gender of the child. In his revision of Freud's Oedipal theory, Lewes (1988) laid out 12 possible outcomes of Oedipal rivalries—6 homosexual and 6 heterosexual. Using this model, the desired caregiver is usually an opposite-sex caregiver among children who will later be straight; in children who later define themselves as gay or lesbian, the desired caregiver is generally a same-sex caregiver (Isay, 1989).

Freud's theory of the Oedipus complex suggests the following: within the three-person relationship of middle childhood, the child might want the desired caregiver all to themselves but may be afraid that this could make the rival caregiver angry. The child might then struggle with the **conflict** between (a) wanting to exclusively possess the desired caregiver, and (b) relinquishing closeness with the desired caregiver in order to appease the rival. The child might then **resolve** the conflict by doing a little bit of both. Where there is conflict, there is anxiety, and where there is anxiety, there is defense (see Chapter 15):

$$\text{Conflict} \rightarrow \text{Anxiety} \rightarrow \text{Defense}$$

It was traditionally thought that the major defense that helps children here is **identification**. They may identify with the rival caregiver, realizing that they can become like the rival some day and ultimately have their own intimate relationship, just like the rival's. In this case,

$$\text{Conflict} \rightarrow \text{Anxiety} \rightarrow \text{Identification}$$

The ease with which children negotiate these conflicts is thought to depend on the way their caregivers participate. Caregivers who overly welcome being desired may make it difficult for a child to relinquish the wish for exclusivity, while caregivers who are made uncomfortable by this desire may inhibit a child's nascent sexuality. Similarly, caregivers who are overly competitive may inhibit a child's willingness to compete, while caregivers who don't compete at all may foster a child's guilt about "winning."

Relationships with siblings

Some of the development of middle childhood may occur in the context of relationships with **siblings**. Siblings can be companions and competitors, playmates and roommates, helpers and hinderers. The presence of siblings means that others are vying for the love and attention of the primary caregivers, but it also affords the potential for alternative sources of affection. When a parent is emotionally or physically absent, a sibling may play a major role in the child's three-person relationship. Too often, when we think about the competitive relationships of middle childhood, we forget siblings, but they are crucial to this period and throughout life.

Development of values

Although children begin to recognize right and wrong at a very early age, their sense of values undergoes tremendous development during their middle childhood (Lewis & Volkmar, 1990). In classical psychoanalytic theory, one of the ways that children resolve the conflicts of the three-person relationships of middle childhood is by internalizing their caregivers' rules and ideals. These rules become part of what Freud called the developing **superego** (Freud, 1923/1990; see also Chapter 20). The internalization of the caregivers' rules is thought to help children further develop their own internal set of behavioral guidelines. The first set of internalized guidelines is often very strict: Children who are aged 3–6 years are often acutely sensitive to rules and sometimes become outraged if the rules are violated (Roiphe & Roiphe, 1985). This preoccupation with rules is seen as a normal and universal aspect of navigating this period of development (Piaget, 1965).

Adult problems and patterns that suggest origins in middle childhood

Adult problems and patterns that suggest origins in middle childhood tend to be more circumscribed than those originating in the earliest years. Recall that more circumscribed problems are ones that affect one part of a function (such as self-esteem) rather than every aspect of it. Nevertheless, they can cause significant pain and suffering. Middle childhood fantasies that are not resolved early in life often come to the fore once people are ready to begin their own sexual and romantic relationships. The following sections illustrate a few ways that might happen.

Difficulty committing to a relationship

In people with clearly developed capacities for trust, attachment, and self-esteem regulation, difficulties with commitment may suggest that they had challenges negotiating the three-person relationships of middle childhood. For example:

> *Monique tells her therapist, "At age 32, I've finally found a man I think I could share my life with. So, why am I so anxious? It started when he started to talk about shopping for rings. How many times have I walked by that jewelry store and hoped I'd have a diamond some day? What's wrong with me? My parents are so happy together—I've always wanted what they have. And they like him, although they are worried that he won't make money as a community organizer. My dad says he could do the same work in law, and they'd probably take him into the firm. Maybe I should have dad talk to him?"*

Persistent fantasies about idealized parents may impede adults' ability to have committed relationships of their own.

Sexual inhibitions

> *At Kyle's suggestion, he and his girlfriend Jeanine consult a couples' therapist. Kyle explains, "It's hard to talk about, but I'm really confused about our relationship—particularly related to sex. Things were so good when we started dating. I love Jeanine—she's beautiful and seemed so comfortable with her body at the beginning. But now that we're living together, I feel like she's turning away from me every night. I need to know what's going on—am I doing something wrong?" Jeanine says, "I'm not sure what's going on either. I love you, too, but in our bed together I feel like I have no space. Am I just supposed to have sex every night?" With encouragement, Jeanine talks about her relationship with her parents: "My mother is pretty cool, but my father is my rock. He'd come into my room every night—even when I had a toddler bed—to tuck me in and to give me a back rub. He told me he missed it when I went to college."*

Although Jeanine loves her father, she was likely conflicted about the closeness of their relationship. Later, when sharing a bed with Kyle, this unconscious conflict may have contributed to her sexual inhibition. When children have been overstimulated during middle childhood, potentially appropriate relationship situations in later life may feel *as if* they are incestuous. This can affect the child who was simply adored by a parent, and can be profound when there was sexual abuse.

Fear of competition and inhibited ambition

When the competition between a child and their rival caregiver seems too dangerous, potentially competitive situations later in life may feel as if they are fraught with the same dangers. Consider the following:

> *Enrique tells his therapist that he was very anxious after a recent meeting at work. "My boss had an idea," he says, "and it made me think of something even better. I brought it up and everyone loved the idea. Then the next day, my boss cancelled a meeting with me that we had on the calendar. I think I'm going to get fired." When his therapist notes that he had a similar fear a few months ago—with no job loss—Enrique comments, "I think that people don't like it when I have good ideas. I generally keep them to myself. My father was like that. He'd say, 'if you're so smart, why don't you pay the bills in this house?' He was a smart guy who never went to college—his family didn't have the money. He could never be proud of my good marks in school. He'd grumble and say, 'I would have done even better if I'd been given half a chance'."*

Enrique learned that being smart and having good ideas felt threatening to his bitter, disappointed father. This remains with him, leading him to overly fear later life situations that have some element of competition.

Learning about the life story of middle childhood

Adults should have at least some memories of their middle childhood period. Their life story is likely to be a mix of their own memories and stories they have been told. You will undoubtedly learn new historical information as the psychotherapy proceeds. Here are some guidelines for reviewing this period.

What was the quality of the relationships with the primary caregivers during this period?

Were there changes in your relationships with your primary caregivers as you grew a little older—say ages 5 or 6?

Was there new closeness with a different caregiver?

Did your primary caregiver change in any way?

Has the family environment changed in any way?

Was there any concrete change in the environment, such as in your family's financial situation or where you lived?

Were new siblings introduced? Are they older or younger? What was your relationship with them like? What is it like now?

Did grandparents or other new adults (such as stepparents) move into the household?

Was there any trauma during this period?

Were there any illnesses during this period? Major separations from caregivers? Divorce or other type of loss? Physical or sexual abuse?

Any early experiences processing societal marginalized identities?

What messages did you receive during this period with regard to gender, ethnicity, religion, or race?

How did you see your primary caregivers experience their gender and racial identities?

Beyond middle childhood

Once in school, the child's world expands exponentially as bonds with peers take on greater importance. These relationships, and the potential difficulties associated with later childhood, are the subject of Chapter 15.

Suggested activity

Can be done by individual learners or in a classroom setting

Read the following vignette and think about these questions:

1. Is there a three-person relationship?
2. If yes, what's happening in that relationship?
3. What issues from this period might persist into adulthood?
4. What kinds of problems might this lead to in later relationships?

> Abby, who is six years old, is the elder of two birth-assigned girls. Abby insists on dressing as a boy and wants to be called Adam. Abby's father is a college professor and Abby's mother, an ex-professional ballet dancer, runs a dance studio for children. The children are taken to work with their mother and expected to sit quietly until it is time for their classes. Abby hates dance and begs the father to go to work with him instead. "You're making it difficult for your mother," the father tells Abby. "You'll like dance—it's also a sport—just keep at it."

Comment

Abby's parents are having difficulty allowing the child to express themself and to understand their own gender. There is a triadic relationship, in which Abby is trying to identify with the father, but is being told to identify with her mother. Abby may have difficulty consolidating a gender identity and may have inhibited self-expression.

References

1. Derman-Sparks, L., Tanaka Higa, C., & Sparks, B. (1980). Children, race, and racism: How race awareness develops. Interracial Books for Children Bulletin, 11(3 and 4). Council on Interracial Books for Children.

2. Drescher, J., & Byne, W. (2017). Gender identity, gender variance and gender dysphoria. In B. J. Sadock, V. A. Sadock, & P. Ruiz (Eds.), *Kaplan and Sadock's comprehensive textbook of psychiatry* (10th ed., pp. 2023–2039). Wolters Kluwer.

3. Dunham, Y., Baron, A. S., & Banaji, M. R. (2008). The development of implicit intergroup cognition. *Trends in Cognitive Sciences, 12*(7), 248–253. https://doi.org/10.1016/j.tics.2008.04.006

4. Freud, S. (1962). The neuro-psychoses of defense. In J. Strachey (Ed.), *The standard edition of the complete psychological works of Sigmund Freud, volume III (1893–1899), early psycho-analytic publications* (pp. 41–61). Hogarth Press. (Original work published 1894).

5. Freud, S. (1968). Three essays on the theory of sexuality. In J. Strachey (Ed.), *The standard edition of the complete psychological works of Sigmund Freud, volume VII (1901–1905): A case of hysteria, three essays on sexuality and other works* (pp. 123–246). Hogarth Press. (Original work published 1905).

6. Freud, S. (1990). The ego and the id. In J. Strachey (Ed.), *The standard edition of the complete psychological works of Sigmund Freud, volume XIX (1923–1925): the ego and the id and other works.* W.W. Norton. (Original work published in 1923).

7. Isay, R. (1989). *Being homosexual: Gay men and their development.* Farrar Straus Giroux.

8. Kinzler, K. (2016, October 23). How kids learn prejudice. *New York Times.*

9. Lewes, K. (1988). *The psychoanalytic theory of male homosexuality.* Simon and Schuster.

10. Lewis, M., & Volkmar, F. (1990). *Clinical aspects of child and adolescent development.* Lea and Febiger.

11. Piaget, J. (1951). The development of children of the idea of the homeland and of relations with other countries. *International Social Science Bulletin, 3*, 561–578.

12. Piaget, J. (1965). *The moral judgment of the child.* The Free Press.

13. Roiphe, H., & Roiphe, A. R. (1985). Your child's mind: The complete book of infant and child mental health care. St. Martin's/Marek.

14. Stoute, B. J. (2019). Racial socialization and thwarted mentalization: Psychoanalytic reflections from the lived experience of James Baldwin's America. *American Imago, 76*(3), 335–357. https://doi.org/10.1353/aim.2019.0025

15. Sullivan, J., Wilton, L. S., & Apfelbaum, E. (2020). Adults delay conversations about race because they underestimate children's processing of race. https://doi.org/10.31234/osf.io/5xpsa

15 Later Childhood

Key concepts

During later childhood (ages 6–12), children develop cognitive skills and expand their ability form relationships outside the family.

Adult patterns and problems that suggest origins in this period include problems with

- Diagnosed or undiagnosed learning disabilities
- Self-esteem related to learning disabilities
- Peer relationships

Development beyond the early years

When we think about psychodynamic formulation, we often think about reviewing development during early and middle childhood, particularly with respect to relationships with caregivers. However, development continues throughout life. Patterns are rarely stable until early adulthood, and major changes can even occur later in life.

Erik Erikson was a psychoanalyst who thought about development as occurring throughout life. He conceptualized the life cycle as being divided into eight phases and specified the key ways in which people grow and develop during each phase (Erikson, 1995). Using this idea, we can think of certain problems of adulthood as being connected to difficulties that might have developed during a particular phase. In the next few chapters, we will

- Briefly review aspects of development that often occur during later childhood, adolescence, and adulthood
- Highlight adult problems that suggest connections to difficulties occurring during each of those periods.

Psychodynamic Formulation: An Expanded Approach, First Edition. The Psychodynamic Formulation Collective.
© 2022 John Wiley & Sons Ltd. Published 2022 by John Wiley & Sons Ltd.

Development during later childhood (ages 6–12)

Cognitive development and building ego function

Leaving aside unusual circumstances, school is the center of life for most children between the ages of 6 and 12. During this time, children must learn **skills** (Piaget, 1929). They also must learn how to practice those skills—everything from penmanship to arithmetic to violin—in order to improve and grow. They gain hobbies and other interests, learning to use these pastimes to handle anxieties and impulses and to build self-esteem. Skill building is generally the biggest growth area for children during this period. Those who have difficulty with the games and activities of the elementary years may be at a disadvantage once the tidal wave of hormones and other changes hit them in adolescence.

Relationships outside of the family

Forming relationships outside of the family—with both adults and other children—is another major task of this period (Leventhal & Dawson, 1984). Primary caregivers remain central figures in later childhood, and they are especially needed during times of stress or transition. In addition, connections to adults in school can have a major effect on development. For the child who has neglectful or abusive primary caregivers—or no primary caregivers at all—a caring mentor, teacher, or coach can have positive, ameliorative effects. Even a best friend can help. A central developmental task of this period is establishing oneself in the world of peers. Peer life can blossom during this time (Rubin, 1980), while bullies and cliques can be devastating (Espelage & De La Rue, 2012). Abusive school relationships, be they with teachers or peers, can impair development of self-esteem. This can be particularly detrimental when related to marginalized aspects of identity, such as race. Racial grouping among children often begins during this time, so for a child of color in a mostly White school the effect on developing peer relationships can be devastating (Tatum, 2017).

Changes in the family

As children get older, the probability that their families will change increases. By the time children are school-age, their caregivers may have been together a while, which means that the probability of family ruptures (e.g., divorce) increases. Changes in the caregivers' finances and family relocations may also occur as caregivers experience their own life changes. Siblings may be added to the family, and deaths of relatives may occur. All these events are likely to affect the developing child. When discussing these events, it is important to ask not only about the *child's* response but also about the *caregivers'* responses, for example, a father's depression after a grandparent's death, or a mother's worsened drinking after a job loss.

The wider world

As children interact more with the world, cultural differences of all sorts become apparent to them. Consider children who are bussed into neighborhoods where they find themselves in the racial or ethnic minority, after spending their early childhood in a more homogeneous community. Role expectations may vary from culture to culture (e.g., whether girls should excel in school or boys can take ballet) and recognition of these differences may affect children's experiences of themselves. Additionally, in later childhood, group peer influences begin to shape prejudiced thoughts and actions. Children with societally marginalized identities, (e.g., sexual, racial, or ethnic) may become targeted and traumatized by such experiences, adversely affecting development. Consider James:

> James, an 11-year-old African-American male, attends a predominantly White middle school in a middle-class suburb to which his family has recently moved. Although initially excited about the prospect of switching schools, halfway into the school year James' grades have significantly declined compared to prior honor-role performance. James has also become more withdrawn from his parents who don't understand the change. In the process of engaging in therapy, James' therapist discovers that he has been excluded from peer groups, teased for being a "Black boy who can't play basketball," and a "know-it-all." James has also been intermittently insulted with racial slurs. James begins to talk about feeling isolated and struggling to deal with not having friends. "I had plenty of friends in my old school," he tells his therapist. "Everyone was like me." James wonders if continuing to pull back academically and shifting to activities of which his peers approve will make it easier to make friends. He continues to struggle with how to manage the possibility that his race and how he speaks might be contributing to the marginalization he is experiencing with peers.

Having fared well in early and middle childhood, James is thrown into a new environment in later childhood. Here, he experiences himself as marginalized for the first time, leading to difficulties with identity, academic performance, and peer group relationships.

Adult problems and patterns that suggest origins in later childhood

Cognitive difficulties and related self-esteem issues

Adults who present with cognitive difficulties, and who are not suffering from dementia or other neurodegenerative disorders, may have had difficulties during later childhood that affected their ability to build cognitive skills. Children who have difficulties during later childhood may struggle academically throughout their lives. Consider the adult whose difficulty with reading or basic arithmetic affects their ability to excel at work. Such difficulties may also affect self-esteem (Kita & Inoue, 2017), leading people to feel perennially incompetent and to have difficulty using intellectual endeavors to bind anxiety.

Problems with building cognitive skills in later childhood could be related to the following:

- A recognized or unrecognized problem with attention or a learning disability which appeared in elementary school
- Other problems during later childhood that may have interfered with cognitive development

For example, trauma that occurs during this period can adversely affect learning, as can psychiatric disorders (Bosquet Enlow et al., 2012). Consider a child with bipolar disorder or ADHD who is trying to consolidate cognitive function in the face of problems with attention or mood regulation. We want not only to know what the child's cognitive development was like, but also how it was responded to by the child and their caregivers. Caregivers and teachers who respond constructively to a severe learning disability may mitigate its effects on self-esteem development, while those who are highly critical or disappointed might worsen the effects (Clark, 1997). School function and the expectations of self and others can have a major effect on self-esteem development and may contribute prominently to the development of shame. Consider a parent who, feeling ashamed of their limited cognitive ability, becomes distant once their child begins to exceed their math or reading skills. This could affect not only the parent but the child as well.

Peer relationships

Adults who have difficulty with peer relationships may have had challenges during later childhood. Difficulties such as autism spectrum disorder, social anxiety, and psychotic disorders should be considered as well. However, if children miss the chance to learn to easily engage in friendships, flexibly interact with peers, and socialize in groups because of difficulty in later childhood (e.g., psychiatric or medical illness, being bullied or marginalized on the basis of a minority identity, frequently relocating, and/or experiencing trauma/loss), they may have difficulty with peer relationships as adults. Here's how this may sound from three adult patients:

Patient 1: I'm OK one-on-one but in a group I'm lost.

Patient 2: I'm terrified of being transferred to a new department—it's impossible for me to break into a new group.

Patient 3: I can only connect if someone reaches out—I'm never the first to initiate.

Learning about these adults' peer relationships during later childhood may reveal important difficulties.

Learning about the life story of later childhood

Many adults have clear memories of later childhood and are able to give a clear developmental history of this phase. Major memory gaps for this time could indicate a history of trauma, medical illness, or substance misuse. Here are some suggested questions to help you learn about this important time in life:

How was your time in school?

Did you have any learning problems? Were you ever tested for learning disabilities? If yes, how did people in your life respond?

Do you remember having friends?

What kinds of activities were you involved in?

Were there any changes in your family during this time?

Do you remember this as a time when you were particularly anxious or depressed?

Did you have any illnesses during this period? Take any medications?

Did you ever get into any serious trouble during this time?

Did anything especially disturbing or traumatic happen?

Did you experience any incidents of discrimination or bias during this period?

Although people may not know whether they had a psychiatric disorder during these years, they will usually remember their general difficulties. For example, a patient might deny having had ADHD, but may be able to say that they had great difficulty in school, were constantly in trouble for not being able to sit still, and could never finish reading a book. Remember, though, that there is about a one-in-six chance that an adult patient had some form of a diagnosable psychiatric disorder dating back to childhood. (Center for Disease Control [CDC], 2021). A history of early cognitive and/or emotional difficulties may shed light on the origins of a patient's current problems. The following types of questions will help you to learn about an adult patient's history of early symptomatology:

When you were growing up, did you ever see a psychiatrist, therapist, or school counselor? If so, for what type of problem?

Were you told that you had a behavioral problem? If so, what type?

Did you have to go to a special school? Do you know what kind of school it was?

As a child, did you ever take medication for a behavioral or other problem?

Do you remember being very sad or nervous as a child? Do you think that you were like that for a long time? For how long?

Were you ever so sad or nervous that it prevented you from doing things like going to school or playing with friends?

Did you have difficulty in school? If so, what kind of difficulty?

Did teachers tell your parents about any particular problems they noticed in you in school?

Did you tend to get in trouble in school? If so, for what kind of behavior?

Suggested activity

Can be done by individual learners or in a classroom setting

Choose one of these children, and write a few sentences about how the challenges of their later childhood might manifest as difficulties in their adult lives:

The youngest of three boys, Kofi struggled to learn to read. "You're so like your brothers," he was told by teachers. "You probably just don't work as hard as they do."

Having overstayed their visa, Ming's parents told him not to say anything about his family to anyone. They were so overprotective—they did not allow him to have playdates or to accept invitations to the birthday parties of classmates.

References

1. Bosquet Enlow, M., Egeland, B., Blood, E. A., Wright, R. O., & Wright, R. J. (2012). Interpersonal trauma exposure and cognitive development in children to age 8 years: A longitudinal study. *Journal of Epidemiology and Community Health*, 66(11), 1005–1010. https://doi.org/10.1136/jech-2011-200727
2. Center for Disease Control. (2022). *Data and statistics on children's mental health*. https://www.cdc.gov/childrensmentalhealth/data.html (accessed 7 May 2022).
3. Clark, M. D. (1997). Teacher response to learning disability. *Journal of Learning Disabilities*, 30(1), 69–79. https://doi.org/10.1177/002221949703000106
4. Erikson, E. H. (1963). Childhood and society. W.W. Norton.
5. Espelage, D. L., & De La Rue, L. (2012). School bullying: Its nature and ecology. *International Journal of Adolescent Medicine and Health*, 24(1). https://doi.org/10.1515/ijamh.2012.002
6. Kita, Y., & Inoue, Y. (2017). The direct/indirect association of ADHD/ODD symptoms with self-esteem, self-perception, and depression in early adolescents. *Frontiers in Psychiatry*, 8. https://doi.org/10.3389/fpsyt.2017.00137
7. Leventhal, B. L., & Dawson, K. (1984). Middle childhood: Normality as integration and interaction. In D. Offer & M. Sabshin (Eds.), *Normality and the life cycle: A critical integration* (pp. 30–75). Basic Books.
8. Piaget, J. (1929). *The child's conception of the world*. Harcourt.
9. Rubin, Z. (1980). *Children's friendships*. Harvard University Press.
10. Tatum, B. (2017). *Why are all the black kids sitting together in the cafeteria?* (Rev ed). Basic Books.

16 Adolescence

Key concepts

Adolescence (ages 13–18) is a critical period of development, particularly for identity formation.

Identity formation during adolescence is strongly affected by

- Hormonal/body changes
- The effects of culture and society
- Cognitive and emotional difficulties

Encountering bias and discrimination can adversely affect sense of self and relationships, even when early attachments are secure.

Adult problems and patterns that suggest origins in adolescence generally involve difficulty with identity.

What develops during adolescence?

If ages 6–12 are mostly about acquiring skills, age 13–18 are mostly about **identity** (Erikson, 1963). School is prominent as well, but adolescence is the time when people really begin to figure out who they are, particularly in relationship to others and the world. It's a time of wildly fluctuating ways of thinking about oneself. For example, one day a teen loves a certain music group and the next day hates them; one day they have a best friend and the next week it's someone else. Every day is something new. This is the norm for adolescents. Yet, by the end of this period of life, young people generally start to have a cohesive, consistent sense of self that helps them figure out their place in their world.

Body changes: gender and sexuality

For adolescents, the new changes happening in their bodies can be overwhelming. Like an enzyme added to a chemical reaction, hormones can cause dramatic changes. Many things must be considered in a psychodynamic formulation that come to the

---

Psychodynamic Formulation: An Expanded Approach, First Edition. The Psychodynamic Formulation Collective.
© 2022 John Wiley & Sons Ltd. Published 2022 by John Wiley & Sons Ltd.

fore in adolescence. For example, one's sense of gender is generally consolidated much earlier; however, continued or even a new onset of questioning may occur during this period. Sexual identity may be somewhat fluid for adolescents, and experimentation is the norm; however, if differences are not accepted by important others, both can be traumatizing, and at times, even devastating. (Drescher, 2002; Pruitt, 1999). Masturbation becomes frequent during adolescence, but it may be prohibited or discouraged in some cultures and by some religions. Inhibitions and fears about masturbation and sexuality can be particularly painful during adolescence, as the growing individual may be unsure about their sexuality and more vulnerable to shame and harsh moral judgments.

Identity development

We can think of **identity** as the aspect of our self-perception that "specifically includes an individual's sense of self in relation to the surrounding culture." (Auchincloss & Samberg, 2012, p. 109). Thus, our identity is shaped by our evaluations of ourselves in comparison to our social surroundings and how others percieve us. Erik Erikson noted that identity formation takes place on all levels of mental functioning, and is crucially determined by how we are seen in comparison to cultural, social, gender, and racial norms (Erikson, 1963). We are evaluated relative to the societal norm, which, for many in the United States, persists as White, heterosexual, and gender conforming. This can inevitably lead to confusion or shame, as a sense of belonging and sameness is crucial to one's identity. This process begins earlier in childhood, far before the development of a capacity to reflect on or question what is occurring or how to intervene. In adolescence, the capacity to self-reflect emerges, enabling adolescents to begin to engage in the questions of who they were, who they are, and who they will be. These decisions, couched in social, cultural, and societal scrutiny and pressures, ultimately shape the individual's choices, which, in turn, will influence their sense of belonging and determine the type of life they lead.

Identity formation in adolescents from nondominant groups

As identity forms within the process of cultural socialization, adolescents can receive conflicting messages. These messages can become internalized; that is, they can both consciously and unconsciously assimilate attitudes from others and society as their own, which can contribute to conflicting self-perceptions and identifications. For example, portrayals of racial minorities in culture are often degraded, presented in stereotyped form, or completely absent. This can lead members of minority groups to internalize a message that their race is undervalued and that they are inferior. Negative, internalized attitudes toward a person's race, ethnicity, class, gender expression, sexual orientation, or socio-economic status can lead a developing adolescent to locate the source of their problem(s) within themselves, leading to feelings of self-hatred, social invisibility, shame, anger, and self-doubt. While many facets come together to inform a person's identity, the predominantly negative messages that these groups receive from their environments profoundly affect their sense of themselves, sense of worth, self-definition, place in the world, and sense of belonging. The **double consciousness** in Black Americans, described by W. E. B. Dubois, refers to a dichotomy in which Black Americans simultaneously view themselves from a White (i.e., degraded) perspective, in which they cannot hope to achieve their ideals; and from a non-White (i.e., valued) perspective, in which they can hope to achieve their ideals. (DuBois, 2021). Other writers have similarly argued that a person's identity with respect to race is not only relative to a White dominant culture, but also relative to a person's own non-White culture (s) and value systems (Erikson, 1963; Yi & Shorter-Gooden, 1999).

Microaggressions—the overt or covert everyday insults that send denigrating messages to individuals because of their group membership or identities—are painful to adolescents in the moment and can have a lasting effect on identity (Sue et al., 2007). Such messages may lead adolescents to deny, or negate, emerging ideas about their identities; for example, consider the teen who is beginning to question their cisgender identity, but who is subject to insults as they try out subtle changes to their appearance. Such insults could delay or arrest identity formation, leading to years of pain and later life-identity issues. Discrimination can also affect the formation of identity (Cronholm et al., 2015; Khan et al., 2017). For example, adolescents of color exposed to educators' biased perceptions of misbehavior and stories that perpetuate a "failure narrative," may internalize this as part of their identity despite a solid early foundation. Consider a Latinx adult who, despite early academic success, was told by a high school guidance counselor that they would "never make it" at an elite college and who now identifies as being "not that smart."

Cognitive and emotional difficulties

Adolescence may also be the time when cognitive and emotional difficulties first appear. Early signs of depression often occur and are too frequently ignored or minimized as normal "teen brooding" (Walsh, 2008). Eating disorders and suicidal ideation are common, as are first experiments with substance use (Kosten, 2008; Suarez-Orozco, 2001). All of these may affect the teen's sense of self and self-esteem, as they can affect one's nascent feeling of mastery over one's environment. Consider the adolescent who is just adjusting to a self-esteem blow of not being as smart as an older sibling, and who then develops new-onset depression. This person will need to work twice as hard to maintain their already vulnerable sense of self. Good early development helps here, but is not necessarily fully protective against the blows of adolescence. Regressions are common and normal as new experiences and difficulties challenge the developing self.

Many factors can disrupt identity consolidation in adolescence. As always, traumas, family strife, and losses must be considered. A very common source of trouble in this area is drug and alcohol use disorders (Newcomb, 1993). Trying to consolidate identity under the influence of substances that alter mood and self-experience is like trying to set Jell-O in a blender. It simply doesn't happen. The same is true for the influence of other cognitive and emotional difficulties, such as bipolar disorder and panic attacks.

Adult problems and patterns that suggest origins in adolescence

Adults who present without a good sense of identity are likely to have had difficulties during their adolescent years. People who are still "finding themselves" in their 30s and beyond may not have had an adequate chance to experiment with different ways of thinking about themselves and the world, or they may have gotten lost during that period of experimentation as a result of trauma or cognitive and emotional difficulties. Consider Flora:

> *Flora, who is married, has two teenage children, and is a well-regarded nursing administrator, presents saying she feels "unfulfilled in her life." Although she is not depressed, she states she is "just going through the motions" at work and dreams of having a different kind of life. She flirts with running off to a writers' colony, or traveling to India to study yoga. She continuously changes her hairstyle and color, and is easily bored with her wardrobe. She reports that her family emigrated from Mexico when she was 10 years old, and that the family was essentially homeless in the United States for the next 6 years, staying with various relatives and moving frequently. She says that without documentation, her parents were forced to work constantly at poorly paying jobs, and she was left to care for her younger brother who had fairly severe asthma. Told by everyone that she was a "good little nurse," she chose to study nursing when she attended community college and has been rapidly promoted throughout her career.*

Forced to assume adult responsibilities early, and potentially traumatized by emigration, poverty, and homelessness, Flora was not able to try out different choices during adolescence; this need re-emerged later, perhaps as Flora's own children began their teenage experimentation.

Learning about the life story of adolescence

Adult patients are likely to have strong memories of adolescence. Here are some questions that can help us to learn about this critical part of the life story:

> *How do you remember your teenage years? Do you remember it as a happy time? A stormy time?*
>
> *What was your relationship like with your parents during this time?*
>
> *Can you remember when you began to develop physically? Was it around the same time as your peers? If early or late, how did this affect you?*
>
> *Did you have any new difficulties during this time like anxiety or depression?*
>
> *Did you try any substances as a teenager? If yes, was this sporadic, or did you use any substances on a regular basis? Which one(s)?*
>
> *Did you date/have any romantic experiences during this period?*
>
> *What kind of sexual experiences did you have during this time?*
>
> *Were there any changes in your family or living situation during this time?*
>
> *Any illnesses or traumatic situations?*

Suggested activity

Can be done by individual learners or in a classroom setting

Consider Jocelyn:

> *Jocelyn is a 15-year-old girl who has grown up with her parents, grandparents, and siblings in a tight-knit community of recent immigrants. A talented ballet dancer, her life has revolved around school and hours of ballet classes. Her family is very involved in their church, and her community stresses strict rules for young people—no drugs or alcohol, no premarital sex, and dating only among people of their ethnic group. Recognizing her extraordinary talent, her teachers recommended that she audition for an elite ballet school in a nearby city, and she has just been accepted. With great trepidation, her parents will allow her to attend the school and live in a dormitory.*

What challenges might Jocelyn face in the next few years? How might they affect her identity and development during adolescence? How might her family's reaction to these challenges lead to different outcomes? How might these challenges manifest in her adult life? If you are an individual learner, try writing a few sentences in response to these questions; in class, discuss as a group.

References

1. Auchincloss, E. L., & Samberg, E. (2012). *Psychoanalytic terms & concepts*. Yale University Press.
2. Cronholm, P. F., Forke, C. M., Wade, R., Bair-Merritt, M. H., Davis, M., Harkins-Schwarz, M., Pachter, L. M., & Fein, J. A. (2015). Adverse childhood experiences. *American Journal of Preventive Medicine*, 49(3), 354–361. https://doi.org/10.1016/j.amepre.2015.02.001
3. Drescher, J. (2002). Invisible gay adolescents: The developmental narratives of gay men. *Adolescent Psychiatry*, 26, 73–94.
4. DuBois, W. (2021). *The souls of black folk*. Chelsea House.
5. Erikson, E.H. (1963). *Childhood and society*. Norton.
6. Khan, M., Ilcisin, M., & Saxton, K. (2017). Multifactorial discrimination as a fundamental cause of mental health inequities. *International Journal for Equity in Health*, 16(1). https://doi.org/10.1186/s12939-017-0532-z
7. Kosten, T. R. (2008). General approaches to substance and polydrug use disorders. In A. Tasman, J. Kay, & J. A. Lieberman (Eds.), *Psychiatry* (3rd ed., pp. 957–970). Wiley Blackwell.
8. Newcomb, M. D., Scheier, L. M., & Bentler, P. M. (1993). Effects of adolescent drug use on adult mental health: A prospective study of a community sample. Experimental and Clinical Psychopharmacology, 1(1-4), 215–241. https://doi.org/10.1037/1064-1297.1.1-4.215
9. Pruitt, D. B. (1999). *Your adolescent: Emotional, behavioral, and cognitive development from early adolescence through the teen years*. HarperCollins.
10. Suarez-Orozco, C. (2001). Afterword: Understanding and serving the children of immigrants. *Harvard Educational Review*, 71(3), 579–590. https://doi.org/10.17763/haer.71.3.x40q180654123382
11. Sue, D. W., Capodilupo, C. M., Torino, G. C., Bucceri, J. M., Holder, A. M., Nadal, K. L., & Esquilin, M. (2007). Racial microaggressions in everyday life: Implications for clinical practice. *American Psychologist*, 62(4), 271–286. https://doi.org/10.1037/0003-066x.62.4.271
12. Walsh, B. T. (2008). Eating disorders. In A. Tasman, J. Kay, & J. A. Lieberman (Eds.), *Psychiatry* (3rd ed., pp. 1609–1625). Wiley Blackwell.
13. Yi, K., & Shorter-Gooden, K. (1999). Ethnic identity formation: From stage theory to a constructivist narrative model. *Psychotherapy: Theory, Research, Practice, Training*, 36(1), 16–26. https://doi.org/10.1037/h0087723

17 Adulthood

Key concepts

When formulating psychodynamically, we must consider the totality of someone's lived experience.

Adults continue to change and develop in many ways—they gain new responsibilities, consolidate relationships with others, and develop their identities over time.

Self and identity consolidation during adulthood may be challenging for adults who are marginalized or who experience discrimination.

Trauma, medical/psychiatric problems, economic stressors, loss, and the aging process are all part of the landscape in which adults continue to develop.

At age 70, after the death of her partner and 5 years into her retirement, Wanda made her first trip to her mother's country of origin and began feeling connected to her mother's culture.

At age 45, after adopting a son, Nils experienced a deep sense of purpose and a newfound interest in young children.

After a fairly uneventful early life, Drew joined the army at age 19, was deployed in a war zone, and returned wary of relationships.

Although we sometimes think of development as synonymous with childhood, we all continue to develop throughout our lives. Everything we do affects the growth and evolution of our conscious and unconscious minds, and adults often have myriad life-changing experiences. Consider adults who

- Give birth to or adopt children
- Raise families
- Are deployed in the armed forces
- Immigrate and/or suffer discrimination
- Have long-term relationships and lose loved ones
- Have a lifetime of medical issues

Psychodynamic Formulation: An Expanded Approach, First Edition. The Psychodynamic Formulation Collective.
© 2022 John Wiley & Sons Ltd. Published 2022 by John Wiley & Sons Ltd.

These are profound experiences, and all adults experience one or more of them. There is good evidence that our sense of self and identity (Fadjukoff & Kroger, 2016), relationships with others and values (Sparrow, 2000), modes of adapting (Diehl & Blohm, 2001), and patterns of cognition change dramatically during our adult years. Thus, problems and patterns with which adults grapple may well have their origins in this critical part of the life story.

A new place in the world

Minors no longer, many young adults have newfound freedoms and responsibilities. For the first time, some may leave home and be challenged to function as adults. How does their sense of self hold up? Can they self-regulate? Remain organized? Care for themselves? While this may be a time of tremendous growth and excitement for some, for others it may be full of terror. Some create and grow, yet others have difficulty and disappointment.

For the young adult who has financial support and opportunities and who does not have to navigate obstacles like discrimination in education/work, it can be a time of seemingly unlimited possibilities. It can also be a time ripe for anxiety and depression if their ambitions exceed achievements, which can be due to external factors, such as mounting debt or a lack of opportunities. However, it can also be due to internal factors, such as emotional dysregulation, mental or emotional difficulties (including substance misuse), or discrepancies between ambitions and capabilities. Negotiating these discrepancies in a realistic way is a key challenge of this time period—those who handle it well gain focus, while others may struggle with fragile self-esteem and despair. Identity consolidation continues during young adulthood, as young people choose partners and career paths. The fluid identity common in 14-year-old teens is less common in 24-year-old adults as people gain a more stable sense of self and of their place in the world.

Cultural variations and norms are important to consider when attempting to understand a young adult's development. For example, in many cultures, unpartnered young or older adults are expected to remain in their parents' home until they start their own family. Yet, in other cultures, adults may be considered developmentally immature if they do not live independently. Young adults living in multicultural communities, or who are first-generation citizens, may need to navigate environmental and cultural norms that differ from those of their families of origin. We can often learn about the cultural differences that shaped someone by asking them about the expectations of their parental figures.

Intimate relationships and sexuality

Emerging from adolescence with a nascent sense of self, the young adult may be ready to share that self with another person (Erikson, 1963). The capacity for love relationships, built on the numerous years of relationships with family members and friends, can help an individual to consolidate their identity. Even people whose familial relationships have been less than ideal can have their self-esteem positively reinforced by mutually satisfying relationships with lovers and friends during this time. However, if the wounds of earlier life have left the person unable to form intimate relationships, this time can be lonely and full of disappointment. The ability to form love relationships can also be affected by marginalization and discrimination, on the basis of characteristics such as sexuality, physical appearance, or disability.

Sexuality and intimate relationships continue to evolve throughout an adult's life. With increased confidence and independence, many adults discover aspects of their gender and sexual identity, about which they were either unaware earlier in life or were unable to share with others. This can bring excitement and freedom as well as anxiety and interpersonal difficulties. Sometimes, within a long relationship, sexual attraction and activity can change over many years. Psychiatric and medical problems can also complicate sexual activity and satisfaction.

Self and identity development—the challenge of being marginalized

Self and identity development during adulthood may present particular challenges to people who are marginalized or who experience discrimination. For example, a young adult who experiences same-sex attraction may have difficulty consolidating their sexual identity in an environment that only values monogamous heterosexual relationships. The ability to integrate multiple important aspects of one's identity, including sexuality, ethnicity, and religion (Cass 1979), can be exceedingly difficult when one experiences intersectional forms of systemic oppression with multiple in-group and out-group challenges.

Racial identity formation continues during adulthood as well. Younger people who are navigating their relationship to racism may initially idealize the cultural or racial norms of the dominant or privileged racial group, subscribing consciously and unconsciously to racist notions, and seeking acceptance from the dominant racial group. Later, however, some individuals may develop awareness of the irrationality of racist ideas and the untenability of seeking acceptance. This may prompt them to prioritize relationships with people from their own racial group or other minority groups, and to seek out activities or cultural norms associated with those groups. Still later in adulthood, people may accept more nuanced concepts of identity: for example, that there is no such thing as a singular identity; that heritage, family, traditions, and history inform one's racial and ethnic identity; and that individuals have the opportunity to define themselves as distinct from outside stereotypes and classifications (Cross, 1978; Phinney, 1999).

Middle and later adulthood

The tasks of middle and later adulthood are myriad and diverse (Erikson, 1963). Though it is commonly believed that people often find meaning in work and love, it is important for us, as psychotherapists, to put aside our own personal judgment to discover what is important to each individual. For example, one person might be content to be an accomplished artist who has always lived alone, while another might be content having a healthy family and no career. Adulthood can be an exciting time of productivity and procreation, but it can also be a time of disappointment and unfulfilled dreams. Asking not only about what people are doing and with whom they have relationships, but also how they feel about "how things turned out," can help us to learn about this part of their life story.

Later adulthood can bring the joys of a life well-lived, or the bitterness of a difficult journey. Older adults may lose many things, including physical and mental capacities, opportunities for productivity, daily work routines, and loved ones. Trauma (see Chapter 18) and marginalization/discrimination (see Chapter 20) can continue to affect development during this time (Boulanger, 2002; Fink, 2003). Although the earliest years are far away, the capacities developed during those years (such as trust, a sense of self, and secure attachments) continue to play a role during times of loss, often buoying older adults through difficult waters. Relationships based on trust, attachment, and a healthy sense of self and others may be the best predictor of mental health during the older years (Vaillant, 2003).

Adult problems and patterns that suggest origins in young adulthood

Difficulty assuming responsibility for oneself during young adulthood can leave some people feeling overly dependent on their family of origin as they enter their third and fourth decades of life. This can lead to mood and anxiety symptoms if the young adult feels unable to mature alongside their peers. For example, a person who becomes depressed after graduating from college may need to take time off from work, or live with family, leading to delays in their career and relationship development. The following sections list some questions that can help us understand development during this period.

Learning about the life story of young adulthood

How far did you continue in school? Did you attend college or graduate school?

Did you continue to live at home? If not, where did you live? With whom? Is this common in your family/community?

What were your aspirations at this point in your life? How did you try to realize them?

How do you remember this time? Fulfilling? Disappointing? Frustrating?

Were you involved with anyone romantically during this period of your life? Sexually? What were these relationship(s) like?

Tell me about your social life during this time. Did you have friends? How close did you feel to them? Did you tend to socialize one-on-one or in groups?

Did you support yourself during this period? If so, how? If not, who was supporting you?

If you were working, what type of work did you do? Was this what you wanted to do?

Did you find time for leisure? If so, what did you like to do during this time?

Did you have any particular difficulties during this time, such as anxiety, depression, or substance misuse? Traumatic situations?

Learning about the life story of middle and later adulthood

Tell me about what you did for work as an adult. Are you/have you been satisfied with what you are doing? Have you been able to support yourself (and your family, if applicable)?

Who is in your family (or families)? If you have started your own family, when did you do this? How do you find your family life?

How do you spend your leisure time? Is this satisfying to you?

Have you had any medical or psychiatric difficulties in your adult life? Substance misuse?

Are you currently sexually active? Can you tell me about this?

Have you lost any people with whom you were close?

As you look at your life, do you feel you have been happy with the choices you have made? Can you tell me more about that?

Remembering the whole life story

Many changes that occur after adolescence can affect the way people regulate self-esteem, have relationships with others, and adapt to stressful situations. New problems emerge, old problems may reemerge in new way, and new experiences and relationships can breed new traumas as well as the hope of repair. All of these things must be considered as we review the life story of our adult patients.

Suggested activity

Can be done by individual learners or in a classroom setting

How might Nico's experiences as an adult have affected his development?

Nico, a 56-year-old man, has worked in the library of a famous museum for 30 years. Nico's coworkers admire him for his encyclopedic knowledge of Etruscan archaeology, but fear Nico's biting sarcasm and don't want to interact with him. Although he graduated with high honors from a PhD program in art history, Nico was never able to land a tenure-track position at a college or university. Nico has never had a relationship and lives in very modest circumstances. "No one is producing anything in academia anymore," Nico grumbles. "I'm glad that I never got into that rat race."

Comment

Nico seems to have had difficulty in **young adulthood**. Although his relationship difficulties may predate this time, his inability to find an academic job after his educational success left him unable to realize his talents and led to bitterness and isolation.

References

1. Boulanger, G. (2002). Wounded by reality. *Contemporary Psychoanalysis, 38*(1), 45–76. https://doi.org/10.1080/00107530.2002.10745806
2. Cass, V. C. (1979). Homosexual identity formation: A theoretical model. *Journal of Homosexuality, 4*(3), 219–235. https://doi.org/10.1300/j082v04n03_01
3. Cross, W. E. (1978). The Thomas and Cross models of psychological nigrescence. *Journal of Black Psychology, 5*(1), 13–31. https://doi.org/10.1177/009579847800500102
4. Diehl, C., & Blohm, M. (2001). Apathy, adaptation or ethnic mobilisation? On the attitudes of a politically excluded group. *Journal of Ethnic and Migration Studies, 27*(3), 401–420. https://doi.org/10.1080/136918301200266149
5. Erikson, E.H. (1963). *Childhood and society*. Norton.
6. Fadjukoff, P., & Kroger, J. (2016). Identity development in adulthood: Introduction. *Identity, 16*(1), 1–7. https://doi.org/10.1080/15283488.2015.1121821
7. Fink, K. (2003). Magnitude of trauma and personality change. *The International Journal of Psychoanalysis, 84*(4), 985–995. https://doi.org/10.1516/350u-fhq2-rtdb-6hw8
8. Phinney, J. S. (1999). Ethnic identity development measures: Multigroup ethnic identity measure. *Encyclopedia of Multicultural Psychology*. https://doi.org/10.4135/9781412952668.n97
9. Sparrow, L. M. (2000). Beyond multicultural man: Complexities of identity. *International Journal of Intercultural Relations, 24*(2), 173–201. https://doi.org/10.1016/s0147-1767(99)00031-0
10. Vaillant, G. E. (2003). *Aging well: Guideposts to a happier life*. Warner.

Putting It Together—REVIEW a Life Story

Now, we're ready to REVIEW a full life story. Let's consider how we might do this for Nia:

Presentation

Nia is a 25-year-old single, African-American cisgender woman who identifies as heterosexual and Catholic and works as an ICU nurse. She presents with mounting depression, anxiety, and thoughts like, "sometimes I wish I could just go to sleep and stay asleep"—all symptoms she hasn't experienced since her teens. She says that she has no wish to die. Nia describes "slipping into a black hole" starting three months ago when her mother began calling more frequently, pleading with Nia to help care for her mentally and physically disabled father. Nia had been planning to leave her ICU job in a year or two to fulfill a lifelong dream of working in a developing country, but now feels obligated to stay to help support her family. She feels increasingly nervous, exhausted and irritable, but does not have difficulty with sleep or appetite.

Life story

Genetics and prenatal development

Nia is an only child born to initially unmarried parents in a predominantly African-American neighborhood in a southern state. She is unaware of any problems with her mother's pregnancy or delivery, but assumes her mother drank during the pregnancy since she was hospitalized for depression and alcohol abuse after Nia's birth. There is also a history of depression in numerous relatives on her mother's side of the family. Nia's father developed irritability with temper control issues over the course of her childhood but never sought psychiatric treatment until he was diagnosed with Parkinson's disease 12 years ago. He is now cognitively impaired and chronically psychotic on anti-Parkinsonian medications.

Earliest years (birth–age 3)

Shortly after delivery, Nia was placed in the care of her maternal grandmother. Nia presumes that this was because of her mother's hospitalization but is unsure why her father could not care for her.

Her grandmother told her she was a healthy, relaxed, "easy" baby who almost never cried and was generally slow to warm up with other children. Nia has very warm memories of her early childhood with her grandmother but few memories of her parents during these years—she was told by her grandmother that they were working hard to save money so they could take care of her again.

Middle childhood (ages 3–6)

When Nia was four years old, her parents married and moved with her to a neighboring town where her father joined a private investigation company. He made a good living, and the family lived a comfortable middle-class life. However, her father became more short-tempered and, harshly critical, slammed doors, frequently yelled at and struck her mother in front of Nia, and occasionally threatened Nia with a belt. Nia remembers feeling frightened of her father as a child and hiding in a closet when her parents argued. She remembers her mother as irritable and depressed, especially when she was drinking, Once, when intoxicated, Nia's mother told her she was an "unwanted pregnancy" and that she would have had an abortion if she hadn't been Catholic. This made Nia feel she was the reason for her parents' unhappy relationship. The only good memories she has of these years were the occasional weekends and holidays she spent with her grandmother.

Later childhood (ages 6–12)

Nia's parents placed her in an all-girls' Catholic parish school starting in kindergarten. Most of the students in the school were African American. She loved the school and says, "it saved my life." She remembers being shy and well-behaved and having close relationships with the nuns and priests. Although she had few friends, she had one close friend to whose home she went most days after school. In middle school, at the urging of one of the nuns, Nia started confirmation classes and began going to Mass every Sunday by herself, as she used to do with her grandmother. When her father and mother said they were too busy to be involved, her friend's parents offered to stand in as her sponsors.

Adolescence (ages 13–19)

When she was 14, Nia's parents said they could no longer afford the parish school and placed her in a large co-ed public high school where African-American students were in the minority. She missed her friends and the nuns at her old school, and was taken aback when White classmates began making comments about her clothing and her style of hair, and treated her as if she was less intelligent than they. It was her first exposure to overt racism, from which she had been largely shielded in her previous school and neighborhood. Her grades slipped, and she had thoughts of suicide. She also experimented with self-starvation and lost 15 pounds but stopped when no one noticed. In 10th grade, a coach encouraged her to try out for the basketball team, and she says she went from "feeling like an outsider to being the star player." She started feeling better about herself and made an effort to eat a healthier diet because she felt she had a "responsibility to the team." She loved sports, although her mother told her it was "unfeminine." She avoided parties, immersed herself in schoolwork and athletics, and excelled at both. During the summer between 11th and 12th grade, Nia volunteered as a candy striper at a local hospital and "just knew" she would ultimately pursue a career in the helping professions. In hindsight, she thinks her father's nascent Parkinson's disease may have influenced her decision: "The more disabled he became, the less angry I felt. He went from scary to needy and pathetic. I also hated seeing how much my mother seemed to enjoy tormenting him and felt like I had to protect him."

Young adulthood (ages 18–23)

When it came time to apply for colleges, Nia's mother was preoccupied with her father's health issues and financial worries, and informed her that if she wanted to go she'd have to handle the tuition costs on her own. Consolidating a strong identity as a strong Black woman, she chose to attend a historically Black university that offered her a full scholarship. She says, "I felt at home again," and she devoted herself to schoolwork and sports. Although she joined a sorority, she tended to shy away from weekend partying and had limited dating experiences. She had a number of short-lived relationships with men who "wouldn't take no for an answer," but none of these lasted more than a year. Nia was initially a pre-med major but because of her frequent trips home to help care for her father, she "never had the time to master organic chemistry and physics," and eventually switched to nursing.

Later adulthood (ages 23–present)

Once she began working, Nia was drawn to Intensive Care Nursing because of the "challenge of life-and-death moments." She also felt that the additional training helped her to maintain status in her predominantly White teaching hospital. She quickly rose through the ranks, taking on leadership and teaching positions in the medical center, with salary increases that enabled her to take on more of her parents' financial burdens and medical bills. In the last few years, she has distanced herself from friends, only dated sporadically, and concentrated on her work, family, and cat.

Suggested activity

Can be done by individual learners or in a classroom setting

As you did after DESCRIBE, try to take time now to REVIEW the life story of one of your patients. Again, classroom learners will benefit from reading the REVIEWS that their classmates write. As in this example, try using the headers from each developmental phase—prenatal, earliest years, middle childhood, later childhood, adolescence, young adulthood, and adulthood. Even if you think that you have a sense of your patient's life story, challenging yourself to review it systematically is likely to help you learn more about your patient and to identify things about which you might want to ask.

PART FOUR: LINK

Introduction

Key concepts

The final step in collaboratively creating a psychodynamic formulation is to LINK the problems and patterns to the life story to form hypotheses about a person's development.

To LINK, we focus what we have DESCRIBED and REVIEWED to focus on the patient's major difficulties and key points in their life story. We then connect these using the following organizing ideas about development:

- Trauma
- Early cognitive and emotional difficulties
- Culture and society
- Conflict and defense
- Relationships with others
- The development of the self
- Early attachment patterns.

When we create psychodynamic formulations, our language should indicate that the links we make are hypotheses, and not facts.

The way we LINK guides the treatment.

By this point in the book, you've learned how to DESCRIBE problems and patterns, and how to REVIEW a patient's full life story. We can now **focus** what we've described and reviewed to hone in on the person's greatest areas and periods of difficulty, and connect these to form hypotheses about a person's development.

LINK using organizing ideas about development

To form these hypotheses, we need to connect the major difficulties to the key points in a person's life story. This is the all-important step—the point at which we turn a patient's history into a formulation by hypothesizing about causation. For this crucial step, we rely on **organizing ideas about development**. These organizing ideas are ways of conceptualizing how what happens during life could lead to the problems and patterns that we see in our patients. They help us to answer questions such as:

> *How might early trauma lead to problems with affect regulation?*
>
> *How might depression in childhood lead to problems with self-esteem management?*
>
> *How might an absent mother lead to interpersonal problems in adulthood?*
>
> *How might being in a marginalized group lead to issues with self-esteem?*
>
> *How might having an attuned mother help someone to grapple with a breakup in college?*
>
> *How might an overly close relationship with a parent lead to sexual inhibitions?*

Numerous developmental ideas can help us link a person's life story to their patterns of thinking, feeling, and behaving. Each idea offers a different way to explain how a person's lived experience—including nature and nurture—could result in the problems and patterns that we see in the adult. We can link problems and patterns to history by thinking about the effect of

- Trauma,
- Early cognitive and emotional difficulties,
- Culture and society,
- Conflict and defense,
- Relationships with others,
- The development of the self, and
- Early attachment patterns.

When we LINK, we scroll through these organizing ideas and choose the ones that will help us to make useful connections between the patient's patterns and their life story. We can use several ideas for a single formulation, and we can use different ideas in different formulations. Each chapter in Part Four presents one of these organizing ideas about development, so that you can begin to have a library of ideas to choose from when you create your formulations.

So many organizing ideas—how do we choose?

Just as there are many ideas about development, there are many ways to link a patient's patterns to their life story. The way the clinician does this in a psychodynamic formulation depends on many variables, including the way the patient tells their story and the needs of the clinical situation. Some clinical situations can be explained well using particular organizing ideas about development, and we outline such situations with examples in each of this Part's chapters. For example, consider two people with difficulty regulating affect—one who had an abusive parent and one who had early bipolar disorder. Despite the similarity of their difficulties, their psychodynamic formulations might require two different ideas about development. It generally makes sense to lead with the information from DESCRIBE and REVIEW and *then* to choose ideas about development, rather than beginning with a favored idea. Try to avoid "looking for history" that suits an idea about development—it can skew the formulation and, as we discussed in Chapter 4, introduce bias.

Writing a psychodynamic formulation

Even though not all psychodynamic formulations are written, we suggest trying to write some chronological narratives as you learn to DESCRIBE, REVIEW, and LINK. As you write, think about how things that happened during the person's life might have affected development—for example, how problems with self-esteem from the earliest years might have affected identity consolidation in adolescence, how trust consolidated during a primary dyadic relationship might have helped someone through a later trauma, or how problems with competition from middle childhood might have affected career development in young adulthood. Begin with a summary outlining your focal points, then try to comment on the way the person developed during each life phase. At the end of Part Four, you can listen in as two therapists consider how to "put together" full psychodynamic formulations, and you can then read the narratives.

When you write *your* formulations, remember that the links we make between life story and adult patterns are hypotheses—best guesses based on developmental research and empirical work with patients. They are not proven facts. They are designed to help us understand our patients, to help our patients to understand themselves, and to guide our treatments. Thus, the language of linking should reflect this. When we link, we use words like "perhaps" and "maybe", and phrases like "it could be" and "it is likely." Saying

> *Marco's problems with self-esteem were caused both by his chronic mood disorder and by his lack of acknowledgment by his father.*

is very different than saying,

> *Marco's report of both a lifelong history of low mood and a consistent lack of mirroring by his father suggests that these may have contributed to the development of his difficulties maintaining and managing self-esteem.*

The second statement clarifies that the links between Marco's difficulties with self-esteem and the elements of his history are hypotheses, not established facts.

Using ideas about development over time

As you gain comfort with formulating, you will not necessarily always consciously think about and apply different ideas about development. They will become a part of the way you automatically think about patients. However, while you are learning to formulate, we suggest that you carefully consider all of these organizing ideas with each patient to decide which ones can best aid you in forming hypotheses about the individual's development.

Linking guides treatment

The way we link our adult patients' problems and patterns to their life stories guides our treatment. If we link problems to early trauma, we must help our patients understand their traumatic experiences and repair their disrupted development. If we link problems to unconscious conflicts and defenses, we must help our patients develop more beneficial ways of dealing with stress. If we link problems to the effects of culture and society, we must help our patients understand how they have internalized society's negative views about them and how to uncouple them from their own. If we link problems to relationships with others, we must help our patients develop new relationship templates. Our formulations guide our goals for treatment, the way we listen to our patients, and the way we choose our interventions (see Chapter 3). Generally, we can help our patients by

- making them aware of a problematic aspect of their development or function
- helping them to develop new more satisfying ways of functioning.

We discuss how to accomplish both in each of the chapters in Part Four.

Looking ahead

In each of the chapters in Part Four, we present one organizing idea about development, outlining the following:

- The basics of the organizing idea
- Clinical situations for which the organizing idea is particularly useful
- A sample formulation using the idea
- Ways in which linking to that idea guides treatment

Note that our sample formulations in these chapters present DESCRIBE and REVIEW sections that have already been focused on, and thus only contain the major difficulties and key developmental points. Now, let's move on to our first organizing idea about development—linking problems and patterns to trauma.

Suggested activity

The following can be done by individual learners or in a classroom setting:

Use the DESCRIBE domains (self, relationships, adapting, cognition, values, work/play) to outline the patterns of a patient with whom you are working. What is your focus question? Where would you focus and why? If working in a classroom setting, consider sharing in pairs or in larger groups.

18 Trauma

Key concepts

Trauma is an experience of extraordinarily stressful and disturbing events or an accumulation of events that overwhelms a person or group of people.

There are different kinds of trauma:

- **Personal trauma** affects an individual
- **Collective trauma** overwhelms a group of people *and* the individual members of the group
- **Traumatic stress** may include distressing and/or frightening events that, even if not life-threatening, have adverse and lasting psychological consequences
- **Systems of oppression** can cause traumatic stress for individuals and/or groups in an ongoing, lifelong way

When trauma is prominent in a person's history, we may be able to LINK the development of the adult's problems and patterns to the impact of trauma.

Trauma can affect the development of all aspects of functioning.

Linking to the impact of trauma is particularly useful when creating formulations for patients who have problems with

- Self-experience
- Affect regulation and impulse control
- Adapting to stress
- Forming and maintaining secure attachments

Trauma has always been a part of human experience, ranging from personal traumas (e.g., childhood abuse and neglect) to collective traumas affecting whole populations (e.g., the Holocaust, enslavement, ethnic cleansing, war, the events of September 11, systemic oppression, and natural disasters). We take for granted that traumatic experiences have a psychological effect on people. But why is this true? Ideas about the impact of trauma on development can help us make the link between traumatic events in a person's history and their characteristic problems and patterns.

Psychodynamic Formulation: An Expanded Approach, First Edition. The Psychodynamic Formulation Collective.
© 2022 John Wiley & Sons Ltd. Published 2022 by John Wiley & Sons Ltd.

What is trauma?

Trauma can be defined as the experience of extraordinarily stressful, disturbing, or violent events, which overwhelm the victims' psychological and biological capacity to cope (Herman, 2015; van der Kolk & McFarlane, 2007). DSM-5-TR defines traumatic events as those in which "the person experienced or witnessed an event or events that involved actual or threatened death, serious injury, or sexual violence." (DSM-5-TR, 2022). Trauma can involve

- a single event or experience
- a protracted period of suffering, marginalization, or victimization
- a repeated series of traumas that relate to one another

The concept of **traumatic stress** is broader than this definition of trauma, and can take many forms, including neglect and abuse. It can also encompass more widespread societal stressors related to racism, sexism, xenophobia, and other forms of systemic oppression or marginalization. The brain is differentially vulnerable to stress in different stages of a person's lifespan. In particular, traumatic stress during early childhood can lead to impairment in emotional, behavioral, and cognitive function. Also, as discussed in Chapter 12, research is beginning to suggest that the neurobiological effects of traumatic stress may be passed on from parents to children via epigenetic mechanisms, leading to the phenomenon of **transgenerational transmission of trauma** (Bowers and Yehuda, 2016; Jawaid et al., 2018; Yehuda & Lehrner, 2018).

Systems of oppression, such as racism, sexism, heterocentrism, homophobia, ageism, and ableism (see Chapter 20) can cause traumatic stress for individuals and groups via experiences such as being othered, misunderstood, stereotyped, excluded, subject to bias, discriminated against in the workplace or legal system, and targeted for harassment or violence. These experiences may often contribute to the problems and patterns that lead people to treatment (Tummala-Narra, 2016). Along with other traumatic experiences within the family, mounting evidence shows that systems of oppression can also lead to depression and anxiety, health problems via the activation of the Hypothalamic-Pituitary-Adrenal (HPA) axis, family conflict, posttraumatic stress symptoms, career difficulties, internalized stereotypes, low self-esteem, problems in identity, difficulty establishing intimate relationships, harassment, and violence (Bor et al., 2018; Paradies et al., 2013; Sirin et al., 2013; Sutter & Perrin, 2016; Tummala-Narra & Claudius, 2013). Although these kinds of experiences have not traditionally been considered as falling under the category of trauma, they are critical to understand when meeting a patient and co-creating a psychodynamic formulation.

Basic ideas about how trauma can affect development

People who study mental health have long grappled with the question of how trauma affects development. One of the earliest psychodynamic ideas about this was Freud's hypothesis that childhood sexual abuse could lead to physical or "conversion" symptoms in adulthood (Breuer & Freud, 1893/1971). Though he later decided that his patient's descriptions of abuse were fantasy rather than reality, today we know that real trauma is widespread in society. Just as there is no single type of trauma, there is no unified idea about how trauma shapes a person's characteristic problems and patterns. In addition, all current theories suggest that there is no one-to-one correlation between trauma and psychological difficulties. Multiple variables, such as the following, may affect how people process traumatic events:

Extent and severity of trauma

Extreme and protracted traumatic experiences, such as internment in a concentration camp, severe physical and sexual abuse in childhood, or prolonged combat exposure, are likely to leave lasting psychic scars on the victims. More circumscribed traumatic events, such as surviving a natural disaster, a severe accident, or a violent crime, may have more variable outcomes.

Age at which trauma occurs

Trauma in childhood affects the developing brain and can cause a global disruption of function. It is associated not only with post-traumatic stress disorder (PTSD) and other anxiety disorders but also with mood disorders, emotional dysregulation, attachment disorders, substance use disorders, and problems with academic performance and social relationships (Carlson et al., 1989; Cicchetti & Toth, 1995; Edwards et al., 2003; MacMillan et al., 2001; Paolucci et al., 2001; Stovall-McClough & Cloitre, 2006). Childhood abuse has been correlated with abnormalities in neural systems involved in regulation of affect and response to stress (Bremner et al., 1997; Heim & Nemeroff, 1999; Stein et al., 1997; Teicher, 2000; Teicher et al., 2003; Yehuda, 2001). Animal studies suggest that early maternal loss or deprivation of care can disrupt neural systems that are normally regulated by close physical and emotional contact between infant and mother, resulting in lasting perturbations in stress response systems and an increased susceptibility to stress and disease later in life (Bremner, 2003; Hofer, 1996). Research using rodent models suggests that stress early in life can potentially cause shifts in neuronal development that correlate with accelerated maturation of behaviors that might be adaptive for responding to that stressful environment (Bath et al., 2016; Gee et al., 2013). The cost/benefit of these behaviors may change throughout life, or in other contexts.

Resilience

Trauma affects some individuals more, or in different ways, than it does others. For example, the prevalence of PTSD is lower than that of trauma itself (McFarlane & de Girolamo, 2007; Yehuda, 1998). Though it is not fully understood why this is, individual differences in vulnerability and resilience in the face of trauma may reflect neural and/or genetic predispositions and may influence the likelihood of developing symptoms of PTSD (see Chapter 12; Foa et al., 2006; Horn et al., 2016; McFarlane & Yehuda, 2007). Rodent models suggest that exposure to some types of early life stress can potentially lead to adaptive behaviors in adulthood or even, via epigenetic mechanisms, in offspring. (Gapp et al., 2014) A "three-hit model" of vulnerability and

resilience to traumatic stress has been proposed, which includes genetic predisposition, early-life environment, and later-life environment (Daskalakis et al., 2013).

PTSD, as it is currently defined by the DSM-5-TR, captures only some aspects of
human response to trauma, namely, a specific set of symptoms involving re-
experiencing the traumatic event(s), avoidance and numbing, and hyperarousal.
Researchers in this area have proposed that a new diagnostic category be created,
called **complex PTSD**, which more fully describes the impact of protracted trauma
on self-experience, self-regulation, and relationships with others (Herman, 2015).
This disorder, also referred to as Disorders of Extreme Stress Not Otherwise Specified
(DESNOS), posits that people with a childhood history of repeated interpersonal
trauma manifest a typical pattern of problems with regulation of affect and impulses,
memory and attention, self-perception, interpersonal relations, somatization, and
systems of meaning (Kilborne, 1999). The debate over the validity of DESNOS as a
diagnostic category is beyond the scope of this book, yet when we are creating psychodynamic formulations it is useful to remember how pervasive the impact of
trauma can be.

Linking problems and patterns to the impact of trauma

Whenever there is a history of trauma, using ideas about the way trauma affects
development helps us to link the life story to adult problems and patterns. When we
formulate using ideas about the impact of trauma on development, we trace problems and patterns to the individual's reactions to traumatic events and situations.
The following sections discuss some clinical situations for which linking to trauma is
particularly useful.

Problems with self-experience

Traumatized children may experience significant impairment in the development of
a coherent and stable sense of self, particularly when trauma occurs early in life and
involves chronic abuse at the hands of parents or trusted adults. Children who have
been victims of abuse tend to blame themselves, rather than accept that their caregivers are unreliable, exploitative, or violent. Such a misattribution of blame may reflect
the cognitive limitations or omnipotent thinking of a young child, and may also be a
child's way of trying to make sense of an otherwise terrifying situation—a bid to feel
in control of it even if they also feel bad as a result. This misattribution may persist
and lead to self-deprecating or masochistic patterns later in the adult (see Chapter 4).
The deep feelings of guilt and shame that often accompany trauma can persist into
adulthood and profoundly affect an adult's self-esteem (Lansky, 2000; van der Kolk
et al., 2005).

Trauma that occurs in adulthood can disrupt a previously well-established sense of
self (Boulanger, 2002; Fink, 2003). Even when it occurs later in life, trauma may result
in a sense of having two distinct experiences of oneself and the world—the "traumatic" and the "nontraumatic," or the "before-the-trauma" and the "after-the-
trauma" perspectives. These may be difficult to integrate. Consider Matthew:

Matthew, a 53-year-old Native American man who identifies as heterosexual, sought psychotherapy for long-standing problems with self-esteem and difficulty forming romantic relationships. Despite living in a community of people from his tribe, Matthew describes chronic feelings of being an "outsider," different from the rest of his family and most peer groups. He feels easily ashamed, humiliated, or guilty, particularly when he experiences himself as not living up to his own very high standards or when he is unsuccessful socially. He and his therapist have been exploring possible origins of these patterns in his early family life. Matthew was a quiet, bright, and motivated student, unlike his parents and siblings, who were extroverted and athletic and did not emphasize intellectual pursuits. He also did not receive much validation for his academic pursuits from his peer group on the reservation. Although his family members are quite religiously observant, Matthew stopped attending church in his 20s and considers himself an atheist. Six months into psychotherapy, Matthew discloses to his therapist that, from the ages of 9–11, a clergyman in his family's church sexually abused him. He says he has been too ashamed to discuss this with anyone, but realizes that many of the painful feelings he has been exploring originated during that time.

The problems and patterns with which Mathew struggles may have multiple roots in development and his socio-cultural environment. However, the experience of having been sexually abused by a trusted adult, along with years of harboring a shameful secret, is likely to have intensified his feeling of "otherness" and his difficulty with self-esteem (Gartner, 1999).

Problems with regulation of affect and impulses

Trauma can also lead to persisting problems with emotional regulation and impulse control. Traumatic stress during childhood is associated with the development of psychiatric symptoms and disorders in adulthood, including depression, suicidality, PTSD and other anxiety disorders, and personality disorders, as well as difficulties regulating anger and sexual impulses (Edwards et al., 2003; MacMillan et al., 2001; Paolucci et al., 2001; van der Kolk et al., 2005).

Patients with PTSD often suffer either from intense emotional and physical hyperarousal, or from emotional blunting or numbing. In patients who do not necessarily meet PTSD criteria, or who have an unacknowledged trauma history, these forms of emotional dysregulation may be diagnosed as a primary affective disorder or borderline personality disorder. Judith Herman, in her landmark book, *Trauma and Recovery*, argues that many patients diagnosed with borderline personality disorder have histories of abuse, and that the emotional lability seen in that disorder may be better conceptualized as the aftereffects of chronic trauma (Herman, 2015).

Another clinical phenomenon seen in trauma survivors that may be linked to trauma-induced emotional dysregulation is deliberate self-harm or self-mutilation. Typically involving cutting or burning of the skin, this behavior is more common in those with a childhood abuse history and often serves the purpose of relieving states of emotional distress, such as anxiety, depression, or dissociation (Briere & Gil, 1998; van der Kolk, 2007). Consider Claudia:

Claudia, a 23-year-old gay, Colombian-American woman, is referred for ongoing psychiatric treatment after a brief hospitalization following a suicide attempt. She describes overwhelming feelings of hopelessness and despair following a breakup with her girlfriend that led her to impulsively swallow a bottle of her roommate's antidepressant medication. Claudia reports that since early adolescence she has had a history of "mood swings," alcohol and drug abuse, skin cutting, and bulimia. Despite these symptoms, Claudia has worked as a computer programmer since graduating from college a year ago. She describes a history of repeated sexual abuse by her stepfather between the ages of 6–12. He warned her that if she ever told anyone about "their secret" he would kill her. Years later, after her mother and stepfather had separated and Claudia and her family immigrated to the United States, Claudia finally told her mother what had happened. While she was being abused, Claudia had frequent physical complaints and performed poorly in school. She started experimenting with drugs in early adolescence and had multiple sexual partners. Claudia describes her emotional life as "a roller coaster," alternating between extremes of anger and sadness, anxiety and numbness, or emptiness. Unaccustomed to talking about her feelings or personal thoughts, she says she usually "takes action" to handle painful emotions.

The experience of protracted sexual abuse early in life may have affected Claudia's ability to tolerate and regulate painful or uncomfortable feelings. Being forced to keep her experiences secret may have led her to adapt to stress by acting rather than talking. This trauma-informed approach to psychodynamic formulation is very useful in clinical situations like Claudia's.

Problems with relationships with others

Traumatic experiences can also affect the ability to establish relationships with others in a variety of ways. The ability to trust is particularly vulnerable to trauma that is perpetrated by others. Early childhood abuse, especially at the hands of a family member, caregiver, or trusted other adult (such as clergy), can affect a developing child's ability to form secure attachments (see Chapter 24; Carlson et al., 1989; Cicchetti & Toth, 1995; Stovall-McClough & Cloitre, 2006). Interactions with caregivers who are consistent, loving, and empathic lay the groundwork for a child's healthy relationships in later life. Children whose caregivers were violent or neglectful, or who were unable to protect them from other violent adults (e.g., during wartime), may be unable to trust others and form secure attachments. As adults, they may have difficulties along a continuum from a pervasive sense of mistrust or paranoia to more circumscribed problems with intimacy. Consider Jerome:

Jerome, a 90-year-old Jewish man, is referred to the clinic when he refuses to have further diagnostic studies to evaluate a suspicious nodule on his chest X-ray. Jerome tells the psychiatrist that he knows it could be cancer, but says, "If it's cancer, what could they do for me? There's no help for that, so why should I find out?" Jerome's son, who has accompanied him to the appointment, says that his father will never ask for help or rely on others and that he prides himself on his business successes as a self-made man. As a young child growing up in Germany during World War II, Jerome remembers their neighbors watching as Nazis dragged the family out of their apartment and sent them to a concentration camp. In the camp, he was separated from his parents and siblings, all of whom were killed.

Jerome, who survived the Holocaust and built a successful life for himself, has a deep-seated belief that other people cannot help him or save him from danger. The horrible reality of his early life makes it difficult for him to believe that people in the present may be able to help him. Linking Jerome's difficulty with trust to his early trauma is a useful way to create a formulation about his development.

Problems with adapting

Difficulty adapting to stress can often be usefully linked to trauma. In fact, one of the hallmarks of PTSD is an abnormal set of responses to external stimuli. Patients with PTSD may be hyperreactive to stimuli that remind them of traumatic experiences (e.g., the sound of a low-flying airplane, a car backfiring, or a face they perceive as angry). What might be *ordinary* stress for a non-traumatized individual is often experienced as *extraordinary* stress for someone with a trauma history. For example, consider Kiri:

> Kiri, a 50-year-old Cambodian-American woman and the mother of a 14-year-old daughter, presents for treatment complaining of severe insomnia, anxiety, getting into frequent arguments with her daughter, and difficulty concentrating in her job as the director of a human rights non-profit organization. She describes "falling apart" after her husband left her for another woman approximately three years ago and now says, "My daughter's behavior is going to push me off the edge. I just can't cope with it." Kiri feels she should be better at handling their relationship and says, "I'm not as strong as my mother was after she left my father, and I don't want to fight with my daughter." Kiri's father, who was persecuted by the Khmer Rouge, physically abused her mother and older brother after he was released. Her mother fled not only from her husband but also the country, emigrating as a refugee from Cambodia to the United States with her two children when Kiri was 7 years old. Kiri says that although she knew that her father was violent, she also has memories of feeling very attached to him as a young child before the Khmer Rouge came to power. She also says she had difficulty with conflict in her marriage as well.

While many parents struggle with their teenage children, Kiri's extensive history of trauma and loss make her especially vulnerable to strife with her daughter.
Childhood abuse can also disrupt the development of object constancy (see Chapter 13), leading to a reliance on splitting-based defenses later in life. By splitting off the negative aspects of an abusive or neglectful caregiver, mistreated children can continue to believe in the goodness of those upon whom they depend, albeit at the cost of seeing people as all good or all bad. This tendency may persist into adulthood and lead to problematic responses to stress and interpersonal conflict (Briere, 2006; Briere & Runtz, 1988; van der Kolk, 2007).

A sample formulation—linking to trauma

Presentation

> Maxine is a 44-year-old woman who seeks psychotherapy for long-standing difficulties maintaining relationships with other people and chronic feelings of low self-esteem. She says that she would like to have a long-term relationship with a man and perhaps marry. Although her romantic relationships always start out passionately, they have never lasted longer than a year. Maxine, who supports her middle-class lifestyle by working as a high school principal, states that she has an active social life that is tied mostly to the school. With some sadness, however, she says, "I don't have any real friends; there's no one in whom I can confide." She describes herself as "naïve" when it comes to choosing friends and lovers, saying, "I keep picking the wrong people who turn out to be really manipulative, cruel, and selfish." She tends to end relationships abruptly once she feels betrayed or rejected. Maxine has "tried therapy" several times in the past, but became disillusioned

or angry with each therapist after a few months. At the end of the second session, she tells the therapist, "I can tell you're different from other therapists I've seen—you're really smart and you understand me perfectly."

DESCRIBE the problems and patterns

*Maxine's greatest difficulty seems to be in maintaining **relationships with others**. She has trouble with **intimacy**, rapidly entering into intense but shallow relationships with friends and lovers, and then becoming quickly and easily hurt or angry. She has a **poor sense of self and others** and at times is unable to tolerate the slightest imperfection or shortcomings in other people. She often chooses people who take advantage of her desperate-seeming need to connect, and thus, her relationships **lack mutuality**. She is **overly trusting** of people who give her little reason to have confidence in them. The short-term quality of her relationships suggests that her **attachments are generally not secure**. Her relationship with the present therapist begins with idealization; at the same time, she devalues previous ones. Nevertheless, her **identity** as an educator is fairly consolidated, and she is able to socialize on a superficial level with colleagues.*

REVIEW the life story

Maxine is an only child. Her mother has been intermittently psychotic since Maxine was in her mid-teens and has been diagnosed with schizophrenia. Maxine's father worked long hours and was often absent from the home. Maxine describes her mother as being "different people at different times." While her mother was sometimes loving and attentive, she could also be violent and abusive, shouting insults or obscenities at Maxine, locking her in her room for long periods of time, and often hitting her. The family lived in near isolation, with no extended family and infrequent contact with friends or neighbors.

LINK the history and problems/patterns to the impact of trauma

Maxine's difficulty maintaining relationships with others may be related to her trouble integrating good and bad qualities in herself and in others, which may have resulted from her traumatic childhood experiences with her mother. Her mother's wildly inconsistent and frightening behavior may have made it hard for Maxine to develop a well-functioning internal sense of self in relation to a generally consistent and positive other. Maxine may have needed to keep good and bad aspects of her mother separate in her mind to adapt to the bewildering fluctuations in her mother's behavior. Her tendency to gravitate to people who are cruel or emotionally abusive may be related to expectations, instilled in her by childhood experiences, that abuse is the price one has to pay for having some sense of safety and security with others.

Linking to trauma guides treatment

Understanding the relationship between a patient's problems/patterns and history of trauma is crucial for formulating a diagnosis and treatment plan. Patients can benefit enormously from being able to discuss their experiences with a mental health professional who can listen to them in an empathic, nonjudgmental way. Often, we are the first people with whom our patients discuss their traumatic experiences.

If we give them time, our patients will generally tell us their stories bit by bit. By acknowledging the effects that trauma may have had on them, and showing that we can bear to hear about it, we can establish an atmosphere of safety and trust that is crucial in helping them begin therapy. Over time, their trust in us may also help them to increase their general ability to trust, form secure attachments, and have a more integrated sense of self and others. Sharing our formulations with them may increase their understanding of the way their traumatic experiences have affected their current functioning.

Suggested activity

Can be done by individual learners or in a classroom setting

How would you describe the ways in which the two people described below have reacted to the traumas they experienced?

Alma is a 30-year-old gay woman who presents for therapy saying, "My girlfriend is alarmed at how frequently I have nightmares." Alma tells you that, as a child, she would lie awake at night, listening to her father physically abuse her mother. Alma says that although her father never physically harmed her, he threatened her with violence and was verbally abusive. Alma's current relationship is the first that she would call "long term;" she reports generally having shorter term, casual relationships that she broke off when they "got too deep."

Dev is a 35-year-old man who presents to a mental health clinic with loneliness, anxiety, and depression. He tells a therapist upon intake that he is devastated after his girlfriend broke up with him due to his excessive marijuana use. Dev says that he smokes marijuana in the morning before work and in the evening after work to "numb" his worries. He reports that his ex-girlfriend wanted him to look for another job because of difficulties he has with his boss. "My boss is constantly asking me to take on too much extra work. And if I refuse, he calls me outside of work hours to dress me down." The younger of two boys, Dev explains that his older brother was a "real bully." "To my parents, he was the golden boy," he says, "But to me he was a terror. He bullied me all the time—even broke my arm once. We told my parents I fell out of a tree."

Comment

Although both Alma and Dev have histories of being traumatized in their childhoods, their reactions to their experiences have been different. Alma has held people at a distance, perhaps in part because she saw the violence in the intimacy of her parents' relationship. Dev may use marijuana to numb the dysregulation triggered in the relationship with his boss, who may remind him of his abusive older brother.

References

1. American Psychiatric Association. (2022). *Diagnostic and statistical manual of mental disorders* (5th ed., *Text Revision (DSM-5-TR)*). Washington, DC: American Psychiatric Press.

2. Bath, K. G., Manzano-Nieves, G., & Goodwill, H. (2016). Early life stress accelerates behavioral and neural maturation of the hippocampus in male mice. *Hormones and Behavior, 82*, 64–71. https://doi.org/10.1016/j.yhbeh.2016.04.010

3. Bor, J., Venkataramani, A. S., Williams, D. R., & Tsai, A. C. (2018). Police killings and their spillover effects on the mental health of Black Americans: A population-based, quasi-experimental study. *The Lancet, 392*(10144), 302–310. https://doi.org/10.1016/s0140-6736(18)31130-9

4. Boulanger, G. (2002). Wounded by reality. *Contemporary Psychoanalysis, 38*(1), 45–76. https://doi.org/10.1080/00107530.2002.10745806

5. Bowers, M. E., & Yehuda, R. (2016). Intergenerational transmission of stress in humans. *Neuropsychopharmacology, 41*(1), 232–244. https://doi.org/10.1038/npp.2015.247

6. Bremner, J. D. (2003). Long-term effects of childhood abuse on brain and neurobiology. *Child and Adolescent Psychiatric Clinics of North America, 12*(2), 271–292. https://doi.org/10.1016/s1056-4993(02)00098-6

7. Bremner, J. D., Randall, P., Vermetten, E., Staib, L., Bronen, R. A., Mazure, C., Capelli, S., McCarthy, G., Innis, R. B., & Charney, D. S. (1997). Magnetic resonance imaging-based measurement of hippocampal volume in posttraumatic stress disorder related to childhood physical and sexual abuse—A preliminary report. *Biological Psychiatry, 41*(1), 23–32. https://doi.org/10.1016/s0006-3223(96)00162-x

8. Breuer, J., & Freud, S. (1971). On the psychical mechanism of hysterical phenomena: Preliminary communication. In J. Strachey (Ed.), *The standard edition of the complete psychological works of Sigmund Freud (1893–1895): Studies on Hysteria, Volume II* (pp. 1–17). Hogarth Press. (Originally published in 1893).

9. Briere, J. (2006). Dissociative symptoms and trauma exposure. *Journal of Nervous & Mental Disease, 194*(2), 78–82. https://doi.org/10.1097/01.nmd.0000198139.47371.54

10. Briere, J., & Gil, E. (1998). Self-mutilation in clinical and general population samples: Prevalence, correlates, and functions. *American Journal of Orthopsychiatry, 68*(4), 609–620. https://doi.org/10.1037/h0080369

11. Briere, J., & Runtz, M. (1988). Symptomatology associated with childhood sexual victimization in a nonclinical adult sample. *Child Abuse & Neglect, 12*(1), 51–59. https://doi.org/10.1016/0145-2134(88)90007-5

12. Carlson, V., Cicchetti, D., Barnett, D., & Braunwald, K. (1989). Disorganized/disoriented attachment relationships in maltreated infants. *Developmental Psychology, 25*(4), 525–531. https://doi.org/10.1037/0012-1649.25.4.525

13. Cicchetti, D., & Toth, S. (1995). A developmental psychopathology perspective on child abuse and neglect. *Journal of the American Academy of Child & Adolescent Psychiatry, 34*(5), 541–565. https://doi.org/10.1097/00004583-199505000-00008

14. Daskalakis, N. P., Bagot, R. C., Parker, K. J., Vinkers, C. H., & de Kloet, E. R. (2013). The three-hit concept of vulnerability and resilience: Toward understanding adaptation to early-life adversity outcome. *Psychoneuroendocrinology, 38*(9), 1858–1873. https://doi.org/10.1016/j.psyneuen.2013.06.008

15. Edwards, V. J., Holden, G. W., Felitti, V. J., & Anda, R. F. (2003). Relationship between multiple forms of childhood maltreatment and adult mental health in community respondents: Results from the adverse childhood experiences study. *American Journal of Psychiatry, 160*(8), 1453–1460. https://doi.org/10.1176/appi.ajp.160.8.1453

16. Fink, K. (2003). Magnitude of trauma and personality change. *The International Journal of Psychoanalysis, 84*(4), 985–995. https://doi.org/10.1516/350u-fhq2-rtdb-6hw8

17. Foa, E., Stein, D., & McFarlane, A. (2006). Symptomatology and psychopathology of mental health problems after disaster. *Journal of Clinical Psychiatry, 67*(Suppl 2), 15–25.
18. Gapp, K., Jawaid, A., Sarkies, P., Bohacek, J., Pelczar, P., Prados, J., Farinelli, L., Miska, E., & Mansuy, I. M. (2014). Implication of sperm RNAS in transgenerational inheritance of the effects of early trauma in mice. *Nature Neuroscience, 17*(5), 667–669. https://doi.org/10.1038/nn.3695
19. Gartner, R. B. (1999). *Betrayed as boys: Psychodynamic treatment of sexually abused men.* Guilford Press.
20. Gee, D. G., Gabard-Durnam, L. J., Flannery, J., Goff, B, Humphreys, K. L., Telzer, E. H., Hare, T. A., Bookheimer, S. Y., & Tottenham, N. (2013). Early developmental emergence of human amygdala-prefrontal connectivity after maternal deprivation. Proceedings of the National Academy of Sciences of the United States of America. Retrieved November 13, 2021, https://pubmed.ncbi.nlm.nih.gov/24019460.
21. Heim, C., & Nemeroff, C. B. (1999). The impact of early adverse experiences on brain systems involved in the pathophysiology of anxiety and affective disorders. *Biological Psychiatry, 46*(11), 1509–1522. https://doi.org/10.1016/s0006-3223(99)00224-3
22. Herman, J. L. (2015). *Trauma and recovery: The aftermath of violence: From domestic abuse to political terror.* Basic Books.
23. Hofer, M. A. (1996). On the nature and consequences of early loss. *Psychosomatic Medicine, 58*(6), 570–581. https://doi.org/10.1097/00006842-199611000-00005
24. Horn, S. R., Charney, D. S., & Feder, A. (2016). Understanding resilience: New approaches for preventing and treating PTSD. *Experimental Neurology, 284*, 119–132. https://doi.org/10.1016/j.expneurol.2016.07.002
25. Jawaid, A., Roszkowski, M., & Mansuy, I. M. (2018). Transgenerational epigenetics of traumatic stress. *Progress in Molecular Biology and Translational Science*, 273–298. https://doi.org/10.1016/bs.pmbts.2018.03.003
26. Kilborne, B. (1999). When trauma strikes the soul: Shame, splitting, and psychic pain. *American Journal of Psychoanalysis, 59*, 385–402.
27. van der Kolk, B. A. (2007). The complexity of adaptation to trauma: Self-regulation, stimulus discrimination, and characterological development. In B. van der Kolk, A. McFarlane, & L. Weisaeth (Eds.), *Traumatic stress: The effects of overwhelming experience on mind, body, and society* (pp. 182–213). Guilford Press.
28. van der Kolk, B. A., & McFarlane, A. C. (2007). The black hole of trauma. In B. van der Kolk, A. McFarlane, & L. Weisaeth (Eds.), *Traumatic stress: The effects of overwhelming experience on mind, body, and society* (pp. 3–23). Guilford Press.
29. van der Kolk, B. A., Roth, S., Pelcovitz, D., Sunday, S., & Spinazzola, J. (2005). Disorders of extreme stress: The empirical foundation of a complex adaptation to trauma. *Journal of Traumatic Stress, 18*(5), 389–399. https://doi.org/10.1002/jts.20047
30. Lansky, M. R. (2000). Shame dynamics in the psychotherapy of the patient with PTSD: A viewpoint. *Journal of the American Academy of Psychoanalysis, 28*(1), 133–146. https://doi.org/10.1521/jaap.1.2000.28.1.133
31. MacMillan, H. L., Fleming, J. E., Streiner, D. L., Lin, E., Boyle, M. H., Jamieson, E., Duku, E. K., Walsh, C. A., Wong, M. Y. Y., & Beardslee, W. R. (2001). Childhood abuse and lifetime psychopathology in a community sample. *American Journal of Psychiatry, 158*(11), 1878–1883. https://doi.org/10.1176/appi.ajp.158.11.1878
32. McFarlane, A., & de Girolamo, G. (2007). The nature of traumatic stressors and the epidemiology of posttraumatic reactions. In B. van der Kolk, A. McFarlane, & L. Weisaeth (Eds.), *Traumatic stress: The effects of overwhelming experience on mind, body, and society* (pp. 129–154). Guilford Press.
33. McFarlane, A., & Yehuda, R. (2007). Resilience, vulnerability and the course of posttraumatic reactions. In B. van der Kolk, A. McFarlane, & L. Weisaeth (Eds.), *Traumatic stress: The effects of overwhelming experience on mind, body, and society* (pp. 155–181). Guilford Press.

34. Paolucci, E., Genuis, M. L., & Violato, C. (2001). A meta-analysis of the published research on the effects of child sexual abuse. *The Journal of Psychology, 135*(1), 17–36. https://doi.org/10.1080/00223980109603677

35. Paradies, Y., Priest, N., Ben, J., Truong, M., Gupta, A., Pieterse, A., Kelaher, M., & Gee, G. (2013). Racism as a determinant of health: A protocol for conducting a systematic review and meta-analysis. *Systematic Reviews, 2*(1). https://doi.org/10.1186/2046-4053-2-85

36. Sirin, S. R., Ryce, P., Gupta, T., & Rogers-Sirin, L. (2013). The role of acculturative stress on mental health symptoms for immigrant adolescents: A longitudinal investigation. *Developmental Psychology, 49*(4), 736–748. https://doi.org/10.1037/a0028398

37. Stein, M. B., Koverola, C., Hanna, C., Torchia, M. G., & McClarty, B. (1997). Hippocampal volume in women victimized by childhood sexual abuse. *Psychological Medicine, 27*(4), 951–959. https://doi.org/10.1017/s0033291797005242

38. Stovall-McClough, K. C., & Cloitre, M. (2006). Unresolved attachment, PTSD, and dissociation in women with childhood abuse histories. *Journal of Consulting and Clinical Psychology, 74*(2), 219–228. https://doi.org/10.1037/0022-006x.74.2.219

39. Sutter, M., & Perrin, P. B. (2016). Discrimination, mental health, and suicidal ideation among LGBTQ people of color. *Journal of Counseling Psychology, 63*(1), 98–105. https://doi.org/10.1037/cou0000126

40. Teicher, M. (2000). Wounds that time won't heal: The neurobiology of child abuse. *Cerebrum, 2*(4), 50–67.

41. Teicher, M. H., Andersen, S. L., Polcari, A., Anderson, C. M., Navalta, C. P., & Kim, D. M. (2003). The neurobiological consequences of early stress and childhood maltreatment. *Neuroscience & Biobehavioral Reviews, 27*(1–2), 33–44. https://doi.org/10.1016/s0149-7634(03)00007-1

42. Tummala-Narra, P. (2016). *Psychoanalytic theory and cultural competence in psychotherapy.* American Psychological Association. https://doi.org/10.1037/14800-000

43. Tummala-Narra, P., & Claudius, M. (2013). Perceived discrimination and depressive symptoms among immigrant-origin adolescents. *Cultural Diversity and Ethnic Minority Psychology, 19*, 257–269. http://dx.doi.org/10.1037/a0032960

44. Yehuda, R. (1998). *Psychological trauma.* American Psychiatric Publishing, Inc.

45. Yehuda, R. (2001). Biology of posttraumatic stress disorder. *Journal of Clinical Psychiatry, 62*(Suppl 17), 41–46.

46. Yehuda, R., & Lehrner, A. (2018). Intergenerational transmission of trauma effects: Putative role of epigenetic mechanisms. *World Psychiatry, 17*(3), 243–257. https://doi.org/10.1002/wps.20568

19 Early Cognitive and Emotional Difficulties

Key concepts

Understanding the way our patients' early cognitive and emotional difficulties have affected the development of their conscious and unconscious thoughts, feelings, and behavior can help us to LINK problems and patterns to their history.

Cognitive and emotional difficulties are very common in childhood and adolescence, and can disturb whatever development is occurring at that time. They include problems that both do and do not meet the criteria for DSM disorders.

The responses of caregivers and early treatment can alter the extent to which cognitive and emotional difficulties affect development. Social determinants can limit access to care and affect outcomes.

Adult patients may not be aware that early cognitive and emotional difficulties (particularly those that were not recognized or treated) played a role in their development.

We should consider linking problems and patterns to early cognitive and emotional difficulties when there is

- An apparent "mismatch" between what we DESCRIBE and what we REVIEW
- A history in childhood or adolescence of a sudden delay or unexpected interruption in development
- A personal or family history of cognitive and emotional difficulties

People with early cognitive and emotional difficulties often experience disadvantage and discrimination.

Like adults, children and adolescents have problems with mood and anxiety, as well as other cognitive and emotional difficulties, that can profoundly affect their development. Some of these may be diagnosed and treated, but many are not; in fact, adults who had these kinds of problems may never have conceptualized them in this way. Nevertheless, as we create psychodynamic formulations, we must remain alert to the possibility that a problem of this nature may have been a factor in our patients' early lives. In this chapter, we review some of the cognitive and emotional difficulties

Psychodynamic Formulation: An Expanded Approach, First Edition. The Psychodynamic Formulation Collective.
© 2022 John Wiley & Sons Ltd. Published 2022 by John Wiley & Sons Ltd.

that commonly occur during childhood and adolescence, and then suggest clinical situations for which linking to them may be helpful.

Why talk about difficulties rather than disorders?

While some of the cognitive and emotional difficulties that people experience during development reach the level of being a disorder, many do not. Think of the child who tends to procrastinate during elementary school, but who does not meet criteria for attention deficit disorder (ADD); or perhaps the teenager who is often sad, but does not meet criteria for major depression or dysthymia. Despite the fact that these are not disorders, such difficulties can affect the development of all aspects of function, including self-experience, relationships with others, adaptation, cognition, values, and work/play. Consequently, we think that it's important to broadly consider our patients' cognitive and emotional **difficulties** as well as their disorders.

Basics related to the impact of cognitive and emotional difficulties on development

Cognitive and emotional difficulties are quite common in children and adolescents. Data on a representative population of American children growing up in the 1990s indicates that about one in three had at least one psychiatric disorder by age 16 (Costello et al., 2003), and frequently, they had more than one psychiatric diagnosis (Arcelus & Vostanis, 2005; Mineka et al., 1998; NIH/National Institute of Mental Health, 2005). Among all adults with psychiatric illness, about three-quarters of these adults had received a diagnosis before age 18 and half before age 14 (Kessler et al., 2005; Kim-Cohen et al., 2003; New Freedom Commission on Mental Health, 2003).

Whenever cognitive and emotional difficulties occur, they have the capacity to disturb development happening during that period, as well as functioning that will develop later. For example, difficulties in later childhood that interfere with performing school tasks and developing friendships with peers (such as ADD or childhood bipolar disorder) powerfully predict work struggles in adulthood (Collins & van Dulmen, 2006; Hyson, 2002). Thus, when we hear that someone has a history of cognitive and emotional difficulties in childhood or adolescence, it's important to determine when those problems emerged, what often develops during that phase of life, and whether development may have been compromised.

To think about this further, let's consider some specific cognitive and emotional difficulties that arise during different phases of development.

Cognitive and emotional difficulties in childhood

Cognitive and emotional difficulties that commonly emerge during the childhood years (0–12) include the following:

- Autism spectrum disorders
- Academic/learning difficulties (including learning disorders)
- Attentional difficulties (including Attention Deficit Hyperactivity Disorder (ADHD))

- Anxiety (including obsessive compulsive disorder, phobias, and separation anxiety disorder)
- Enuresis/encopresis
- Motor/verbal tics
- Mood difficulties (including depression)
  (Costello et al., 2003; Kessler et al., 2005).

Some of these difficulties may even begin at birth and be related to inherited disorders, prenatal development, or temperamental traits (see Chapter 12). When they begin in early childhood (before age 6), they can have profound and pervasive effects on emotional, cognitive, and physical development, and may predict a lifetime of problems, especially in the absence of early detection and intervention (National Advisory Mental Health Council Workgroup on Child and Adolescent Mental Health Intervention Development and Deployment, 2001). For example, early undiagnosed depression, as well as subthreshold mood disorders, can affect everything from the development of self-esteem to relationships with others. Hearing that a patient has had lifelong difficulty with relationships and seems emotionally disconnected during early visits could raise the possibility of an undiagnosed autism spectrum disorder. Recognizing that these problems may have been at play can help us to better understand our patients and can help our patients to better understand themselves.

The ways in which children adapt to their cognitive and emotional difficulties can further affect development. For example, learning disabilities or ADHD may compromise school performance, self-esteem, and the ability to form friendships. If children then isolate themselves to avoid social rejection, they may compound the effect of the original problem. Even if someone was never formally diagnosed with a learning problem or ADHD as a child, lifelong problems with self-esteem coincident with poor academic achievement should suggest that this was—or may continue to be—a difficulty. The lack of understanding and an ableist response of others to a child's learning disabilities during childhood may compromise the development of the child's sense of self and contribute to patterns of responding to self-esteem threats with avoidance or grandiosity.

Cognitive and emotional difficulties in adolescence

Across cultures and centuries, adolescence has always been a time of dramatic change in body and behavior (see Chapter 16). During the teen years, enormous changes also take place in the neural systems that control higher cognitive functions, interpersonal interactions, self-regulation, and motivation. As such, it is a time of high risk because brain systems appear to be most vulnerable when they are evolving (Douaud et al., 2009; Giedd et al., 2008).

Despite bumps in the road, most adolescents eventually manage to navigate the transition from dependent children to self-sufficient young adults. However, the turbulent teen years can be even more challenging if the adolescent is also contending with cognitive and emotional difficulties. Problems that typically emerge or worsen during adolescence include difficulties with the following (Costello et al., 2003; Kessler et al., 2005; New Freedom Commission on Mental Health, 2003):

- Anxiety (including panic disorder, generalized anxiety disorder, and PTSD)
- Eating (including anorexia nervosa and bulimia)

- Conduct (including conduct and oppositional defiant disorders)
- Emotional regulation and impulse control
- Mood (including major depression and bipolar disorder)
- Psychosis (including schizophrenia)
- Substance misuse and addiction

Adolescents with difficulties in any of these areas may miss out on the opportunity to develop and strengthen the skills their peers are practicing, including the ability to regulate affect, control impulses, exercise self-restraint, and consolidate identity. They may continue to have trouble in these areas even during periods when their cognitive and emotional difficulties are less problematic. Consider an adult who presents for therapy saying, "I don't know what I want to do with my life," and who notes spending most of adolescence battling anorexia. It's likely that when peers were consolidating their identities and building careers, this person was dealing with an eating disorder. Now, free of symptoms for over 25 years, they are left without a clear sense of what they enjoy doing and without skills that might help them negotiate the next phase of life.

Cognitive and emotional difficulties in adulthood

Although our focus in this chapter is on the effect of cognitive and emotional difficulties in childhood and adolescence, development doesn't stop at age 18 (see Chapters 16 and 17). Thus, emotional and cognitive difficulties that arise in adulthood can also affect development. Take, for example, a woman who presents with fears that she is a bad mother and who says that she cried for weeks after having her child. It is likely that this woman had an untreated postpartum depression, which has left her feeling that she is a terrible mother and that she couldn't handle having a second child. These are new patterns that evolved in adulthood that we can usefully link to the effects of a problem with mood on her sense of self.

Parental response and access to care

The extent to which early cognitive and emotional difficulties affect development depends on various factors, including

- The nature, timing, and chronicity of the difficulty
- The child's early relationship with primary caregivers, including the caregivers' responsiveness to the difficulty
- General family stress and the child's social environment
- Peer relationships
- Limited access to early care
- Adequate early treatment, and the way the difficulty is conceptualized by the caregivers and, ultimately, by the child
  (Aneshensel & Sucoff, 1996; Jessor, 1993; Rutter, 2000, 2005)

Parental response to a child's cognitive and emotional difficulties and early treatment intervention can make an enormous difference in the way those problems affect development (Sroufe et al., 2000). Early and aggressive behavioral treatment, sensitive parenting, and a supportive school environment can all contribute to limiting the duration and impact of early cognitive and emotional difficulties. It is important to remember that although positive responses from caregivers and early recognition/treatment may help mitigate adverse consequences, they are not necessarily protective against the disruptive effects of these early difficulties, particularly when they reach the level of being psychiatric disorders.

The effect of limited access to early care

Limited access to money, medical/psychiatric care, and special education can restrict access to early care, drastically changing the outcome of early cognitive and emotional difficulties (Compton & Shim, 2015; Shim & Vinson, 2021). Consider the following two people:

> *Jackson, a 35-year-old White man who was born to married parents, began having academic difficulties in the second grade. The teacher in his exclusive private school immediately phoned his parents and arranged a conference that included a school counselor. His parents, wealthy college graduates, were easily able to arrange and pay for extensive and expensive neuropsychological testing. Jackson was found to have dyslexia and several learning differences. Jackson began tutoring and counseling and was soon back to his grade level. He excelled in school, graduated from high school, and gained admission to a prestigious college where he continued to receive help from the learning center. He is now a self-supporting middle-class professional.*

> *Henry, a 35-year-old African-American man, began having academic difficulties in the second grade. One of seven children raised by a single mother receiving government assistance, his reading problems were neither noticed at home nor in his overcrowded school. By fourth grade, he was skipping classes and was frequently in trouble with the principal. Ashamed by his inability to read fluently, he was disparaging of students who did their work, and began to hang out with older kids who had dropped out of school. He never finished high school and was intermittently involved in the juvenile justice system. He remains only intermittently employed at a minimum wage job.*

Jackson and Henry both had early cognitive problems but had completely different outcomes. Life stories like Henry's should make us consider the linkage to early cognitive and emotional difficulties, particularly in those disadvantaged by systemic oppression.

Linking problems and patterns to the impact of early cognitive and emotional difficulties

Although some patients can tell us that they had early cognitive and emotional difficulties, many cannot. How, then, can we know when to usefully hypothesize about links to early emotional problems? The following sections present some guidelines.

"Mismatch" between what we describe and what we review

Sometimes, what we describe and what we review just don't seem to match. For example, someone may present with global disruption of function but describe having grown up in a very supportive, functional early environment with siblings who do not have the same difficulties. Some patients might describe having had "terrible" caregivers who "ruined" their lives, but again, this might not seem to match what you have learned about the caregivers over time. Consider Elaine:

> Elaine is a 21-year-old college student who is referred by her college dean after roommates noticed that she had multiple cuts on her arm. Elaine admits that she started cutting herself "again" after discovering that her boyfriend was communicating with other women on social media. She says, "I've always been all over the place—up, down—I don't know what's wrong with me. Nothing bad ever happened to me—my parents are good people who try to help, but they just don't get where I come from. My brother and sister never had these problems. Why can't I get it together?"

Elaine's pervasive problems with mood and self-harm, in the setting of what sounds like a "good enough" family situation, suggests that she has likely been suffering from lifelong problems with mood and self-regulation. Although it is always possible that one family member is treated differently from the others, it is also possible that Elaine may have had an early cognitive or emotional problem. Of course, it's not always one or the other—a child with early difficulties may, in fact, be treated differently from other children in the family, either with more or less attention, empathy, and patience.

History in childhood of unexpected interruption of previously normal development

Hearing about sudden or unexpected interruptions in development should trigger the thought that early cognitive or emotional difficulties may have played a role—even if this is not the way this was conceptualized at the time. For example:

> Arthur is a 35-year-old man who presents for help negotiating social issues in his new company. "I started at a small firm, and this is a real step up—but the place is huge! I feel a little lost and don't know how to find good mentors." Although Arthur denies current symptoms of anxiety or depression, he admits to feeling a little "off-kilter." Over time, the therapist learns that Arthur was an excellent student with many friends, ". . .except for sixth and seventh grade. I don't know what happened. I was in a new school, and I just imploded or something. I spent all my time in my room playing video games. My grades plummeted. My parents were constantly angry with me, telling me to get on the stick. But by eighth grade, I was OK again. Maybe it was the new school. That experience has always made me worried about new situations."

The sudden interruption of function in later childhood, with social isolation and disruption of school performance, suggests that Arthur might have had a mood or anxiety disorder—perhaps an undiagnosed major depression—at the beginning of middle school. However, this is not the way he or the people around him conceptualized it. That episode led to conflicts with his parents and affected his confidence about entering new situations. In this situation, linking to early emotional difficulties can enhance the way Arthur understands himself and his current problems at work.

Personal or family history of cognitive and/or emotional difficulties

It almost goes without saying that early cognitive and emotional difficulties should be suspected as contributing to the current problems and patterns when there is a personal or family history of this, as illustrated in this example:

> *Hayden is a 28-year-old woman who works in the restaurant industry. She presents saying that she needs to feel better about herself. "Everyone at work is smarter or more interesting than I am," she states." And I need to be stronger when my partner gives me a hard time." Hayden denies current symptoms of depression, but says that she was always a "quiet" child who kept to herself. She did not volunteer for things at school, and she generally presumed that she would not be chosen for parts in school plays and sports teams. "I'm kind of like my mom," she says. "She was pretty low energy." Although she doesn't know the details, she says that she thinks that her maternal grandmother once took something for depression.*

Although Hayden doesn't complain of depression, her family history suggests that some difficulties with mood—either depression or dysthymia—may have played a role in her development. It has likely affected the way she consolidated her sense of self and her ability to manage self-esteem.

People with early cognitive and emotional difficulties are often disadvantaged by structural discrimination

It's important to remember that people with cognitive and emotional difficulties are historically marginalized, have suboptimal educational opportunities, and may suffer in the workplace (Shim & Vinson, 2021). Additionally, resources are likely to affect the impact that early cognitive and emotional difficulties have on the individual, and is an example of **intersectionality** (Shim & Vinson, 2021), or the compounding of disadvantage. A wealthy family may be able to hire tutors or access special educational opportunities not available to families with fewer resources. These early interventions can be deciding factors in the way that early difficulties affect an individual's sense of self, others, and the world.

A sample formulation—linking to the impact of early cognitive and emotional difficulties

Linking problems and patterns to the impact of early cognitive and emotional difficulties is about more than making diagnoses. It's about trying to understand the ways that those early problems affected our patients' development, including their conscious and unconscious ways of thinking about themselves, relating to others, adapting to stress, thinking, conceptualizing values, working, and playing. When you suspect that an early cognitive or emotional problem existed, don't stop there—think about the way it affected both the person and the person's environment throughout development. Here's an example:

Presentation

Krista, a 45-year-old married woman has, until recently, worked as a part-time secretary at a real estate company. She comes in with her husband saying that she is "exhausted." She explains that she "had to quit" her job because it's "too much." Her husband explains that she has quit a series of temporary jobs that she'd taken on since he went on disability for a back injury a year ago. Previously, Krista had been supported by her husband and never worked outside the home. Her husband complains she is "acting like a sad sack" and is "lazy and unmotivated." "She knows what she needs to do.and if she'd quit surfing the internet at work, she'd be great."

Interviewed alone, Krista states that she had been "keeping up OK" at work at first, but when she was asked to cover several brokers and things became more hectic, she felt increasingly depressed and anxious, was unable to concentrate, slept poorly at night, felt tired and apathetic on awakening, and had trouble getting to work on time. She feels ashamed and frustrated about her "collapse," but can't understand why she keeps "losing it," stating, "I'm just one of those people who can't seem to get it together."

DESCRIBE the problems and patterns

*Krista is overwhelmed by tasks at work, leading her to quit jobs repeatedly. She has particular **difficulty staying focused and organized**, and she finds it hard to prioritize tasks, tending to flit from one thing to the next without finishing anything. In the wake of having quit her most recent job, she is also feeling depressed and anxious, with some difficulty sleeping. Krista **identifies** herself as a "housewife"and states she has no trouble keeping up with household tasks, shopping, and paying bills "as long as I take my time."She has a good sense of herself in this role but feels that she is "limited"in her abilities and intelligence. She tends to defer to her husband and often feels bullied by him. She has **few other leisure activities**. She explains, "it generally takes me twice the time to do whatever other people are able to do, so it's hard to find time to relax."*

REVIEW the life story

Krista is the only child born to a single mother whom she describes as "loving but depressed—she had a hard life but she did the best she could to give me a better life." Her mother worked two jobs and was rarely home for dinner but tried to make up for lost time by devoting herself to her daughter on the weekends. Krista states that she had "always loved school" until the fourth grade when she suffered a head injury in a fall while ice-skating with her mother. She doesn't recall much about the incident but was told by her mother that doctors said her X-ray reports were fine. Soon after, Krista began to throw tantrums as her mother tried to dress her for school and was disciplined for hitting other girls. She had more trouble paying attention in class, had trouble keeping up with math, and could only read a few sentences at a time before losing track of the overall gist of the text. She needed help organizing herself to do homework and tended to procrastinate to the last minute before completing assignments. Krista started to slip into worsening depression and anxiety toward the end of high school but would not accept any psychological help. She "limped" through secretarial school, but after meeting her future husband, she was relieved that she wouldn't have to look for a job.

LINK the history and problems/patterns to the impact of early cognitive and emotional difficulties

> *Krista's current work-related difficulties are likely related to long-standing cognitive problems, which may date back to an episode of head trauma in childhood that was never defined or treated. The lack of diagnosis or treatment was in part due to limited financial resources and being raised by a single mother who was often working to support the family. Krista's cognitive difficulties have likely contributed to her lifelong difficulties with self-esteem, which includes feelings of intellectual inferiority that have likely impaired her relationships with others. Her contentious relationship with her mother may have stemmed from her cognitive problems but may also have contributed to the development of poor self-perceptions and difficulty with self-esteem management. All of these are likely to have contributed to her choice of spouse, as well as her choice to remain at home.*

Linking to early cognitive and emotional difficulties guides treatment

If we suspect that a person's development and current difficulties may have been influenced by early cognitive and/or emotional difficulties, this can influence treatment in several ways:

- Further testing (e.g., neuropsychological testing) may be needed to define the nature and severity of cognitive problems
- Taking a family history for cognitive and emotional difficulties should be a part of every evaluation, but it may need to be reviewed in greater depth
- Appropriate interventions for concurrent cognitive or psychiatric problems (e.g., cognitive remediation or pharmacotherapy) may be a mainstay of treatment

Recognition and acknowledgment of the presence and impact of early cognitive and emotional difficulties can offer patients the opportunity to create new and often more forgiving life narratives. In addition, treatment of underlying difficulties, such as anxiety and depression, can often substantially improve the patient's quality of life, function, and feelings about themselves. With time, treatment can also help patients to develop new conscious and unconscious ways of thinking about themselves and others.

Thinking back to Krista, let's consider how the formulation might guide the treatment:

> *The therapist refers Krista to a neuropsychologist for further testing and to a psychiatrist for evaluation of her mood and anxiety symptoms. He also offers Krista and her husband psychoeducation, suggesting that her work-related difficulties have nothing to do with laziness or a lack of effort. He explains that bright, motivated people with cognitive problems may abandon tasks not because they are lazy, but because they have lost track of what they are doing, especially if they are working in a hectic, stressful environment like a busy real estate firm. The therapist also expresses optimism that after neuropsychological testing has helped define the nature of her cognitive problems, Krista should benefit greatly from both cognitive remediation to improve her neuropsychological skills and psychotherapy to help her to understand the way she thinks about herself, her abilities, and her relationships with others.*

Helping Krista and her husband understand that her work-related difficulties are related at least, in part, to early cognitive and emotional difficulties (rather than character flaws), may go a long way toward repairing her sense of self and lessening tensions/misunderstandings in their marriage.

Suggested activity

Can be done by individual learners or in a classroom setting

How might the following be linked?

1. *Difficulty asking a boss for a raise—early temperamental shyness*
2. *Difficulty dealing with one's 8-year-old daughter—early learning difficulties*
3. *Difficulty with self-esteem regulation—bed-wetting*

Comments

1. There are many reasons for why a person might have difficulty asserting oneself at work, but early shyness could definitely be a contributing factor. It could be the persistent shyness itself, and/or it could also be other patterns (such as avoidance or self-deprecation) that evolved as a result of the shyness. Identifying this as a temperamental trait could be very important to the formulation and treatment.

2. Having had a learning difficulty himself, a parent could become irritable, anxious, or fearful as their child begins to do classroom work that gave the parent difficulty. Understanding this link could help the parent understand their feelings and could improve the relationship.

3. Any early difficulty that potentially leads to shame, such as bed-wetting, can affect the developing child's sense of self and capacity for self-esteem regulation. This can also affect the adult's ability to regulate self-esteem long after the childhood difficulty disappears.

References

1. Aneshensel, C. S., & Sucoff, C. A. (1996). The neighborhood context of adolescent mental health. *Journal of Health and Social Behavior, 37*(4), 293–310.
2. Arcelus, J., & Vostanis, P. (2005). Psychiatric comorbidity in children and adolescents. *Current Opinion in Psychiatry, 18*(4), 429–434. https://doi.org/10.3109/00048670903282733
3. Collins, W. A., & van Dulmen, M. C. (2006). The significance of middle childhood peer competence for work relationships in early adulthood. In A. E. Huston & M. N. Ripke (Eds.), *Developmental contexts in middle childhood: Bridges to adolescence and adulthood* (pp. 23–40). Cambridge University Press.
4. Compton, M. T., & Shim, R. S. (2015). *The social determinants of mental health.* American Psychiatric Association Publishing.
5. Costello, E. J., Mustillo, S., Erkanli, A., Keeler, G., & Angold, A. (2003). Prevalence and development of psychiatric disorders in childhood and adolescence. *Archives of General Psychiatry, 60,* 837–844. https://doi.org/10.1001/archpsyc.60.8.837
6. Douaud, G., Mackay, C., Andersson, J., James, S., Quested, D., Ray, M. K., Connell, J., Roberts, N., Crow, T. J., Matthews, P. M., Smith, S., & James, A. (2009). Schizophrenia delays and alters maturation of the brain in adolescence. *Brain: A Journal of Neurology, 132,* 2437–2448. https://doi.org/10.1093/brain/awp126
7. Giedd, J. N., Keshavan, M., & Paus, T. (2008). Why do many psychiatric disorders emerge during adolescence? *National Review of Neuroscience, 9*(12), 947–957. https://doi.org/10.1038/nrn2513
8. Hyson, D. (2002). Understanding adaptation to work in adulthood: A contextual developmental approach. *Advances in Life Course Research, 7,* 93–110. https://doi.org/10.1016/S1040-2608(02)80031-4
9. Jessor, R. (1993). Successful adolescent development among youth in high-risk settings. *American Psychologist, 48,* 117–126.
10. Kessler, R. C., Berglund, P., Demler, O., Jin, R., Merikangas, K. R., & Walters, E. E. (2005). Lifetime prevalence and age-of-onset distributions of DSM-IV disorders in the National Comorbidity Survey Replication. *Archives of General Psychiatry, 62*(6), 593–602. https://doi.org/10.1001/archpsyc.62.6.593
11. Kim-Cohen, J., Caspi, A., Moffitt, T. E., Harrington, H., Milne, B. J., & Poulton, R. (2003). Prior juvenile diagnoses in adults with mental disorder: Developmental follow-back of a prospective-longitudinal cohort. *Archives of General Psychiatry, 60*(7), 709–717. https://doi.org/10.1001/archpsyc.60.7.709
12. Mineka, S., Watson, D., & Clark, L. A. (1998). Comorbidity of anxiety and unipolar mood disorders. *Annual Review Psychology, 49,* 377–412. https://doi.org/10.1146/annurev.psych.49.1.377
13. National Advisory Mental Health Council Workgroup on Child and Adolescent Mental Health Intervention Development and Deployment. (2001). Blueprint for change: Research on child and adolescent mental health. https://www.nimh.nih.gov/about/advisory-boards-and-groups/namhc/reports/blueprint-for-change-research-on-child-and-adolescent-mental-health
14. New Freedom Commission on Mental Health. (2003). *Achieving the promise: Transforming mental health care in America.* DHHS Pub. No. SMA-03-3832. www.mentalhealthcommission.gov
15. NIH/National Institute of Mental Health. (2005). *Mental illness exacts a heavy toll, beginning in youth.* https://www.eurekalert.org/news_releases/646485
16. Rutter, M. (2000). Psychosocial influences: Critiques, findings, and research needs. *Development and Psychopathology, 12*(3), 375–405. https://doi.org/10.1017/S0954579400003072

17. Rutter, M. (2005). Environmentally mediated risks for psychopathology: Research strategies and findings. *Journal of the American Academy of Child and Adolescent Psychiatry*, 44(1), 3–18. https://doi.org/10.1097/01.chi.0000145374.45992.c9
18. Shim, R. S., & Vinson, S. Y. (2021). *Social (In)justice and mental health*. American Psychiatric Association Publishing.
19. Sroufe, A. L., Duggal, S., Weinfield, N., & Carlson, E. (2000). Relationships, development, and psychopathology. In A. J. Sameroff, M. Lewis, & S. M. Miller (Eds.), *Handbook of developmental psychopathology* (2nd ed.). Kluwer Academic/Plenum Publishers.

20 The Effects of Culture and Society

Key concepts

Traditionally, psychodynamic organizing ideas about development have focused on the influence of the immediate environment (i.e., primary caregivers and family) on the development of a person's conscious and unconscious mind.

The Ecological Systems model (Bronfenbrenner, 1977) is an organizing idea that suggests that human development is influenced by many different social environments. These include:

- The immediate environment or **microsystem**
- The community environment, or **mesosystem**
- The society at large, or **macrosystem**

The macrosystem includes structural systems of privilege/advantage and oppression/disadvantage based on race, gender, sexual orientation, gender identity and gender expression, physical and mental ability, age, class, religion, and indigenous status (Hays, 2016).

In people who are disadvantaged by the structures of society, patterns such as mistrust, self-hatred, shame, otherness, and anger may be linked to the effects of those systems.

In people who are advantaged by the structures of the society, patterns such as entitlement and fragility may be linked to the effects of those systems.

Linking to the effects of culture and society involves collaboratively understanding the way that structures related to privilege and disadvantage/oppression have shaped a person's lived experience. They should be considered in the psychodynamic formulations of all patients.

It stands to reason that

- If your society wants to kill you, you may become afraid and mistrustful
- If your culture calls you loathsome, you may feel othered and self-hating
- If laws and policies keep you from power and resources, you may become angry

Psychodynamic Formulation: An Expanded Approach, First Edition. The Psychodynamic Formulation Collective.
© 2022 John Wiley & Sons Ltd. Published 2022 by John Wiley & Sons Ltd.

Thus, when we think about how people develop, we must factor in the impact of culture and society's "economic, social, education, legal and political systems" (Bronfenbrenner, 1977, p. 515). This chapter offers conceptual ways to incorporate the effects of culture and society into our psychodynamic formulations.

Basics of psychodynamics and the ecological systems model

Over the years, researchers who study human development have increasingly understood that culture and society influence development in myriad ways throughout life. In the 1970s, Bronfenbrenner outlined the ecological systems model to help explain these broader, lifelong effects. This model, which we introduced in Chapter 1 and in the Introduction to Part 3, posits that there are three major social environments that affect development:

1. The **microsystem** is "the complex of relations between the developing person and environment in an immediate setting containing that person (e.g., home, school, workplace, etc.)" (Bronfenbrenner, 1977, p. 514).

   Example: A child grows up feeling "less than" after a sibling was overtly favored by their parents.

This effect originated in the child's immediate environment—his family—and is thus a microsystem effect.

2. The **mesosystem** "comprises the interrelations among major settings containing the developing person at a particular point in his or her life. Thus, for an American 12-year-old, the mesosystem typically encompasses interactions among family, school, and peer group; for some children, it might also include church, camp, or workplace. . ." (Bronfenbrenner, 1977, p. 515).

   Example: A devout member of a religious organization feels excluded and with diminished support after being shunned for deciding to become a single parent.

This effect originated in this person's local community, and thus can be considered a mesosystem effect.

3. The **macrosystem comprises** "the overarching institutional patterns of the culture or subculture, such as the economic, social, educational, legal, and political systems, of which micro [and] mesosystems . . . are the concrete manifestations. Macrosystems are conceived and examined not only in structural terms, but as carriers of information and ideology that, both explicitly and implicitly, endow meaning and motivation to particular agencies, social networks, roles, activities, and their interrelations" (Bronfenbrenner, 1977, p. 515).

   Example: An African-American man living in the United States might understandably feel unsafe when walking alone in predominantly White neighborhoods. He finds that he feels safer if he whistles classical music, trying to signal to White people that he is culturally assimilated.

This kind of situation has its basis in the structures of society at large, and thus can be considered a macrosystem effect.

The hierarchies of society

What we think of as the "structures" of the macrosystem include the explicit and implicit systems of domination, privilege, and advantage that exist in society. Many of these systems are **hierarchical**, enabling those few at the top of the hierarchy to have the majority of the resources/privilege/power, while the rest of the group has less or none at all (Moane, 2011). In this model, one group is dominant, and the rest are dominated. We can consider these systems using the **ADDRESSING** framework (Hays, 2016):

- **A:** Age and generational influences
- **DD:** Developmental or other disability
- **R:** Religion
- **E:** Ethnicity or race
- **S:** Socio-economic status
- **S:** Sexuality
- **I:** Indigenous heritage
- **N:** Nation of origin
- **G:** Gender

These hierarchies affect us whether we are consciously aware of them or not, helping to shape the way we think about ourselves and others, and how we adapt to the vicissitudes of life. **Intersectionality** occurs when we are disadvantaged by more than one system of oppression (Crenshaw, 2017). Examples include people who are lesbian and Latinx, Black and undocumented, or female and disabled.

Systems of oppression and the maintenance of society's hierarchies

The hierarchies of society are maintained by the following means of control:

- Violence (e.g., murder, genocide, rape, female castration)
- Political exclusion (e.g., voting restrictions, inability to participate in government)
- Economic exploitation (e.g., slavery, poverty, lack of a minimum wage, inadequate social services such as health insurance and education)
- Cultural control (e.g., control of educational systems, inability to practice religion or speak a native language, propaganda)
- Control of sexuality (e.g., bans on contraception and abortion, sodomy laws, prostitution)
- Fragmentation (e.g., ghettoization) (Moane, 2011).

Because these means of control are often oppressive, these hierarchical structures have been called **systems of oppression**. The Smithsonian defines systems of oppression as:

> *The combination of prejudice and institutional power which creates a system that discriminates against some groups (often called 'target groups') and benefits other groups*

(often called 'dominant groups'). These systems enable dominant groups to exert control over target groups by limiting their rights, freedom, and access to basic resources such as health care, education, employment, and housing (National Museum of African American History and Culture, 2020).

Systems of oppression create a hierarchy of in-groups and out-groups (e.g., White/of color, male/female, cis/trans, young/old, rich/poor) in which one group is treated as the socially desirable one, and the other as a less desirable alternative, or even suspect, alien, or **other**. Being the other is not neutral but negative and less than. Those of us in advantaged in-groups may be unaware of, unreflective about, or even vehemently opposed to the idea that being part of an in-group has positively advantaged us in life. Those of us in disadvantaged out-groups are often extremely and constantly aware of the ongoing effects of discrimination, marginalization, and being disadvantaged relative to others in daily life, and of the daily microaggressions directed at us because of our perceived status.

Implicit bias and the transmission of cultural and societal effects

When we internalize the hierarchical attitudes of society, they become automatic attitudes defined as **implicit bias** (FitzGerald & Hurst, 2017). Systems of oppression are often unconsciously transmitted from generation to generation via implicit bias (Banaji & Greenwald, 2016). Examples of implicit bias include unconsciously associating Blacks and weapons, or boys and science, despite a conscious understanding of the prejudicial and irrational basis of such associations.

Societal hierarchies can also be transmitted from generation to generation consciously and intentionally. By internalizing the verbal and nonverbal attitudes of their parents, children can be indoctrinated to hate and fear others who are unlike them or who are othered by their parents from earliest life. Studies indicate that children begin to develop implicit bias about traits such as skin color as early as six months of age (Winkler, 2009).

Social determinants of mental health and societal hierarchies

Because economic exploitation and cultural control are two of the means by which society's hierarchies are maintained, the **social determinants of health**, defined as the "conditions in which people are born, grow, live, work and age" (World Health Organization, 2008), are mediated by the individual's relationship to these structures. Advantaged children reap the benefits (e.g., money, power, resources) of being born into privilege, while disadvantaged children suffer from lack of resources and the chronic stress and strain of their caregivers (Shim & Compton, 2015). Being in a disadvantaged or othered group can affect access to basic needs like food, medical care, and parental attention, all of which are known to affect cognitive and emotional development (Compton & Shim, 2015). Preliminary data supports that a mother's exposure to discrimination when pregnant may affect her children's brain development (Sonderlund et al., 2021). Early impact may also depend on whether the caregiver and children belong to the same advantaged or disadvantaged group.

For example, an immigrant child raised by immigrant parents will have a different experience of systems of oppression than will an LGBTQ+ child born to a family of straight individuals. Belonging to the same disadvantaged group as one's caregivers could offer support, or could compound stress and strain.

Basic ideas about how culture and society affects psychological development throughout life

During development, people become aware of society's hierarchies implicitly as bias, and explicitly as prejudice, discrimination, and privilege. The means by which these hierarchies are maintained (e.g., discrimination, violence, war, poverty, political disenfranchisement) affect every member of society. Researchers in the fields of critical race theory, feminist theory, colonial oppression, LGBTQ+ mental health, and ableism as well as others have proposed various mechanisms by which the implicit and explicit transmission of society's hierarchies of dominance affect our psychological development throughout life.

Younger children may be consciously unaware of these systems, but may experience their impact in the form of lack of access to economic/societal resources and chronic stress/strain. At the same time, they may be absorbing parental and societal attitudes toward themselves and other groups through the transmission of their parents' implicit and explicit biases.

Once they venture out of the home to attend school, children consciously and unconsciously absorb and internalize the rules of the macrosystem. These internalized rules can affect many domains of psychological function, such as sense of self, relationships with others, and adaptation to stress. Hypotheses about how this happens (Christian et al., 2021; Edwards & Hanley, 2021; Moane, 2011; Shim & Compton, 2015), including the minority stress model (Meyer, 1995), suggest the following as potential psychological mechanisms:

- **Internalization** of the culture's negative attitudes toward the individual or individual's minority group, leading to self-hatred and self-doubt as well as hatred and devaluation of others in the dominated group
- **Isolation** from the individual's culture and history and from other parts of society, leading to difficulty with identity formation and otherness
- **Inhibition of expression** of personal needs, of aspects of the self, and of negative feelings, leading to difficulties with relationships and intimacy
- **Stigma and trauma** related to discrimination and violence, leading to mistrust and fear
- **Decreased access to money, resources, and power**, leading to poor mental and physical health, developmental delays, and compounded stigma

Moane (2011) suggests the internalization of systems of oppression disconnects the disadvantaged individual from their history and culture, diminishing their sense of self and affecting self-esteem and identity formation. This, in turn, affects behavior and mood regulation. Thinking of oneself as belonging to a group perceived as inferior sets the stage for self-esteem issues in the form of self-hatred and shame.

For those advantaged by society's hierarchies, internalization of the culture's positive attitudes toward the individual and expectation of access can lead to conscious and unconscious feelings of entitlement and superiority, which may manifest in patterns of behavior, such as entitlement or self-esteem fragility.

Linking problems and patterns to the effects of culture and society

Being disadvantaged by the hierarchical structures of society can affect all aspects of function, including every dimension of mental life. Thus, any conscious or unconscious pattern in a person who has suffered (or who continues to suffer) from discrimination can be linked to the impact of society's hierarchies. We can use the mechanisms of impact proposed above to link problems and patterns to the effects of culture and society. Several patterns may particularly suggest this linkage:

Self-experience

Sense of inferiority, self-doubt and shame

> You were born into a society which spelled out with brutal clarity, and in as many ways as possible, that you were a worthless human being (Baldwin, 1963, p. 7).

When the sense that one is worthless is internalized, the effect can devastate self-esteem. The **feeling of being less than,** as well as **self-hatred** of one's nondominant qualities, can affect identity formation and self-esteem as well as relationships with others. This can take the form of self-hatred, depression, self-inflicted physical or emotional punishment, or masochistic/submissive behavior (Moane, 2011). For example, consider Paula:

> Paula, who is 40 years old, consults a therapist for stress at work. "I'm just not cut out to be a manager," she explains. "I'm letting everyone down all the time." Although she says that she was recently promoted, she says, "They just don't know. I'm not doing enough for my family either." When asked about her early life, Paula says that she emigrated with her parents to the United States from El Salvador when she was 4 years old. "My parents had a visa at first, but then we just stayed. We had no papers until I had finished college. My mother cleaned houses, and my father did odd jobs. They are proud of me, but they still can barely speak English. I lived my whole childhood in the shadows, afraid of being sent home. I always felt like all eyes were on me—like I was a criminal."

Having internalized society's suspicion of and anger at undocumented immigrants, Paula was unable to develop a sense of self that matched her talents.

Embodying traits that are deemed negative by the dominant group can also lead to **shame**. Aspects of the self that are sometimes not readily apparent by looking at someone (e.g., sexual orientation, gender identity) may be experienced as parts of the self that need to remain hidden lest they trigger dislike, discrimination, or rejection from family, peers, or one's community (Drescher, 1998). Aspects of the self that are readily apparent by looking at someone (e.g., race, physical ability, gender atypicality in childhood) may feel like they are always on display such that one's other qualities can never be seen. This can inhibit self-expression, affecting both sense of self and the ability to enter into and maintain intimate relationships with others.

> *Todd, a 45-year-old trans man, presents with depression and difficulty with relationships. "Hormones saved my life," he tells the therapist. "They made me feel alive. But even with a beard, I still feel like it's a costume. Where I'm from, I was just a weird girl. I watched the boys play on the field and just wanted to run out to them and say 'I'm here!' My parents were always worried about me—they just didn't know how to help. How could I tell them? When kids danced at a party, I cringed—I could barely move my body and I sure didn't want anyone to see me doing it. Now, I barely know who I am—how can I share that with someone else?"*

Todd's inability to live as a man until his 40s inhibited his capacity for self expression, leaving him depressed, unsure of his own identity, and unable to form relationships with others.

Entitlement or sense of superiority

Developing in a culture in which a person or a person's group is advantaged may result in a sense of **entitlement** or **superiority**.

> *Driving over the speed limit when late for a therapy appointment, a White cisgender woman was stopped by a policeman. "I never have problems with the cops," she cheerfully told her therapist. "A White woman with a 'soccer mom' bumper sticker? They never give me a ticket!"*

Fragility

When members of advantaged groups feel that they are not getting what they have come to expect, this is sometimes called **fragility** (e.g., White fragility) (Diangelo, 2018):

> *A White cisgender heterosexual man sought therapy for depression after his son was rejected from his alma mater. "My family has gone to that school for generations," he told the therapist. "Half the buildings are named for my uncle—they could never have built them if not for us. I've given so much money for scholarships there; it feels like such a slap in the face for them not to admit my own son—particularly when we would pay full tuition."*

Relationships with others

Otherness

Being **othered** is an active societal sorting process and an alienating experience in which a person is made to feel less than the mainstream representative. People are often othered for traits outside of their control, such as being trans, queer, female, of color, differently abled, overweight, or older. Being the other is negative, not neutral.

Clinically, this can manifest as isolation, loneliness, feeling different or alien, or not feeling understood:

> Carly, a 40-year-old African-American high school teacher, tells her therapist, "All my friends would tell you that they love me and that I 'fit in.' But all these years later—all those years of being in classrooms with mostly White kids and mostly White teachers, of not being invited to birthday parties, of surprising the guidance counselor when I got into good schools—I still don't just sit down at a table with other teachers without being invited. I'm sure they don't even know it's happening."

The gay teen who is teased and who avoids social events, the child of color who sits alone in the cafeteria, or the young adult who wears a backbrace for scoliosis, may grow up and often continue to feel othered as adults—often unbeknownst to those around them.

Fear and mistrust

> And I am afraid. I feel the fear most acutely whenever you leave me, But I was afraid long before you, and in this I was unoriginal. When I was your age the only people I knew were Black, and all of them were powerfully, adamantly, dangerously afraid. I had seen this fear all my young life, though I had not always recognized it as such (Coates, 2015 p. 14).

Many disadvantaged people are afraid all the time. They have fear of being killed, bullied, shunned, shamed, harmed, discriminated against, exploited, and trapped. It is natural and adaptive that this fear breeds **mistrust**. When the origin of disadvantage is apparent (e.g., color, sexuality), people may feel that they are wearing a target on their back. When it is hidden, people may feel that one false move may lead to exposure and catastrophe. These experiences can lead to fear and mistrust of others and an inability to be open with oneself and one's thoughts and feelings. As we discussed in Chapter 7, individuals can develop trust within their immediate family (microsystem) but have general mistrust as the result of their membership in a marginalized group. This is essential to consider when trying to understand trust and lack of trust in adult patients.

Adaptating

Anger and indignation

> Aggression leaps from wounds inflicted and ambitions spiked. It grows out of oppression and capricious cruelty. It is logical and predictable if we know the soil from which it comes. People bear all they can and, if required, bear even more. But if they are [B]lack in present-day America they have been asked to shoulder too much. They have had all they can stand. They will be harried no more. Turning from their tormentors, they are filled with rage (Grier & Cobbs, 1968, pp. 3–4).

Both single and repetitive experiences of being unfairly treated and discriminated against can lead to feelings of **anger** and **indignation**. This understandable and adaptive response can be channeled into assertiveness, empowerment, and activism (Edwards & Hanley, 2021) but can also manifest as self-criticism, depression, interpersonal aggression, or violence. For example, a patient whose family had been held at a country's border for months might become enraged every time they have to show their ID when they enter the clinic. This anger can also be directed at people from the same disadvantaged group. When this occurs, it is sometimes called **lateral violence** (Maracle, 1996).

A sample formulation—linking to the effects of culture and society

Presentation

Ronni is a 35-year-old biracial lesbian woman who seeks psychotherapy with a White lesbian therapist, saying, "My girlfriend broke up with me. I don't know how to be emotionally intimate with her." Ronni noted that she has always been mistrustful of others in a way that kept her from developing "really deep" relationships, in which she felt that she could reveal her "true thoughts and feelings." She felt this also happened in her two prior psychotherapies, in which she says she "did not feel fully understood." She states she always feels that she does not belong anywhere and that this makes her feel depressed and "empty" inside.

Ronni is very successful at her tech job and has many friends and acquaintances from work who like her "hip and cool" self-presentation, and the fact that she's always the first one tuned into emerging new music. She feels at home and freer in underground clubs and lesbian bars where she says she can "lose myself in the music and just dance." Despite an active social life with friends from work and the clubs, each romantic relationship seems to end in the same way—women are drawn to her but ultimately leave when she is unable to open up sexually and emotionally. "It's like I reach a wall, beyond which I can't really talk to them, and I'm more comfortable working more or watching TV. Then I start to dread that they want me to go deeper and I feel trapped and freaked out, which shuts me down even more." When asked about her initial responses to her new White therapist, she states, "Well, at least you're lesbian. I'm desperate to get better and find a partner who can tolerate me and to be able to have kids someday—I don't want to be so alone. We'll see how it goes."

DESCRIBE the problems and patterns

Ronni fears and **mistrusts** *others, feeling they will not understand her. This prevents her from fully revealing herself to both friends and lovers, interfering with her capacity for intimacy. She also has* **feelings of inferiority** *because she has trouble believing that someone who really knows her will like and accept her fully if she does reveal herself wholly to them. Her strong* **feelings of otherness** *about both her sexuality and her biracial background make her feel she doesn't belong and that people won't understand or accept her. She has a* **sense of shame about who she is***, which is relieved only when she can lose the pervasive sense of otherness by blending into the anonymous and mixed crowd while dancing in a club. At best, she feels she may find a partner who "tolerates" her and a therapist with some overlap in her identity who may at least partially understand her experience.*

REVIEW the life story

Ronni is the only child of an older White father and a mother of Afro-Caribbean descent. Ronni's mother immigrated to the United States for college where she met Ronni's father at a coffee bar: Ronni's father, an executive at a computer company, was getting coffee and her mother was working as a barista. Ronni's mother had a history of abuse and neglect, had experienced food insecurity as a child, and had moved frequently when her family could not afford rent. Ronni remembers her mother as being "disorganized," says she never saw her parents being intimate with one another, and felt that her father treated her mother "like the help." Her parents rarely socialized with other families, and she believes that her mother may have been depressed. Growing up in an affluent, predominantly White suburban town, Ronni was one of a small group of people of color in her class. Identifying as "neither White nor Black, "she felt unable to fit into any group. She was embarrassed to invite friends to what she called her "curry-infested" house, and she was increasingly mistrustful that peers would reject her. When it was time to apply to college, she found her mother and father unable to help her, and she felt her college counselors advised her to "aim too low." She also found her parents unable to help her navigate problems at school or advocate on her behalf when it came time to apply to colleges, and she felt it was racist that her college counselors advised her to apply to lesser schools than she should have. She became aware that she was lesbian when, in high school, she developed a crush on a female peer from her soccer team. This added to her sense of inferiority and otherness, and she hid her interest in women for another decade.

LINK the history and problems/patterns to the effects of culture and society

Ronni's difficulty in intimate relationships and in creating deep friendships may be related to having been treated as the other in multiple ways—her status as an only child, having little family or community interaction, being biracial in an overwhelmingly White town and school, and realizing that she was gay. This sense of otherness may have been internalized, resulting in a feeling of alienation and difference that was not a neutral state of mind, but one that made her feel inferior in comparison to others around her. For their own reasons, her parents may not have been able to connect fully to one another or to their daughter as well, leaving her no model for what an intimate relationship looked or felt like. As a biracial couple in a White suburban enclave, her parents may have experienced discrimination as well, and this may also have contributed to Ronni's internalized sense of inferiority and shame.

Linking to the effects of culture and society guides treatment

Understanding the relationship between a patient's problems/patterns and the effects of culture and society is crucial for creating a formulation and planning treatment. Patients can benefit enormously from being able to discuss their painful experiences of otherness, difference, discrimination, and mistrust with an empathic, nonjudgmental mental health professional who can validate the impact of powerful hierarchies. Developing an atmosphere of safety and trust also requires that clinicians be sensitive to the possibility that patients may feel that therapists cannot or do not want to understand these experiences.

As therapists, we can strive to communicate our appreciation of the effects of culture and society, while not assuming we fully understand them. This requires careful self-reflection, both for those of us from in-groups as well as for those of us from outgroups. Our ability to convey that our patients' experiences of systemic oppression are difficult, unacceptable, and powerful is critical as our patients attempt to feel more deserving of better treatment and as they experience rage and indignation. Collaboratively creating formulations that incorporate ideas about the effects of culture and society can help our patients to feel seen and to better understand how their interactions with the world have affected every aspect of their mental lives.

Suggested activity

Can be done by individual learners or in a classroom setting

How might you describe the ways in which Norma and Scott have been affected by culture and society?

> *Norma, a 47-year-old African-American woman, comes to the attention of the clinic director after refusing to work with the third therapist to whom she was assigned. "They are all idiots," explains Norma. "They think that they are so smart, with all those diplomas on their walls, but they don't know about life. I know about life. I don't need someone to nod at me and hand me a tissue. I need someone to help me get a job. Can they help me get a job?" Norma had been working as a nurse's aide but was recently fired. "Insubordination is what they said," she tells the clinic director. "But I know racism when I see it." After being fired, she had trouble sleeping and was sent to the clinic by her internist. "I've had the same story my whole life. My father left, my mother died young, and I had to raise myself and my sister. No one helped me then, and no one will help me now."*

Norma's life experience as a woman of color and of lower socio-economic status in the United States may have led to her feeling that she is perennially disadvantaged and unable to be helped. This may have contributed to her **anger** and frustration as well to her expectation that she will not be helped or understood. Left alone at a young age to fend for herself and her sister, Norma may also have an avoidant attachment style that may contribute to her difficulty connecting to people who could offer her help.

> *Scott, a 65-year-old White cisgender heterosexual man who was born in the United States, has no disabilities, and owns a consulting firm, presents with depression. He comes at the suggestion of his wife. "She says I'm hard to live with," he reports. "What does she expect?" He says that when he was in college he thought, "the world would be my oyster," but "it hasn't turned out that way." "My dad's generation had it all," he laments. "After they came back from the war, the world just rolled out the red carpet for them. I hardly ever saw my dad—he was always out with his army buddies or golfing at the club. He had a great life." Scott is disappointed in his profession, feeling that he works very hard for "money that will never put me at the top," and says, "There is so much paperwork. It's not why I went to B-school." Although he says he is "fond" of his wife, he wishes she was more interested in entertaining. She, too, works, which means that he has to do more around the house. "We both work hard," he says, "but we'd have to work much harder to have the help we need to really enjoy ourselves when we are off."*

Scott may have a sense of **entitlement**; that is, he may feel that he should be able to "have it all" because of his inclusion in several traditionally dominant groups (e.g., White people, cisgender males, heterosexuals, abled individuals). Although his seemingly **fragile** sense of self may have been contributed to by parental neglect, it is also likely that this may connect to his sense that he is not having the life he was raised to expect.

References

1. Baldwin, J. (1963). *The fire next time*. Dial Press.
2. Banaji, M. R., & Greenwald, A. G. (2016). *Blindspot: Hidden biases of good people*. Bantam Books.
3. Bronfenbrenner, U. (1977). Toward an experimental ecology of human development. *American Psychologist, 32*(7), 513–531. https://doi.org/10.1037/0003-066x.32.7.513
4. Christian, L. M., Cole, S. W., McDade, T., Pachankis, J. E., Morgan, E., Strahm, A. M., & Kamp Dush, C. M. (2021). A biopsychosocial framework for understanding sexual and gender minority health: A call for action. *Neuroscience & Biobehavioral Reviews, 129*, 107–116. https://doi.org/10.1016/j.neubiorev.2021.06.004
5. Coates, T. (2015). *Between the world and me*. One World.
6. Compton, M. T., & Shim, R. S. (Eds.) (2015). *The social determinants of mental health*. American Psychiatric Association Publishing.
7. Crenshaw, K. W. (2017). *On intersectionality: Essential writings*. The New Press.
8. Diangelo, R. (2018). *White fragility*. Beacon Press.
9. Drescher, J. (1998). *Psychoanalytic therapy and the gay man*. Routledge.
10. Edwards, L. L., & Hanley, S. M. (2021). Scale of internalized trans oppression: Measure development and exploratory factor analysis. *Contemporary Family Therapy, 43*(2), 124–139. https://doi.org/10.1007/s10591-020-09564-4
11. FitzGerald, C., & Hurst, S. (2017). Implicit bias in healthcare professionals: A systematic review. *BMC Medical Ethics, 18*(1). https://doi.org/10.1186/s12910-017-0179-8
12. Grier, W. H., & Cobbs, P. M. (1968). *Black rage*. Basic Books.
13. Hays, P. A. (2016). *Addressing cultural complexities in counseling and clinical practice* (3rd ed.). American Psychological Association.
14. Maracle, L. (1996). *I am woman: A native perspective on sociology and feminism*. Press Gang Publishers.
15. Meyer, I. H. (1995). Minority stress and mental health in gay men. *Journal of Health and Social Behavior, 36*(1), 38. https://doi.org/10.2307/2137286
16. Moane, G. (2011). *Gender and colonialism: A psychological analysis of oppression and liberation*. Palgrave.
17. National Museum of African American History and Culture. (2020, June 2). Talking about race. Retrieved November 13, 2021, from https://nmaahc.si.edu/learn/talking-about-race. https://nmaahc.si.edu/learn/talking-about-race/topics/social-identities-and-systems-oppression.
18. Shim, R. S., & Compton, M. T. (2015). Social injustice and the social determinants of mental health. In R. S. Shim & S. Y. Vinson (Eds.), *Social (In)justice and mental health*. American Psychiatric Association Publishing.
19. Sonderlund, A. L., Schoenthaler, A., & Thilsing, T. (2021). The association between maternal experiences of interpersonal discrimination and adverse birth outcomes: A systematic review of the evidence. *International Journal of Environmental Research and Public Health, 18*(4), 1465–1496. https://doi.org/10.3390/ijerph18041465
20. Winkler, E. N. (2009). *Children are not colorblind: How young children learn race*. Retrieved November 13, 2021, from https://inclusions.org/wp-content/uploads/2017/11/Children-are-Not-Colorblind.pdf.
21. World Health Organization. (2008). *Closing the gap in a generation: Health equity through action on the Social Determinants of health - final report of the Commission on Social Determinants of Health*. World Health Organization. Retrieved November 13, 2021, from https://www.who.int/publications-detail-redirect/WHO-IER-CSDH-08.1.

21 Conflict and Defense

Key concepts

An organizing idea about development, called **ego psychology**, suggests that adult problems and patterns can be LINKED to unconscious conflicts and defenses.

According to this idea, unconscious conflict happens when opposing thoughts, feelings, or wishes collide. This conflict, which is out of awareness, causes anxiety, prompting us to use defenses to work out compromises. These compromises result in our characteristic problems and patterns.

Linking the development of problems and patterns to unconscious conflicts and defenses is particularly useful for understanding difficulties related to

- Feeling "stuck"
- Inhibited function
- Difficulties with commitment and sexual intimacy

Picture this: You're a sophomore in college, it's Saturday at 5 p.m., and all your friends are going to a party. You'd love to go, but you know that you have tons of work to do before Monday. What do you do? Part of you feels you need a break after a long week, but another part feels obligated to start that stack of homework. You waffle back and forth, and finally decide to stay home. Once your friends have left the dorm, you sit down at your desk to begin. Before you start, though, you decide to clean your desk. Then your desk looks so clean in comparison to the mess around it, you decide to clean the whole room. While you're doing that, you find a note that your friend from high school called, so you call your friend back, talk for a while, make yourself a sandwich, and by the time you sit down again it's 11:30 p.m. and you haven't done any work! What happened?

Conflict and compromise

What happened to you on that Saturday night is that you were conflicted. Part of you wanted to go out to have fun, and part of you felt you should stay home to do your work. These two parts were in **conflict** (Auchincloss & Samberg, 2012; Cabaniss et al., 2017). Although you thought you had made a choice, the battle continued without your conscious mind being able to see it, and your mind forged a **compromise**

Psychodynamic Formulation: An Expanded Approach, First Edition. The Psychodynamic Formulation Collective.
© 2022 John Wiley & Sons Ltd. Published 2022 by John Wiley & Sons Ltd.

(Cabaniss et al., 2017). The compromise was that you stayed home (partially satisfying the part of your mind that felt obligated to do homework), but you didn't do any work (partially satisfying the part of your mind that wanted to relax after a long week). All of this happened out of awareness, so we call it **unconscious conflict** (Auchincloss & Samberg, 2012; Cabaniss et al., 2017; Kris, 2012). One way of thinking about the way the mind works and develops, called **ego psychology**, suggests that conflicts like this one occur constantly and underlie the way we think, feel, and behave.

Basics of ego psychology

Conflict → Anxiety → Defense

The idea that problems and patterns can be linked to unconscious conflict was originally conceptualized by Freud (Freud, 1923/1990). Freud first thought that the conflict was between *two* parts of the mind: the conscious part and the unconscious part. He called this idea the **topographic model** because it suggested that the conscious mind was "on top of" the unconscious mind (Mitchell & Black, 1996). According to this theory, problems arise when unconscious thoughts and feelings are prevented from reaching consciousness, generally because they are deemed too painful to tolerate. Freud soon realized, however, that conflict could exist between two parts of the mind that are *both* unconscious. This led him to a second theory, which he called the **structural model**, that describes the mind in terms of structures rather than locations (Mitchell & Black, 1996). Freud did not think of these structures as literally anatomical; rather he thought of them as clusters of functions. They are the id, the ego, and the superego. According to this model:

- The **id** represents wishes and feelings that are unconscious because they tend to make people uncomfortable (e.g., anxious, ashamed, or angry). Consequently, they are repressed—that is, they are kept out of awareness.

- The **ego** represents the executive function of the mind—the mediator among the id, superego, and reality. Ego functions include reality testing, defense mechanisms, and the capacity to conceptualize self and other (Cabaniss et al., 2017).

- The **superego** represents the conscience and the ego ideal (i.e., the way people like to see themselves, which includes positive values such as honesty, loyalty, etc.).

The structural model suggests that these parts of the mind are in constant conflict with one another and with reality. Wishes, in the form of unconscious fantasy, are in conflict with the superego, or with reality. Most of this conflict is unconscious (i.e., out of awareness), but it nevertheless affects the individual's conscious life. In this model, unconscious conflict between or among these structures causes **anxiety**, which the ego tries to protect the person from experiencing. We can call this protection **defense** (Cabaniss et al., 2017). Defenses are the unconscious and automatic ways the mind adapts to stress (see Chapter 8). They are the coping mechanisms and internal compromises that limit a person's awareness of painful feelings like anxiety, depression, and envy, and that resolve emotional conflicts.

Compromises and defenses—costs and benefits

In our example of the college sophomore, defenses try to partially satisfy each side of a conflict. The resulting thought, feeling, or behavior is thus a compromise. And, like defenses, some compromises offer more benefit and less cost than others (see Chapter 8).

For example, consider a teenager who is very angry at their controlling, successful older sibling, and who, during this time, takes up karate, becomes a black belt, and feels very accomplished. This person's unconscious conflict might look something like this:

I'm so angry I could kill my sibling.	vs.	It would be wrong to hurt my sibling.

This conflict causes anxiety, which the ego protects against using a defense—in this case, **sublimation** (Auchincloss & Samberg, 2012). Sublimation enables someone to gratify an uncomfortable wish or feeling by doing something useful or socially acceptable. By becoming interested in martial arts, the teenager partially gratifies the wish to attack the sibling by fighting with other people in a controlled way, while abiding by the prohibition against actual violence toward the sibling. The teenager feels good about the accomplishment, doesn't hurt anyone, and thus this defense is, in the balance, beneficial.

Now consider the conflict of a person who had a very physically abusive parent. As an adult, this person continues to idealize the parent, assumes blame in relationships, and tolerates bad treatment from others. This person's unconscious conflict might look like this:

I love my parent and need to feel that they are taking care of me.	vs.	I am angry because my parent is abusive and not taking care of me.

Again, this conflict causes anxiety, which triggers the ego into action. Here, the ego uses a defense called **splitting**, which preserves good feelings about one person by completely devaluing another. Because this child needed the abusive parent, they idealized the parent and devalued themself. This is a compromise that "worked" in childhood because it enabled the person to avoid thinking about the abuse and to lead as normal a life as possible. However, what worked in childhood became problematic in adulthood, leading to unsatisfying relationships and poor self-esteem (see Chapter 8 for more on defenses).

Linking problems and patterns to conflict and defense

When might we choose to link problems and patterns to conflict and defense? This model can be very useful when people feel stuck, when they inhibit themselves, and when they have difficulty with commitment.

Being "stuck"

People often come to therapists because they feel stuck. They might feel stuck in a relationship, in a job, or in a decision. To them, things feel like nothing is moving, and that there is no way to change the situation or make a decision. Very often, the feeling of "stuckness" has to do with conflict. When forces are pulling in equal and opposite directions, it's as if there's no movement, but, in reality, it's an incredibly dynamic situation. Often, we can hear the conflict in the way the person describes the "stuck" situation:

> I've been stuck in this job for too long. I should probably leave, but the pay is too good. I don't know, maybe it's just me. Maybe I'm the problem. But then I think about my boss—I just can't stand him. I don't know. I end up doing nothing.

We can hear the back and forth of the conflict—one part of this person hates the job, while another is afraid to leave the pay and structure. The resulting defenses are self-blame and a lack of action. This kind of problem is often very well understood in terms of conflict and defense.

Inhibited function

Thinking about the mind in terms of conflict and defense generally presumes that people **have** capacities that they defensively inhibit. These could be anything, including but not limited to, athletic/artistic/academic ability, assertiveness, and competitiveness. This kind of inhibition can often be well understood using a conflict/defense model. Consider a person who wants to do really well at work but is afraid their success will make others jealous and angry. The fear that doing well could be dangerous prompts them to inhibit their ambition. One way to think about this is that some children struggle between the wish to do better than their parents did, and the fear that this will cause them to lose their parents' love. This is an unconscious conflict. If it is not resolved in childhood, it may persist into adulthood, causing adults to experience anxiety when they are competitive or assertive.

Difficulties with commitment and sexual intimacy

Conflicts resulting from the three-person relationships (child and two caregivers) of middle childhood can also be useful in terms of understanding adult difficulties with intimacy. As we discussed in Chapter 14, some children may long for closeness with a desired caregiver while fearing punishment for this wish from a rival caregiver. Again, this is a conflict. Getting too close to the desired caregiver may thus cause anxiety, which can persist into adulthood when the person gets close to a romantic or sexual partner. Consider the child of divorced parents whose desired caregiver takes the child to dinner parties in lieu of a partner. While potentially exciting for the child, this situation is also likely to cause anxiety. As an adult, this person might become anxious when more casual dating threatens to become exclusive.

A sample formulation—linking to conflict and defense

A formulation using ego psychology hypothesizes that problems and patterns are linked to unconscious conflicts and defenses. The following is an example:

Presentation

> Ahmet is a 28-year-old man who identifies as heterosexual. He was born in the United States, but his parents were born in Turkey. He presents for treatment saying that recently he has been delaying doing important work projects. Although he is generally able to get his work done on time, when it comes to the big presentations he "freezes up." He is acutely aware of this because he is coming up for a major review that could affect his potential for promotion. He is frustrated with this behavior and would like to change it but does not know how.

DESCRIBE the problem and patterns

> Ahmet reports that he has had a long-standing **problem with procrastination**, particularly when the stakes are high. He is generally very **competent and organized**—he loves biking and routinely takes his bicycle for tune-ups, pays his taxes by the deadline, and arranges complicated vacations. He has a good job that is well matched to his level of education, which he enjoys. He has a **secure relationship** with his partner and has several intimate friendships. He generally uses **defenses that tend to keep emotions conscious and repress thoughts**, and, as above, he uses avoidance as a major adaptive strategy during periods of stress.

REVIEW the life story

> Ahmet recalls having a close and warm early relationship with his mother. He says that his father loved him as well; however, he felt that his father's esteem was much more contingent on performance. "He praised me when I did well, but was really critical and sort of withdrew from me when I didn't do spectacularly." He felt that his father devalued his mother for not being "as smart as we are," and he somewhat guiltily reports that he was favored by his father over his younger sister, who excelled in sports but not academics. Ahmet says that he recalls having a happy childhood and that he had many friends. He was an avid reader and enjoyed math in elementary school. He was eager to please teachers and did not use drugs or alcohol. However, once the pressure of high school and college acceptance felt real to him, he began to have difficulty completing schoolwork. Ahmet wanted to date in high school, but his father felt it would be a distraction. Despite excellent scores on standardized testing, his grades dropped, and he matriculated at a community college before transferring to a state university. His father was disappointed as many other kids in their Turkish-American community matriculated at the university right after high school. He remains close to both parents—his father often wants to have lunch to discuss Ahmet's future career.

LINK the life story and problems/patterns to conflict and defense

> Ahmet's problems with procrastination seem circumscribed. He is able to plan ahead and has considerable intellectual talents. Thus, he has abilities that he seems to be inhibiting, perhaps because of unconscious conflicts and defenses. We can hypothesize that Ahmet, who felt well loved by his parents, had secure dyadic relationships and was able to learn to trust. However, he felt that his

father's esteem for him was in danger if he did not excel. Thus, he may have developed an uncon-scious conflict that was something like this:

I want to excel and do well to receive praise from my father.	vs.	I want to avoid situations in which I could fail, because this could mean loss of my father's love and esteem.

When Ahmet is in situations in which he fears that he could fail—like his senior year in high school and now in his job—this conflict produces anxiety. The anxiety leads to a high-cost defense—avoidance. While he consciously thinks that he wants to move forward, he unconsciously prevents himself from actually doing the work because he fears that he might fail. Although this enables him to avoid the anxiety that these situations create, it also puts him in danger of sabotaging himself despite his considerable talents.

Linking to unconscious conflict and defense guides treatment

If we suggest to our patients that their problems and patterns are linked to uncon-scious conflicts and defenses, we need to help them find more beneficial, less costly ways of reconciling these conflicts and defending against anxiety. We can do this in two basic ways. If they have the ability to tolerate strong affects and are relatively self-reflective, we can help them to become consciously aware of conflicts and defenses that are giving them difficulty. We call this **uncovering** (Cabaniss et al., 2017). On the other hand, if they cannot tolerate strong affects and are unable to self-reflect, we can help them to shift adaptive strategies without becoming aware of their uncon-scious conflicts and defenses. We call this **supporting**. We briefly review these tech-niques here; please refer to *Psychodynamic Psychotherapy: A Clinical Manual* for a more in-depth discussion of these techniques.

Uncovering

Just because a conflict is unconscious does not mean that it disappears. On the con-trary, it continues to exert its effect on the way a person thinks, feels, and behaves. However, if it is out of awareness, the person cannot use their logical, conscious, adult mind to forge the compromise. Instead, a compromise is formed out of aware-ness, based on thoughts and fears that may have originated in childhood. One of Freud's original ideas about treatment was that it was important to "make the uncon-scious conscious" in order to allow the conscious mind to grapple with the conflict, and to create more adaptive solutions. In therapy, we do this by having patients say whatever comes to mind (known as **free association**) in order to enable unconscious thoughts and feelings to become conscious. Once an unconscious fantasy comes to light, and is viewed from an adult perspective, it can be seen as a holdover from childhood and may cease to feel so frightening. A good analogy is the item in a dark bedroom that looks like an intruder but is revealed to be a hat on a chair when the light is turned on—making things conscious helps us to view them in a more realistic way. Consider the person who requires an operation but who, at the last minute, becomes terrified and won't sign the consent form. After spending some time talking about this fear with a therapist, the person remembers being scared during an overnight stay at a hospital after their parents went home. Once this is uncovered, the person is able to go through with the procedure.

Supporting

When we use techniques to support, we are supporting someone who, for one reason or another, is using defenses that are less beneficial than they could be. This could be the result of a chronic problem, such as the persistent effects of early childhood abuse or a severe mental illness, or an acute problem, such as a recent loss or a sudden medical problem. In these situations, we do not try to make the unconscious conflicts and defenses conscious; rather, we try to support the use of more beneficial defenses while decreasing the use of less beneficial defenses. For example, a person might present after almost getting into an altercation with their primary care provider, saying, "It took them four hours to call in that prescription—so irresponsible! If I'd been able to become a doctor, rather than having to take care of my parents, I would have done better than that." We might suspect that a conflict about thwarted ambition might be at the root of this anger, but because the person is having trouble regulating emotions, supporting techniques, such as thinking together about strategies for managing anger, might be more helpful at this moment than uncovering the conflict.

Suggested activity

Can be done by individual learners or in a classroom setting

What unconscious conflicts might be affecting Stephan?

Stephan is a 32-year-old single banker who has been dating Tina, a 31-year-old teacher, for 5 years. Although he feels that he is "in love" and that he wants to spend his life with Tina, he does not feel ready to get married. Tina, who comes from a large family, would like to have several children and feels she's ready to begin. Stephan feels troubled by his inability to commit and presents for therapy to try to understand this issue. He reports that he is from a wealthy family and enjoys spending time at his family's summer home where he frequently goes sailing with his brothers. The brothers also enjoy their yearly camping trips and weekly poker games, at which they are often joined by their father. Stephan has recently been offered a promotion at work, which would offer him the ability to support a family independently, but he is concerned that this might "trap" him in a lifestyle and leave him little ability to make a career change in a few years.

Comment

Stephan says that he wants to spend his life with Tina but does not feel ready for marriage. In addition, he's not sure why he's having difficulty making this commitment. This suggests that one or more unconscious conflicts could be causing him to feel 'stuck.' His closeness to his brothers and family suggests that this could be involved. Here is one conflict that could be operating:

I want to be a grown-up man and start a family of my own.	vs.	I want to remain as a child with my parents and brothers.

This conflict is suggested by Stephan's continued attachment to his brothers and parents. Perhaps the closeness in this family makes it difficult for Stephan to assume a role as father in a family of his own because the gratifications of being "one of the brothers"'is so enormous. Here is another conflict that could be affecting him:

I want to spend my life with another person.	vs.	I want to remain independent.

This way of thinking about Stephan's conflict emphasizes his conflicting wishes about personal autonomy and is suggested by his recent decision at work. Both could be operating simultaneously, making it difficult for Stephan to move forward in his life.

References

1. Auchincloss, E. L., & Samberg, E. (Eds.) (2012). *Psychoanalytic terms and concepts*. Yale University Press.
2. Cabaniss, D. L., Cherry, S., Douglas, C. J., & Schwartz, A. (2017). *Psychodynamic psychotherapy: A clinical manual*. Wiley-Blackwell.
3. Freud, S. (1990). The ego and the id. In J. Strachey (Ed.), *The standard edition of the complete psychological works of Sigmund Freud, Volume XIX (1923–1925): The ego and the id and other works*. W.W. Norton. (Original publication in 1923).
4. Kris, A. O. (2012). Unconscious processes. In G. O. Gabbard, B. E. Litowitz, & P. Williams (Eds.), *Textbook of psychoanalysis*. American Psychiatric Publishing, Inc.
5. Mitchell, S. A., & Black, M. J. (1996). *Freud and beyond: A History of modern psychoanalytic thought*. Basic Books.

22 Relationships with Others

Key Concepts

Another organizing idea about development LINKS problems and patterns to the unconscious repetition of early relationships. These relationships could be with people in the immediate home environment, the extended community, or society at large.

Linking to conscious and unconscious relationship templates is particularly useful for understanding problems that adults have in forming relationships, including:

- Global problems involving trust in their work and personal lives (microsystem)
- Circumscribed problems involving unrealistic expectations of others (mesosystem)
- Difficulties that arise in the context of being mistreated in society (macrosystem)

We do not live in vacuums—we live with others. Everything we do is affected by the people around us, from our earliest development (see Chapters 13 and 14) to our later relationships. It's hard to imagine, then, trying to explain human development without taking into consideration relationships with others—both in terms of our actual relationships and the way we think about or remember those relationships. Feelings of love and anger, for example, seem inseparable from the people to whom they are directed. Many psychoanalysts after Freud began to incorporate this view. Their ideas formed the basis of several theories. **Object relations theory** focuses primarily on early life relationships in the immediate home environment. **Interpersonal theory** addresses relationships throughout the life cycle, both inside and outside one's home, in the broader community, and society at large (Sullivan, 1953a, 1953b). **Social psychologists** have also made an important contribution to the way that we understand the influence of relationships in all social spheres on the developing person (see Chapters 1 and 20) (Bronfenbrenner, 1977).

To begin to think about this, let's consider Cynthia:

> *Cynthia, a Chinese-American woman, who was born in the United States and who works in public relations, had just reached the bus after running six blocks in high heels. Breathlessly, she reaches into her purse to get her prepaid transportation card and realizes she left it at home. Finding only a $10 bill, she asks the driver if he has change. He does not. She quickly scans the other passengers on the bus; to her, none appears to be of Asian descent. They all stare at her blankly, offering no help.*

Psychodynamic Formulation: An Expanded Approach, First Edition. The Psychodynamic Formulation Collective.
© 2022 John Wiley & Sons Ltd. Published 2022 by John Wiley & Sons Ltd.

She is enraged and throws her $10 at the driver, curses, and takes her seat. Later that day, Cynthia feels ashamed about the morning episode and anxious about who might have seen her behave this way. She realizes that having had this kind of outburst throughout her life has sometimes led to bad outcomes, for example, in high school when she had to stay for detention after cursing at a teacher, and recently, when her boyfriend broke up with her after an argument that got out of hand.

Why does Cynthia have difficulty managing her temper? She clearly struggles with her anger, and this might be rooted in conflict. But could it be related to expectations stemming from early relationships, her cultural background, and/or her experience in the broader society? Let's explore ways to conceptualize her difficulty as stemming from her experiences of relationships in her immediate, community and broader environments.

Basics of models about relationships

Object relations theory—relationships in the immediate environment

In the 1940s, a group of analysts including Fairbairn, Winnicott, Baliant, Bowlby, Jacobsen, and Guntrip developed a set of theories later called **object relations theory**. This theory, which builds on concepts initially developed by Melanie Klein, suggests that early interactions with important caregivers help shape the way we come to think, feel, and behave (Fonagy & Target, 2003; Kernberg, 1995). These early relationship experiences are **internalized** and exist in the individual's unconscious as they mature. Internalization is the process by which people take in their experiences throughout development and make them part of themselves. Internalization of experience occurs throughout the life cycle and, as people get older, is more often called **identification** (Auchincloss & Samberg, 2012). Internalized representations of people's earliest relationships become basic **templates** for relationships that affect all subsequent experiences with others.

Object relations theorists focus on the templates that form around children's relationships with their primary caregivers—those people in their **immediate environment**. In most situations, children develop positive relationship templates when caregivers fulfill their needs and negative relationship templates when their needs go unfulfilled (Kernberg, 1992). Children can develop both positive and negative templates about the same caregiver.

Internal relationship 1: Need-fulfilling

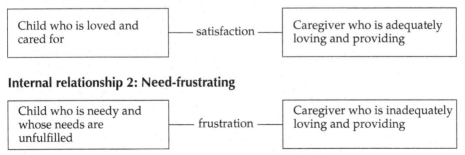

Internal relationship 2: Need-frustrating

If children are more often satisfied than frustrated in their relationships with early caregivers, they tend to learn to trust others and to develop healthy, balanced expectations of future relationships (Winnicott, 1953). On the other hand, if they are predominantly frustrated, children may have difficulty learning to trust others and may develop problematic expectations of future relationships (see Chapter 7). For example, they may come to expect that they will be mistreated or neglected. These expectations, although unconscious, may continue to operate in their adult relationships—even if the here and now situation does not warrant such concerns.

As we have mentioned, children may feel predominantly frustrated by their caregivers either because of the caregivers' limitations, or because of a poor match between what the child needs and what the caregiver can offer. For example, a temperamentally difficult-to-satisfy infant may struggle with a well-meaning caregiver. Alternatively, a resilient infant may thrive despite a caregiver's limitations.

To explore the way early templates can affect adult relationships, let's return to Cynthia, who became upset on the bus. Reviewing her life story, we learn that when she was 2 years old, her mother became depressed after a miscarriage. Using the lens of object relations theory to think about her relationships with people in her immediate environment, we can hypothesize that Cynthia had unmet needs during that time, leading to unconscious anger. Here's how we might depict that template:

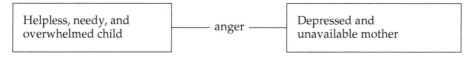

When Cynthia is frustrated as an adult, as she was on the bus, she expects that the people around her (like her mother) will be unavailable and unhelpful. This makes her angry and leads her to behave in a way that might be more appropriate for a frustrated child than for an adult in public. Conceptualizing her outburst in this way helps us to think about how Cynthia's early experience with a depressed mother may have influenced her ability to manage disappointment in her adult life.

For another example, think of Jane, who works for a bank and is responsible for collecting late mortgage payments. When Jane was a teenager, her mother had terminal cancer. Later in life, Jane wished she had spent more time with her mother before she died, rather than remaining focused on her social life. Currently, Jane is struggling at her job because she has a hard time collecting payments from people in hardship, especially when medical problems are involved. Using object relations theory, we wonder if her problem collecting mortgage debt is related to an early template of her relationship with her mother, in which she depicts herself as selfish and inattentive. This idea about herself in relation to her mother makes her feel guilty:

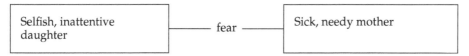

We can then hypothesize that this unconscious template is activated when she has to collect mortgage payments from struggling people—she feels too guilty and is unable to function well in her job. This idea helps us to connect her early experience in her immediate environment to the development of her current problems and patterns at work.

Interpersonal theory and contributions from social psychology—relationships in the community and society at large

Relationship templates can also be based on experiences with people outside the home including teachers, peers, and the community at large. **Interpersonal theory**, developed by analysts including Harry Stack Sullivan, suggests that our relationships are affected by both the early and later social environments in which we live (Sullivan, 1953). For example, the feeling of **otherness** or **outsiderness** in relationships often stems from experiences that occur in the context of our communities (Kanwal, 2020).

Now let's think again about Cynthia, considering her relationships in her community and society at large. When the non-Asian passengers on the bus stare blankly at her rather than offering assistance, she is offended, and her frustration and helplessness expands to include feeling **othered**. While her early experience of neglect by her depressed mother may have played a role in triggering her outrage, the catalyst may also be related to her experiences with people outside of her immediate environment. We may learn, for example, that Cynthia is aware that Asian Americans have been verbally and physically attacked based on erroneous, racist assertions that they spread the coronavirus. This awareness is deeply distressing to her and has put her on edge. She noted that neither the bus driver nor any of the passengers were Asian that morning, and felt othered and vulnerable when no one offered her help. This resonated with her parents' stories of prejudice after first arriving in New York, and with her memories of being taunted upon entering a mostly White private middle school. At the same time, the value her family and culture place on keeping negative emotions private may have exacerbated her shame at becoming publicly angry. Here's how we might depict that template:

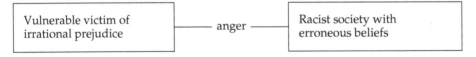

Relationship patterns are multidimensional

Everyone's mind has a wide range of relationship templates. Most are not problematic and are seamlessly integrated into the way we think about ourselves and others in daily life. Templates generally cause problems when they are derived from painful or confusing experiences. One can have positive, need-fulfilling experiences within the home *and* negative, need-frustrating experiences outside of the home. These negative experiences, which can be in the community (e.g., difficulty with peer groups) or in society at large (e.g., structural racism) may cause difficulties with trust, anger, poor self-esteem, and/or depression.

It's also important to remember that we can experience ourselves in either role of a relationship template. In terms of the early relationships of object relations theory, sometimes we feel like the child, and other times we feel like the caregiver (Bollas, 1987). One way to look at this is that, as children, we identify with our caregivers and others in our environment. For example, the mortgage collector we discussed above might sometimes feel like the selfish child and at other times like the needy parent. When she has children of her own, she may identify with her mother and feel angry and neglected when her children exhibit age-appropriate selfishness.

In the broader social context, outsiderness can lead to chronic feelings of isolation, denial of one's origins, and distancing from one's past. For example:

> Byron is a 25-year-old African-American man who grew up in an inner-city housing project and sought treatment for feelings of emptiness and depression. When he was growing up, his mother did in-home childcare, and his father was employed intermittently in construction. While money was often tight, his parents valued education as a means to advance, and spent what they had to support Byron's schooling. In high school, Byron was awarded an academic scholarship to attend a private university. When he arrived there, he felt like an outsider. While there was some racial diversity at the school, he struggled to purchase supplies, books, clothes, and fund the social activities in which his fellow students participated. He ultimately joined the African-American student organization where he found some new friends. He felt ashamed of his class background and took on extra work-study jobs to earn the extra cash he needed. By the start of sophomore year, he felt he had overcome these hurdles, but started to resent having to see his family during breaks, choosing instead to visit the homes of his new friends or staying in the dorm. He felt ashamed of his parents and distanced himself from them, preferring the new identity he was creating for himself. He was often lonely.

Byron alternates between two different relationship templates. When he arrives at college, he experiences significant economic stress and feels like an **outsider** based on these disparities:

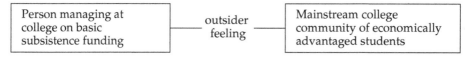

| Person managing at college on basic subsistence funding | outsider feeling | Mainstream college community of economically advantaged students |

Once he gains comfort in his new environment, he distances himself from his family in reaction to both having struggled to fit in and his shame about his class origins. To protect his new feeling of belonging, he keeps his family on the outside. Rather than being *othered*, he does the *othering*. However, this relationship template, in an effort to solve one problem, leaves him feeling empty and depressed, as he is left disconnected from a central part of his identity and his parents.

Linking problems and patterns to relationships with others

Linking problems and patterns to relationship templates is helpful when trying to understand both global and more circumscribed problems with relationships.

Global relationship problems involving problematic relationships from the child's immediate environment

People who, as children, developed problematic relationship templates in their immediate environment, often have tremendous difficulty trusting people in their adult lives. Consider Curtis:

> Curtis is a middle-aged man who has never had a significant love relationship and avoids intimacy by working late hours and weekends. His parents divorced when he was a young boy, and he lived with his mother, a self-involved person who engaged him in helping her dress-up for dates, then left him alone while she went out. Now, when he tries to date online, he experiences all women as self-centered. "They view me as a 'sperm machine,'" he says. "All they care about is becoming pregnant."

Curtis may have difficulty with intimacy and dependency because his earliest relationships have led him to expect little from others. Here is a way to depict one of his relationship templates:

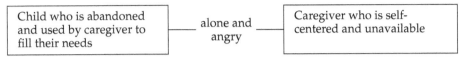

We can hypothesize that this relationship template becomes activated when Curtis meets women, leading him to expect that they will be self-centered and exploitative. This way of linking his difficulties to his early relationship with his mother helps us to understand his current problems and to plan therapy.

More circumscribed relationship problems involving relationships from the community and broader society

People who have already attained **object constancy** (see Chapter 13) and have more balanced views of themselves and other people are less likely to grossly distort interpersonal experiences. Nevertheless, they may still suffer when they have unrealistic expectations of themselves and others, which are often based on templates from relationships in the community and beyond. For example, consider Edward:

> *Edward is generally very content with his work and his family life and tends to be a stable, reliable partner. When his father-in-law developed a terminal illness, his husband, Niles, became preoccupied and unavailable. As the months wore on, Edward felt angry with Niles, but was unable to express these feelings because, as he said, "what he is doing is understandable." He felt ashamed that he couldn't just be a better partner and put his needs aside. Edward has a younger brother who had childhood leukemia. His whole community knew about his brother's health struggles, and teachers at school would often ask Edward about his brother's condition. He would dutifully respond and communicate with the outside world on his family's behalf and patiently took on his brother's chores around the house during his illness. Edward recalled with pride that he was praised for being so independent, well behaved, and "grown up."*

Edward has a well-integrated sense of himself and his important early caregivers. However, although he has attained object constancy, during the period of his brother's illness he may have developed a relationship template related to the expectation that he prematurely behave like an adult both within his immediate family and in the broader environment of school and his local community:

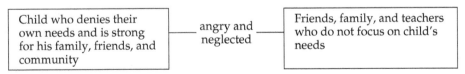

This template, including the feeling of anger toward his parents, teachers, and members of his local community, remained out of awareness while Edward was aware only of his wish to help his family and to be his brother's spokesperson. Now, in his adult life, the similarity of the situation activates this template, causing him to be angry with Niles as if Niles were one of his distracted parents or a teacher focused only on the sick person. Using relationship templates, we can make the link between the feelings Edward had as a young child and his current marriage difficulties. This may offer him the opportunity to see that just because his husband is caring for his father does not mean that he will neglect Edward. It may also help Edward to alter his expectations of others and become more able to ask for what he needs, even when people have competing priorities.

A sample formulation—linking to relationships with others

Formulating links to relationships with others means explaining problems and patterns by tracing them to relationships in the person's immediate, community, and broader environments. Consider Deena:

Presentation

Deena, who is 29-years-old, presents with difficulty in her relationship with her boyfriend of six months. She says that he threatened to break up with her after finding out she had had sex with a male coworker. "I don't even know why I did it," she says. "But after a few months, I always start to feel dissatisfied with the guy I'm with." She says that this also happens in jobs, and that she has had as many as 10 jobs in the past 2 years. She says that the timing is "ironic" because she and her boyfriend had just started to talk about moving in together. "I don't think that he's really in it for the long haul—guys never are." She has few friends and, in the first session, asks if the therapist gives out her home phone number. "My last shrink didn't—what was I supposed to do at midnight after a fight?"

DESCRIBE the problem and patterns

*Deena's greatest area of difficulty is in her **relationships with others**. She **does not trust** others, and she creates situations in which others cannot trust her. Her **relationships are not secure**, and she frequently ends them prematurely. These patterns are global in that they affect her romantic relationships, her friendships, and her work situations. It is even evident in the early relationship with the therapist.*

REVIEW the life story

Deena is the younger of two children born to parents who misused heroin. Her mother died of an overdose when Deena was 2 years old, leaving her in the care of her father. She says that she is not sure whether her mother was misusing drugs while she was pregnant. Her brother, who is 4 years older, corroborates that the two children were left alone—often overnight—when Deena was as young as 3 years old. She depended on her brother but says that he was "wild" and that, beginning when she was about 6 years old, her brother would occasionally get into bed with her and touch her breasts. Deena did well academically but was shunned by others in her extended community who, knowing her parent's difficulties, feared that she would be a bad influence on their children. In school, Deena was exposed to negative images of "drug abusers," reinforced by judgmental stereotypes about people who had drug problems in the media. Her father finally stopped misusing drugs when she was in high school, but he then became depressed and had difficulties maintaining a job. As soon as he was eligible, her brother left home to join the army. Deena often found solace in "hooking up" with boys from her neighborhood, "I knew that they didn't really care, but it felt good to be next to someone." She ultimately finished college and became a social worker to "try to help kids who grew up the way I did," but she has drifted from placement to placement, generally due to interpersonal difficulties with her coworkers.

LINK the life story and problems/patterns to relationships with others

Deena's current difficulties with other people may be related to her earliest relationships. In her immediate home environment, her parents' active misuse of substances may have interfered with her care from birth. Her life story is filled with abandonment, neglect, and abuse.

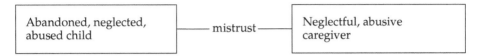

Deena may have an early template in which she expects to be abandoned and abused by people with whom she has relationships. To survive, she has not allowed herself to trust other people, including her romantic partners, friends, and people with whom she works. The closer she comes to imagining that she could trust someone, the more anxious she becomes, which prompts her to rupture relationships, leading to more instability.

Deena's troubled relationship templates also extend to the community and broader society. Isolated by the parents of her peers, she learned not to expect support from her community. And taught by society to be ashamed of her parents, she felt othered and alone.

Linking to relationships with others guides treatment

Linking problems and patterns to relationships with others in the immediate, community, and society at large suggests that our work should involve helping people to identify their problematic templates, understand the origins of those templates, and develop new templates that are more personally beneficial. As we discussed in Chapter 13, children who suffer from abuse and neglect often have trouble achieving object constancy and may adapt by using **splitting** in order to maintain positive images of problematic early caregivers. Object relations theory and interpersonal theory suggest that people will reactivate their relationship templates in their relationship with the therapist (**transference**), which can then be interpreted back to, and understood by, the patient. As people become more aware of their problematic relationship templates in the transference, and, over time experience the constancy of a new object (i.e., the therapist), they often improve their ability to tolerate more ambivalent connections to people. Through this process in therapy, they can develop more complex, nuanced images of important early caregivers and people throughout their lives. As this occurs, the need for splitting may decrease and object constancy improve (Caligor et al., 2007).

In addition to insight, psychodynamic psychotherapy provides a new relationship—the relationship with the therapist. This new relationship can provide the basis for new, more trusting and secure relationship templates (Loewald, 2000). To see how this technique can work, let's first consider Cecelia:

Cecilia is a 30-year-old Latinx publicist who, as a child, was yelled at and punished by her father when she didn't follow instructions. She tried to be perfect and lived in fear of triggering a disciplinary reaction from him. In high school, if a teacher was critical of her homework,

Cecilia trembled as if she were a helpless child about to be punished. She did well in high school and was admitted to a very competitive college, even though her SAT scores were in the lower range for that school. In college, Cecilia was anxious, checking things multiple times, and unable to sleep before exams. She feared that she was granted admission to round out the school's diversity. Now, at work, she still cannot relax and has anxiety attacks before quarterly reviews, thinking that she is about to be fired.

An important relationship pattern for Cecilia may be of an abusive, critical authority figure from both the immediate environment (i.e., family) and her community environment (i.e., school), and an insecure, vulnerable child. These two images are connected by an affect—fear. Cecilia internalized this relationship template and alternately identifies herself as either a frightened child or an aggressive authority:

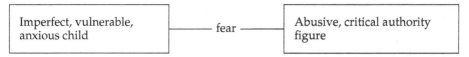

This fundamental template may be activated when relationships resonate with any of these components, even if they are not the same as her early experience. Her self-esteem was additionally challenged at college where she interpreted the largely White university's public mission to recruit students of color as a sign that she was admitted because she was Latinx, rather than because of the strength of her academic work. Similar experiences were exacerbated at work, where she had a demanding boss and a company that also valued diversity. Here's how this could be addressed in treatment:

In therapy, Cecilia was always careful to get everything right in sessions and seemed anxious if she forgot to pay a bill on time or arrived a few minutes late. Her White male therapist noticed this and commented to Cecelia that she acted like she expected him to get angry with her for these minor issues. Over time, Cecelia realized that she had an expectation of her therapist that was based on an early relationship template—she was behaving as if he were a punitive, abusive authority figure. Cecilia then realized that she was also having the same reaction to her boss, who was also a White man. This insight enabled her to rethink whether her boss was really critical, or whether she was just experiencing him as if he were a parent and she were still a helpless child. She began to understand that their adult work relationship had room for constructive criticism and was not actually punitive. She began to experiment with communicating to her boss how she felt about his critiques, and became able to discuss with him which points she thought were warranted and which ones were not. In addition, she learned how to negotiate with the therapist to rearrange her session times when necessary, and to relax when she needed to pay her bills a few days late. She was also able to speak about what the differences in their cultural background meant to her, and to speak more openly about her experiences of racism in college.

These interactions led to the internalization of new relationship templates for Cecilia, ones characterized by more understanding authorities. In object relations and interpersonal theory, the new experience with the therapist is a large part of what is therapeutic.

Suggested activity

Can be done by individual learners or in a classroom setting

What relationship templates might be operating in these people?

> *Phoebe is a 51-year-old single woman who is "always there" for her friends. She'll babysit for their children, pick up groceries for them, and spend endless hours on the phone listening to them complain about their husbands. Recently, she had a colonoscopy. When she arrived, the receptionist asked who would be available to take her home. "No one," she said, "They are all busy. I'll take a cab."*

> *Lawrence is a 45-year-old man who takes his husband out to an expensive restaurant for their wedding anniversary. They are shown to a table that is next to the restroom. He is noticeably disturbed and asks to see the maître d'. "You probably don't want your clientele to be uncomfortable seeing two guys celebrate their love for each other?" he says, raising his voice. "But our money is the same as theirs. I don't see why we can't sit at a good table."*

Comment

Phoebe is very available for others but feels that she cannot ask them for help. She could have a relationship template that looks like this:

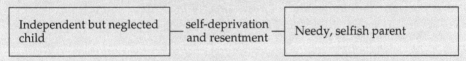

Lawrence assumes that he is being discriminated against. He could have a relationship template stemming from his experience as a gay man in a homophobic society that looks like this:

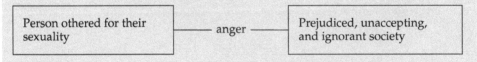

References

1. Auchincloss, E., & Samberg, E. (2012). *Psychoanalytic terms and concepts* (p. 107). American Psychoanalytic Association.
2. Bollas, C. (1987). *The shadow of the object*. Columbia University Press.
3. Bronfenbrenner, U. (1977). Toward an experimental ecology of human development. *American Psychologist, 32*(7), 513–531. https://doi.org/10.1037/0003-066x.32.7.513
4. Caligor, E., Kernberg, O., & Clarkin, J. (2007). *Handbook of dynamic psychotherapy for higher level personality pathology*. American Psychiatric Publishing.
5. Fonagy, P., & Target, M. (2003). *Psychoanalytic theories: Perspectives from developmental psychology*. Brunner-Routledge.
6. Kanwal, G. S. (2020). Outsiderness: A meditation in six visions. *Contemporary Psychoanalysis, 56*(2–3), 330–342. https://doi.org/10.1080/00107530.2020.1756722
7. Kernberg, O. (1992). *Aggression in personality disorders and perversions*. Yale University Press.
8. Kernberg, O. (1995). Psychoanalytic object relations theories. In B. E. Moore & B. D. Fine (Eds.), *Psychoanalysis: The major concepts* (pp. 450–462). Yale University Press.
9. Loewald, H.W. (2000). On the therapeutic action of psychoanslysis. In H.W. Loewald (Ed.), The Essential Loewald Collected Papers and Monographs (pp. 221–256). University Publishing Group. (Originally published in 1960).
10. Sullivan, H. S. (1953a). *The interpersonal theory of psychiatry*. Norton.
11. Sullivan, H. S. (1953b). *Conceptions of modern psychiatry*. Norton.
12. Winnicott, D. (1953). Transitional objects and transitional phenomena. *International Journal of Psychoanalysis, 34*, 89–87.

23 The Development of the Self

Key concepts

Theories about the development of the self also serve as organizing ideas about development to which we can LINK problems and patterns to the development of the self.

Self psychology, an organizing idea about development, suggests that early caregivers perform functions that are essential for the child's development of the self. Called **selfobject functions**, these are experienced by the child as part of the self. They are:

- **Mirroring**—the caregiver's empathic ability to reflect the child's abilities and internal states
- **Idealization**—the caregiver's ability to be idealized by the child

We can also link problems and patterns to self-development that occurs throughout life, particularly when related to being a member of a minority group.

Linking problems and patterns to the development of the self is particularly helpful when constructing formulations for patients who have problems with

- Self-esteem regulation
- Empathy and envy

For centuries, philosophers have pondered the question of how to define the self. We think of the self as the essential attributes of a person that are relatively stable over time, and that make a person unique (Auchincloss & Samberg, 2012). If we have

- a coherent sense of who we are, how we feel about ourselves, and our likes, dislikes, abilities, and limitations, and
- a generally positive sense of self-esteem, characterized by an acceptance of our positive and negative qualities and the capacity to maintain good feelings about ourselves in a variety of contexts, including adversity or criticism from others

then our function in all other domains (e.g., relationships, adapting, cognition, values, work/play, etc.) is likely to be generally more beneficial and satisfying to us.

Psychodynamic Formulation: An Expanded Approach, First Edition. The Psychodynamic Formulation Collective.
© 2022 John Wiley & Sons Ltd. Published 2022 by John Wiley & Sons Ltd.

Cultural variations in ideas about the self

When linking to ideas about development of the self, it is important to consider that psychoanalytic theories about the self are influenced by the cultural context in which they developed (i.e., mid- to late-twentieth century Western European and American culture) (Frie, 2013). For example, this culture may place a higher value on the notion of the self as autonomous and independent than do other cultures, which may view the self as more interdependent on family or a larger social group (Markus & Kitayama, 1991, 2010). It is helpful for us to consider these cultural variations about what constitutes a cohesive authentic self when we formulate collaboratively with our patients.

Basics of models related to self-development

Self psychology

Heinz Kohut, a psychoanalyst who worked in Chicago in the 1960s and 1970s, developed a model of psychological development, which focused on the emerging sense of self and that came to be known as **self psychology**. As with object relations theory, self psychology focuses on the effect of early relationships on development, particularly the way in which parenting fosters the development of a coherent and vital sense of self. It is primarily a theory about the child's immediate environment—specifically, the early caregivers. The center of this model is that the development of the self depends on empathic caregiving. Empathic caregivers are able to accurately sense what their children are thinking and feeling, demonstrate their understanding of these thoughts and feelings, and respond in an affectively attuned and developmentally appropriate way. This is called **mirroring**. This theory also suggests that children need to **idealize** their caregivers to feel strong, good, and safe. In addition to mirroring and idealization, self psychology suggests that **grandiosity** in childhood is essential for the development of healthy self-esteem, and that this must be allowed and encouraged by caregivers (Kohut, 1971, 1978; Mitchell & Black, 1995). Grandiosity includes intense feelings like being powerful, special, or beautiful. Empathic caregivers acknowledge and reflect these feelings back to the child in age-appropriate ways.

Selfobjects

Kohut coined the term **selfobject** (Kohut, 1971, 1978; Mitchell & Black, 1995) to describe critical caregiver functions that young children experience as not completely separate from themselves. Children use selfobjects, such as parents or other caregivers, to regulate their self-esteem and emotional states, as in this example:

> *A 3-year-old girl is playing "house" with her mother. She tells her mother to play the role of the little girl while she plays the mother, and instructs her mother very specifically about everything she is to do and say. The mother complies cheerfully, and in her role as "baby," tells the "mother" how nice and pretty she is. The little girl, imitating her mother's voice, says, "I'm the best mommy in the world."*

In this example, the mother responds empathically to her daughter's age-appropriate wishes to play with, idealize, and control her. The little girl's identification with her mother, whom she feels is "the best," makes her feel strong and powerful, and helps her to build her own sense of self. In addition, the mother's mirroring of the pride her daughter feels helps the little girl to develop self-esteem.

Conversely, children who grow up with caregivers who are preoccupied or distracted, struggling with mental health issues, or psychologically unable to empathize with the emotional states and needs of their young children, may have trouble developing healthy self-esteem. Parents with their own self-esteem deficits may have trouble encouraging or tolerating their child's idealization of them, interfering with the child's developing sense of self. This might occur due to problems in their own early relationships with caregivers, or due to problems in the broader environment (e.g., traumatic stress, systemic oppression, or discrimination).

Similarly, children with caregivers who fail to help them understand their limitations may grow up to have an unrealistically grandiose sense of self that is overly vulnerable to the ordinary slings and arrows of life. Consider this example:

> A 5-year-old boy runs into the house, yelling that he is a superhero who has just beaten the villains in a game of tag. He bumps into a table and knocks a vase full of flowers onto the ground, spattering water and bits of pottery everywhere. His father storms into the room, yelling, "Look at the mess you made! Why can't you watch where you're going? Some superhero you are—if you have special powers, let me see you put that vase back together again! I thought so; you can't do it."

Here, the father does not respond empathically either to his son's need to feel joyful, powerful, and special (playing the role of a superhero), or to the developmentally common occurrence of knocking something over by accident. He is angry with his son and treats him in a humiliating way, teasing him about not having special powers. We can hypothesize that if the father typically treats his son this way, the boy may be at risk for not being able to feel adequately strong and powerful.

Sometimes, mirroring overestimates a child's abilities. For example:

> A 9-year-old girl tries out for the school musical. Although she has never performed before, or taken singing or acting lessons, her parents tell her, "You're the best singer and actress in the whole school, and if they don't cast you in the lead role they're idiots." One of her classmates, who has been studying singing and acting for several years, gets the lead part. The girl, sobbing, tells her parents how unfair it all is. Her parents say, "You should quit the play, that director is incompetent. We'll call the principal to complain."

Here, the parents communicate unrealistic expectations to their daughter. When she does not meet them, they blame the director rather than helping her to understand the role that experience and practice play in achievement. In this way, they hinder her ability to assess her capabilities and limitations in a more realistic way. We can hypothesize that this girl is at risk for developing a falsely elevated sense of self, which may crumble in the face of frustrations, leading to rage and an externalization of blame.

Each of these examples are isolated incidents—even the most empathic and patient caregivers will occasionally get frustrated or lose their temper. Situations like these are likely to have pervasive and enduring effects only if they represent frequent and typical ways in which caregivers interact with their children. In fact, self psychology asserts that all caregivers will, at some point, fail to respond empathically to their children, *and* that this failure is actually necessary for development. When this **empathic failure** happens, in an age-appropriate and not exaggerated way, children learn to **internalize their caregivers' selfobject function**. This is important for helping them learn to buoy their self-esteem, and to realistically assess their capabilities and limitations.

Winnicott

Another important contributor to psychodynamic theories about the self was Donald Winnicott, a British pediatrician and psychoanalyst. Like Kohut, Winnicott emphasized the importance of the primary caregiver's role in mirroring the infant's experience and in providing a "holding environment" that enables the infant to experience a sense of safety and, temporarily, omnipotence (Winnicott, 1960). He was also concerned with the role of play and creativity in the development of an authentic or **true self** (Winnicott, 1971).

This true self reflects the individual's inherent potential, sense of personal continuity, and inner reality. Winnicott defined the **false self** as based on compliance with others' demands and projections (Winnicott, 1965), as illustrated in the following example:

> *Tobi, a 18 year old cisgender gay woman in her first year of college, joins an LGBTQ+ student group on campus. She makes several close friends, comes out to some relatives and childhood peers, and starts to dress and style her hair differently. As the end of the semester nears, she seeks therapy in the counseling center, feeling anxious about returning home for the holidays. She tells her therapist, "My mom and I have always been really close, but I never felt I could be my real self with her. She always wanted me to look and act like a girly girl and was obsessed with me having a boyfriend. I guess I always went along with it because I wanted her love and approval."*

Learning to embrace her sexuality, Tobi realizes the extent to which her sense of self was shaped by her mother's wishes.

Self development and lived experience

The development of self-esteem is thought to depend on inborn characteristics (e.g., resilience and optimism), on relationships with early caregivers, and on lived experience. The community environment (e.g., school, peer group, or neighborhood), as well as society at large, contribute to the development of the sense of self and self-esteem. Factors such as sexuality, racial and ethnic background, and immigration and disability status may affect the development of the aspects of self. For example, being a member of a minority group that is disfavored or discriminated against by the dominant group can adversely affect self-esteem (Akhtar, 2014; Eng & Han, 2000; Stoute, 2019), while feelings of membership in or identification with a larger community or group can bolster self-esteem (Aberson et al., 2000; Cameron, 2004; Layton, 2006; Moualeu, 2019; Woo et al., 2019).

Linking problems and patterns to the development of the self

Linking to the development of the self is most helpful when trying to understand problems related to self-esteem. In addition, difficulty in interpersonal relationships stemming from problems with empathy for or envy of others can be well understood using this idea about development.

Self-esteem regulation

Low self-esteem

Low self-esteem can be usefully understood using self psychology. Adults whose earliest caregivers did not recognize and acknowledge their abilities (i.e., mirroring) may underestimate their capacities and have difficulty feeling good about themselves. Such people may present for therapy with problems related to underachievement and difficulty in their interactions with others, such as being exquisitely sensitive to criticism, feeling easily blamed or attacked, or tending to castigate themselves. They are also often particularly prone to shame. For example, consider Teresa:

> Teresa is a 35-year old Guatemalan-American woman who seeks therapy for chronic low-grade depression and feelings of low self-esteem. She is single, lives alone, has few friends, and works as an administrator at a university—a job she describes as unsatisfying. Teresa says she had wanted to become an immigration lawyer, but didn't have the self-confidence to continue her schooling after community college. She explains, "I never could have competed with all those law students who are so sure of their opinions and not afraid to argue." In describing her social life, she says "I'm not that interesting or outgoing, so I guess that's why people don't want to date me or hang out with me." When the therapist gently points out how self-critical Teresa is, she says, "I'm just telling it like it is." Teresa's parents immigrated to the United States shortly before she was born, fleeing the violence of the civil war in Guatemala; they were undocumented for years before obtaining permanent resident status. She describes her mother, who worked in restaurants during Teresa's childhood, as frequently sad, tearful and nervous, suffering from nightmares and chronic headaches. When a high school guidance counselor suggested to Teresa's parents that her excellent grades could get her into an excellent college, Teresa's mother said, "Don't fill her head with that. I need her at home."

Teresa's difficulties with self-esteem may be linked to her experiences early in life with parents who, having experienced the multiple traumas of violence, immigration, and being undocumented, were likely unable to mirror their young daughter and appreciate her potential. Using self psychology, we might formulate that Teresa's underestimation of her talents and her lack of self-confidence are at least, in part, related to the reverberating impact of traumatic stress on her parents, and through them, on her.

Overly inflated, but fragile, self-esteem

As we've discussed, mirroring can be problematic if it underestimates *or* overestimates a child's abilities. People whose early caregivers overestimated their abilities may have a false sense of self that is outwardly overly inflated but inwardly extremely fragile. These people may seek help because they, like their caregivers, overestimate their abilities and then have trouble tolerating the disappointment of not attaining their goals. Although they may present as overly confident or arrogant, in the face of self-esteem threats they may quickly become anxious, enraged, or devastated. Patients with this type of problem may seek out others to bolster their self-esteem, and thus their relationships often seem shallow and manipulative. They may become easily discouraged when they can't achieve as much or perform as well as they believe they should. This may have happened to Leo:

> Leo, a 33-year-old White man, works as a journalist. He was recently passed over for an important assignment that was given to a junior colleague. Leo was referred to therapy by his internist whom Leo consulted, complaining of "heart palpitations." No cardiac abnormalities were found. Leo reports he feels anxious and angry much of the time. He says he is thinking of leaving the organization because the editors are "obviously idiots for thinking that guy is better than I am. He didn't go to journalism school like I did, and he can't write his way out of a box." He hopes one of his friends, another journalist whose family is "incredibly well connected," will land him a job at a prestigious newspaper. Leo tells the therapist, "My internist is one of the best doctors in the city—I only go to the best—so if he recommended you, then you must be tops."

When the therapist learns about Leo's life story, he finds that Leo is an only child whose father is a wealthy and influential businessman in his hometown. He describes his mother as a "social climber," and says that both parents were very focused on his academic and athletic achievements, showering him with praise when he performed well and contempt when he did not. Using self psychology, we could formulate that his parents' overemphasis on success prevented Leo from developing a realistic sense of himself and a healthy sense of self-esteem. Instead, he developed a fragile sense of self that is overly reliant on superficial markers of success and exquisitely vulnerable to self-esteem threats. His sense of self may also be influenced by his own expectations throughout life, related to his membership in several dominant groups (see Chapter 20).

Problems with empathy and envy

Children who fail to form a strong sense of self may have difficulty developing the capacity for empathy. As adults, they are often preoccupied with protecting their own fragile sense of self and are not attuned to the needs, experiences, or perspectives of others. This can be chronic, or may emerge only during periods of stress (e.g., medical illness or emotional distress). As we've discussed (see Chapters 6 and 7), this can lead to problems in relationships with others. Consider Clara:

> Clara is a 30-year-old woman with a 1-year-old daughter. She comes to therapy with the complaint that "having a child ruined my life." Clara says she no longer has any time to herself to relax, exercise, or socialize. She feels frustrated with and angry at her daughter much of the time, feeling that she is "too needy" and "spoiled." Clara doesn't understand how her friends with children have the patience to sit and play with them. Clara describes her own mother as "really narcissistic," noting that her mother rarely displayed much interest or pride in her.

Self psychology might suggest that growing up with inadequate mirroring, Clara developed a brittle, fragile sense of self, which limits her ability to think about the needs of others, including her child. Needing to offer empathic mirroring to her own child—something she did not receive—may be particularly challenging for her.

Envy can also be well understood using ideas about the development of the self. People who have a balanced but generally positive sense of themselves can tolerate the idea that others have things they lack. However, people who struggle with maintaining self-esteem are often threatened by what others have—possessions, abilities, or relationships. Envy (see Chapter 6) can be aggressive and destructive, and can make it difficult to have relationships with others. For example, consider Shintaro:

> Shintaro, a 24-year-old graduate student, immigrated to the United States from Japan for graduate school and is working in a basic science lab. Despite hard work, his investigations are slow moving and have not engendered much excitement at lab meetings. When his colleague's experiments result in an important discovery, he is publicly derisive of the colleague's results and starts rumors that the colleague "has no ideas of his own—his mentor does all the work." While most children in his community were raised in two-parent homes, Shintaro, whose father left the family when he was age 5, was raised by a single mother. Shintaro was teased by other children at school about this, leading to shame. Although he did not see his father for many years, Shintaro was aware that his father had remarried and lived with his new wife and two children. When he did see him as a teenager, his father bragged about his new family and told Shintaro that he should "take a tip on how to behave from your half-brothers."

Abandoned by his father, and later unfavorably compared to his father's new children, Shintaro likely struggled to consolidate a positive sense of self. He felt ashamed to have been raised by a single mother in his community. It is reasonable to imagine that he had nearly intolerable envy of the new children who had usurped his place with his father. Now, as an adult, he is similarly unable to tolerate the success of his "lab sibling," and his envy leads him to be aggressive in an effort to destroy his colleague's success.

A sample formulation—linking to the development of the self

Presentation

> Evan is a 35-year-old White cisgender gay man who works as a high school music teacher. He is anxious at work much of the time, feeling as if he is always "performing" for his students. He gets good evaluations from students and faculty, but struggles with not feeling good, smart, or funny enough. Although he believes that being a teacher is a "noble" profession, he wishes he had a higher paying, more prestigious job, and he is intensely envious of his friends and acquaintances who do. In his spare time, he plays guitar and harbors secret fantasies of forming a pop band and becoming famous.

DESCRIBE the problem and patterns

> Evan has frequent symptoms of anxiety and **chronic feelings of low self-esteem and envy** of others. He is not able to experience satisfaction at work, despite a belief in the value of his job and evidence that he does it well.

REVIEW the life story

Evan is the youngest of three children whose parents divorced when he was 2 years old. He describes his father, who had been in the military, as frequently depressed, and his mother as irritable and preoc-cupied. He remembers often feeling lonely as a child. His older sisters were outstanding students and very popular, and he felt he always lived in their shadow. His mother effusively praised him when he did well in school or at sports, but he feels "she wasn't really interested in who I was as a person." As a child, he did not spend a lot of time with his father, who wished that Evan would devote more time to sports and other more typically masculine activities. He remembers trying to "cheer him up" by singing or making jokes, which his father either ignored or reacted to "in a negative way." He also remembers when, at age 6, he told his father he wanted to be a musician, his father said, "Don't waste your life- you should think about joining the military like I did."

LINK the history and problems/patterns to the development of the self

Using self psychology, we can postulate that Evan did not have adequate selfobjects in childhood; his parents were not empathically attuned to him, and he was not able to idealize them. Consequently, he was unable to develop a robust sense of self. His efforts to idealize or enliven his father were met with dismissal or lack of response. He felt that neither parent could mirror his interest in music or performing. His father was also dismissive of him for not being interested in traditionally mascu-line pursuits. He felt outdone by his older sisters, and his mother seemed uninterested in his inner life and excessively praised only the achievements she valued. As an adult, he is unable to take appropriate pleasure or pride in himself and his work, feels chronically anxious about how he appears to others, and takes refuge in fantasies about difficult to attain goals.

Linking to the development of the self guides treatment

Linking problems and patterns to the development of the self suggests that the thera-pist's therapeutic strategy should be to help the patient further develop their sense of self. In self psychology, this is thought to happen via the therapeutic relationship itself. Patients look to the therapist to serve selfobject functions—that is, to help stabilize, restore, or enliven their sense of self. Such patients tend to treat therapists not as sepa-rate, independent people, but as extensions of themselves over whom they expect to have control. This signals a reactivation of a developmental process that was never fully or optimally completed in childhood. Essentially, these patients use the therapist to satisfy their unmet developmental needs to idealize and to gain affirmation and validation of their experiences, states of mind, and grandiose sense of self. They want and need to experience the therapist as all powerful, special, or perfect. From a self psychological perspective, this kind of idealization is seen not as a defense but rather as an important phase of the treatment, intended to help shore up a shaky sense of self.

Rather than interpreting these transferences early on, the therapist enables them to flourish. Under the influence of these selfobject transferences, the patient can feel understood and enlivened, and can experience feelings of union with or control over the therapist. Inevitably, however, the therapist will not always respond just as the patient desires, and these **empathic failures** may cause the patient to feel frustrated or angry. If the empathic failure is appropriately timed and not too intense, the therapist can point it out and discuss it with the patient, who can then start to see the therapist as a separate, flawed, but nevertheless good and caring person. Hopefully, patients can then begin to offer themselves what they have needed and desired the therapist to do for them—affirm their feelings of specialness and power, comfort them, and validate their experiences. Here's an example:

> Fred is a 55 year-old man who works as an electrician and has become a weekend triathlete. He spends his sessions regaling his male therapist with tales of his athletic prowess—passing others in the last moments of races, "shocking" younger competitors by telling them how old he is, and having female racers "come on" to him. His therapist listens, hypothesizing that Fred, who reports that his parents were "disappointed" that his "learning disability" precluded him from going to a prestigious college like his siblings, needs to demonstrate his abilities to a new, idealized man. After Fred wins a triathlon, he becomes angry that the therapist "didn't seem very excited about it." He spends several sessions telling his therapist that although he "thought" he was interested in him, he now sees he was wrong. The therapist acknowledges how disappointed Fred is in him. After his next big win, Fred notices that although the therapist may not be giving him the kind of excited reaction he hoped for, he is interested and attentive. Over time, Fred realizes that he is able to feel good enough about himself without the fantasied reaction from the therapist.

The therapist's steady, empathic attunement to the patient, and his interpretation of the perceived empathic failure, helps Fred to internalize the mirroring function he craved. This helps Fred to buoy his sense of self gradually without the continuous congratulations of others, as well as to have a more measured expectation of the people around him. This technique helps people to develop a healthier sense of self that is more resilient in the face of self-esteem threats.

Suggested activity

Can be done by individual learners or in a classroom setting

How might you link the difficulties of these people to problems with the development of the self?

> Victor gets a big bonus at work and comes home with a bottle of wine to celebrate with his husband, Douglas. Douglas, however, has his hands full with the children and has had a long day—he greets the news with, "Great, honey, can you run to the store and get some more milk?" Victor then becomes depressed and has fantasies of seducing his administrative assistant, whom he thinks has a crush on him.

> Liliana invites her coworkers over for a dinner party. For weeks in advance, she discusses her menu—everyone is looking forward to the meal. When they arrive, she is disorganized and prepares a fairly simple dinner of chicken and vegetables. She is enraged when people leave early and are not complimentary.

Comment

When he does not receive immediate kudos from his husband, Victor is deflated and has fantasies about being admired by his assistant. This suggests that he has a continued need for mirroring from a selfobject and that without it he cannot maintain his self-esteem.

Liliana misperceives her abilities to cook and entertain, and then is angry when others do not share her self-assessment. This suggests that she received problematic mirroring as a child—perhaps her talents were overestimated by parents who needed to see her as more capable than she actually was.

References

1. Aberson, C. L., Healy, M., & Romero, V. (2000). In-group bias and self-esteem: A meta-analysis. *Personality and Social Psychology Review*, 4, 157–173.
2. Akhtar, S. (2014). The mental pain of minorities. *British Journal of Psychotherapy*, 30(2), 136–153. https://doi.org/10.1111/bjp.12081
3. Auchincloss, E. L., & Samberg, E. (2012). *Psychoanalytic terms and concepts*. Yale University Press.
4. Cameron, J. E. (2004). A three-factor model of social identity. *Self and Identity*, 3(3), 239–262. https://doi.org/10.1080/13576500444000047
5. Eng, D. L., & Han, S. (2000). A dialogue on racial melancholia. *Psychoanalytic Dialogues*, 10(4), 667–700. https://doi.org/10.1080/10481881009348576
6. Frie, R. (2013). The self in context and culture. *International Journal of Psychoanalytic Self Psychology*, 8(4), 505–513. https://doi.org/10.1080/15551024.2013.825953
7. Kohut, H. (1971). *The analysis of the self*. International University Press.
8. Kohut, H. (1978). The disorders of the self and their treatment: An outline. *The International Journal of Psychoanalysis*, 59, 413–425.
9. Layton, L. (2006). Racial identities, racial enactments, and normative unconscious processes. *The Psychoanalytic Quarterly*, 75(1), 237–269. https://doi.org/10.1002/j.2167-4086.2006.tb00039.x
10. Markus, H. R., & Kitayama, S. (1991). Culture and the self: Implications for cognition, emotion, and motivation. *Psychological Review*, 98(2), 224–253. https://doi.org/10.1037/0033-295x.98.2.224
11. Markus, H. R., & Kitayama, S. (2010). Cultures and selves. *Perspectives on Psychological Science*, 5(4), 420–430. https://doi.org/10.1177/1745691610375557
12. Mitchell, S. A., & Black, M. J. (1995). *Freud and beyond*. Basic Books.
13. Moualeu, N. (2019). *Does racial identity explain the buffering impact of racial socialization on discrimination?* Graduate Theses and Dissertations. 17062. Iowa State University.
14. Stoute, B. J. (2019). Racial socialization and thwarted mentalization: Psychoanalytic reflections from the lived experience of James Baldwin's America. *The American Imago*, 76(3), 335–357. https://doi.org/10.1353/aim.2019.0025
15. Winnicott, D. W. (1960). The theory of the parent-infant relationship. *International Journal of Psychoanalysis*, 41, 585–595.
16. Winnicott, D. W. (1965). *The maturational processes and the facilitating environment: Studies in the theory of emotional development*. International Universities Press.
17. Winnicott, D. W. (1971). *Playing and reality*. Tavistock Publications.
18. Woo, B., Fan, W., Tran, T. V., & Takeuchi, D. T. (2019). The role of racial/ethnic identity in the association between racial discrimination and psychiatric disorders: A buffer or exacerbator? *SSM—Population Health*, 7, 100378. https://doi.org/10.1016/j.ssmph.2019.100378

24 Attachment

Key concepts

Our last organizing idea about development, called **attachment theory**, helps us to LINK problems and patterns to early attachment styles.

According to this idea, early attachment styles affect how people develop their sense of self, relationships with others, ways of adapting to stress, and patterns of self-regulation. These attachment styles are thought to carry over into adult life, affecting the way adults think about themselves, have relationships, and adapt to stress. Adult attachment styles are categorized as

- Secure
- Anxious-avoidant
- Anxious-ambivalent
- Disorganized

Cultural norms may affect the value groups place on attachment styles.

Linking to early attachment styles is particularly useful when creating formulations for patients who have problems with

- Self-regulation, including self-control and affect regulation
- Empathy and mentalization
- Understanding a person's response to separation and loss

Two people go for job interviews. After each interview, the prospective employer gives an equivocal smile and says, "Thank you for coming in. We'll be in touch." The first person shakes off their residual nervous energy by walking around the block, then goes home, talks to a roommate about the interview, watches TV, and goes to sleep. The second person, however, is undone by the interview and its ambiguous end. The person tries to fight the impulse to call the interviewer but fails, ultimately texting to ask about sending more references, incessantly asking a roommate, "What do you think? Do you think I'll get it?" The person then eats a

Psychodynamic Formulation: An Expanded Approach, First Edition. The Psychodynamic Formulation Collective.
© 2022 John Wiley & Sons Ltd. Published 2022 by John Wiley & Sons Ltd.

pint of ice cream and later has two drinks before trying unsuccessfully to sleep. These people had very different reactions to having endured a stressful situation that left them in limbo. Why?

One way to think about this is that the first person is more able to self-regulate as a result of having more secure attachments, while the second person's difficulty with self-soothing resulted from an anxious attachment style. As we discussed in Chapter 13, an enormous amount of development happens in the context of the child's dyadic relationship with their primary caregiver. This relationship has a large role in mediating the development of fundamental capacities that enable the person to develop their sense of self, form relationships with others, adapt to stress and anxiety, and self-regulate. The style with which infants attach to their primary caregivers has been shown to carry over into the way they attach to others as adults. By describing adult attachment styles, **attachment theory** helps us to understand early relationships and how they contribute to the development of a person's problems and patterns.

Basics of attachment theory

Attachment theory starts with the idea that people are born with a predisposition to become attached to caregivers in their earliest years (Bowlby, 1958; Slade, 2000). The sense of safety that children get from their central caregiving relationship helps them to develop the system of emotional regulation they use to handle a wide variety of experiences. This experience of nurturance and protection is encoded in the brain and, over time, helps people develop both the ability to predict and understand their environment and a psychological sense of security (Main, 1993). In addition, these interactions help them to develop relatively stable patterns of adapting to stress and regulating their responses to anxiety and affects (Fonagy & Target, 2002).

These early patterns of connection, which are called **attachment styles**, are classified as secure, anxious-avoidant, anxious-ambivalent or disorganized, and are relatively stable after the first year of life (see Chapter 13 on the **strange situation**; Ainsworth et al., 1978). In research studies on American families, the children who have secure attachments tolerate separations well and are easily soothed by their primary caregivers when reunited with them, while children who have anxious-avoidant, anxious-ambivalent, and disorganized attachments become highly stressed during separations and are not easily soothed after reuniting (Hesse & Main, 2000; Main, 2000). These attachment styles have been shown to predict the comfort with which children experience their environments later in development, and carry over to the way they adapt to stressful situations as adults. In other words, the attachment style that children have by age one is likely to predict the way they will respond to their internal and external environments as adults (Dozier et al., 1999). Anxious attachment styles are not necessarily maladaptive but rather may be *"resilience-promoting adaptations* to specific environments enabling survival under adverse circumstances"* (Holmes & Slade, 2018).

Categories of attachment in adults

To review, the attachment styles of young children are described as:

- Secure
- Anxious-avoidant
- Anxious-ambivalent
- Disorganized

These styles correspond to children's behavior at age one when observed in brief separations from the mother (see Chapter 13; Hesse & Main, 2000; Main, 2000). Not surprisingly, when adults are interviewed about how they cope with stress and anxiety specifically in regard to intimate relationships, their attachment styles generally fall into four similar categories (Fonagy et al., 1991; Hesse, 2008). These adult attachment styles include the way people recall and describe early childhood relationships (particularly those that had significant negative aspects) and the way they describe their current relationships with others (Fonagy, 2001; Lyons-Ruth & Block, 1996; Slade, 1996). Although investigators sometimes name these categories differently, we can usefully think of these styles as discussed below.

Secure

People with this adult attachment style easily remember experiences of others, are able to incorporate painful memories into their discussions, can think about others in three-dimensional terms, and can look at emotions from other people's point of view. They find it relatively easy to become emotionally close to others and are comfortable both depending on others and having others depend on them. People with secure attachment were most often raised in families with strong emotional support and a low level of major life stressors (e.g., illness, socioeconomic difficulties, or racial/ social discrimination (Vaughn et al., 1979; Waters et al., 2002).

Anxious-avoidant

People with this attachment style show less emotional response to separation and tend to remember little of their childhood relationships. They may also offer idealized portraits of people in their current lives. When probed, however, they are often able to remember incidents suggesting parental neglect or rejection. In some instances, these people present as strong and independent but actually struggle internally to face the reality of early disappointments. In other instances, the life stories of people with this attachment style may indicate that it was helpful/adaptive for them to push away negative thoughts about their early life, because they might have become overwhelming. Children raised in cultures that tend to have multiple caregivers (sometimes called kinship cultures) may show little to no reaction to strangers or separation. Here, their behavior is thought to be an adaptive response to their environment, rather than being due to a negative experience (Johow & Voland, 2014).

Anxious-ambivalent

In contrast to those with avoidant style, people with this attachment style hold themselves responsible for problems in their relationships and idealize their early caregivers. They are anxious and worried about relationships with others and how they are perceived. They often find it hard to speak in an organized way about past relationships. They are consciously preoccupied with their early caregivers upon whom they may remain very reliant. In their adult relationships, they seek high levels of intimacy and are often very dependent. Their life stories may suggest that they adapted to having unreliable caregivers by offering them help and assistance.

Disorganized

People with this attachment style often have dramatic fluctuations in their descriptions of others and may be unable to recall past relationships. Many people with this attachment style have a history of trauma or loss of a parent and a high chance of repeating trauma with their own children. Their adult relationships are fairly chaotic; for example, they typically enter quickly into intense relationships, and then become easily mistrustful and withdraw (Sroufe, 2005).

For example, consider the differences in attachment style between these two middle-aged men:

> Milton comes to therapy because he has been anxious since his daughter went away to college. His history reveals that he was an anxious child. He remembers screaming at the chain-link fence in the playground when his mother left him at elementary school. In adolescence, he became despondent after a girlfriend broke up with him. When he talks about his daughter, he speaks haltingly and starts to tear up, saying "I don't know why she couldn't have gone to college closer to home. How could she do this to me?"

> Anthony comes to therapy because his wife complains that he overworks and will not curtail his work life to spend time with their family. Their daughter told his wife that she wishes she had a closer relationship with him. Anthony reports this with little concern and, staring out the window, says, "She's doing fine. I think a daughter's primary relationship is with her mother."

In these examples, Milton likely has an **anxious-ambivalent** pattern of attachment, while Anthony's attachment pattern is best described as **anxious-avoidant**.

Family and attachment styles

Empathy and the development of affect regulation

Why does one adult have one attachment style versus another? Children are more likely to develop a secure attachment style if their caregivers can understand and process their emotional experiences (Bouchard et al., 2008; Coates, 1998). The caregivers' processing of emotion fosters the development of the child's ability to **regulate affect**—that is, the ability to handle basic emotions, such as fear, anxiety, insecurity, and excitement (Schore, 1994, 2001). When caregivers are unable to empathize and respond sensitively, however, children are more likely to develop anxious or disorganized attachments that predispose them to chronic difficulty modulating their sense of self, controlling their impulses, and reacting to anxiety (Fonagy, 2000; Lyons-Ruth, 2002).

Attachment styles are passed on from parent to child

People with each adult attachment style tend to have children with a related attachment style. This process is referred to as **intergenerational transmission of attachment** (Beebe et al., 1997; Fonagy, 1996; Van Ijzendoorn et al., 1999). Thus, people may develop an attachment style related to the trauma of a parent or grandparent, even if they did not experience the trauma themselves.

Social factors that can affect attachment styles

Attachment styles can be affected by the child's experience in the world

Trauma inflicted by society, such as racism, discrimination, migration, war, or persecution, can also result in anxious or disorganized attachment (Davis, 2007). In some situations, attachment patterns may help children adapt to inequities in the community and society at large. For example, anxious-avoidant and anxious-ambivalent attachment patterns have been shown to help secondary school children navigate competition for resources (Chen & Chang, 2012).

Attachment styles may vary depending on cultural background

The majority of research studies from which the above categories were developed looked at White, middle-class families in Western countries (Ainsworth et al., 1978; Main, 1993). Thus, the attachment model has been critiqued as privileging a singular view of parenting with a mother as primary caretaker, and as overly emphasizing secure attachment as a measure of well-being (Otto & Keller, 2014). Cross-cultural theorists and writers, who have looked at a variety of factors that affect attachment (e.g., co-operative care and multiple attachments), suggest that many different relationships can contribute to an individual's attachment patterns (Morelli & Henry, 2013). Potential bias related to culture should be considered when linking to attachment theory.

Attachment styles can change in adulthood

People who develop anxious and disorganized attachment patterns during childhood can achieve secure patterns in adulthood (Holmes & Slade, 2018). This is called

earned security and is thought to be attained through positive relationships, including those established in psychotherapy (Saunders et al., 2011).

Linking problems and patterns to attachment styles

Attachment theory helps us to understand people who struggle with self-regulation and affect management. It can also be helpful in understanding people who have difficulties with empathy and mentalization.

Self-regulation and affect management

Self-regulation and affect management can be usefully understood in relation to attachment style, which is often evident around challenges such as loss, separations, and life transitions. Dealing with divorce, leaving for college, changing jobs, managing illness, and losing a loved one are just a few of the many separations and losses that highlight a person's attachment patterns and bring people to psychotherapy.

> *Sidney and Ryan, both young African-American gay men, started dating in medical school. When they started separate medical internships at different institutions, Sidney became very anxious but adapted by staying in regular contact with Ryan via text messages. As the months of the internship unfolded, Sidney became more panicked and clingy. One day, Ryan could not respond to a text because he was conducting a procedure. Sidney panicked and called 911 to find him. In therapy, Sidney reported that his father died when he was young and his mother coped with her grief and anxiety by staying in almost constant contact with her young son, often worrying about his safety.*

Using attachment theory, we can hypothesize that Sidney developed his anxious-ambivalent attachment style in response to his mother's similar attachment style. In therapy, he realized that his difficulties were connected to his early relationship with his mother, and that her worries had to do not only with her grief but also with the prevalence of anti-Black violence in their predominantly White community. He learned that talking with Ryan about both real and imagined dangers could help him manage his anxieties about their separations.

Difficulty with empathy

Attachment theory is also helpful in understanding people's capacity to empathize with others. Consider the following example:

> *Nallini, who is of South Indian descent, is raising her 5-year-old daughter as a single mother after being left by her husband. She is referred for psychotherapy by the school psychologist, who has noted that Nallini's daughter is having great difficulty separating from her mother. Nallini explains that her daughter has few friends, keeps to herself, and sits on the sidelines while the other children play. She says, "I've recently brought my sick mother to live with us and haven't been as available to my daughter as I usually am. She seems to manage fine, though; she hardly complains." Nallini tells the therapist that her daughter suffers from asthma and was hospitalized several times as a baby. When the therapist asks Nallini about her own childhood, she learns that Nallini was also a withdrawn child who lived in a multigenerational household and was often expected to care for herself.*

Using attachment theory, we could suggest that Nallini's detached attitude toward her daughter is related to her anxious-avoidant attachment style, now emerging in her daughter as well. Offering Nallini other perspectives—for example, that perhaps her daughter is reacting to the early hospitalization, separation from her father, or worry about her grandmother's illness—may help Nallini to become more interested in understanding her daughter's internal experience.

A sample formulation—linking to attachment

Presentation

Patrick, a middle-aged man of Irish-Catholic descent, has become increasingly distraught because his daughter, who previously lived down the block with her husband, announced she was getting divorced. Patrick and his wife are very upset that their daughter will be moving into an apartment farther away. Although he says that he knows that he's overreacting, he talks quickly and loudly in therapy and asks if he can have a "double session" because he has so much he needs to talk about.

DESCRIBE the problem and patterns

*Patrick's major difficulty is in his **relationship to others**. He also has **difficulty adapting to change and loss**. His family has long felt that he smothers them. He didn't allow his children to go more than a car ride away to college and doesn't understand why this bothers them. He thinks his daughter should work things out with her husband who he thinks is "a terrific guy" but who never worked and who is fully supported by his daughter.*

REVIEW the life story

Patrick grew up in a tightly knit family with an anxious mother who currently lives with him and his wife. He recalls having few friends as a child and being kept home by his mother to watch TV with her. His father, who passed away several years before this presentation, was a World War II veteran who had been injured and had fairly severe Post Traumatic Stress Disorder (PTSD). Patrick's only brother moved away years before and was estranged from the family after numerous disappointments related to his not coming home for family events/holidays. Patrick did well academically and had opportunities to pursue college away from home but chose a nearby parochial school so that he could continue to live with his parents. He married young; his wife, who is also anxious, has become devoted to his mother as well.

LINK the history and problems/patterns to attachment styles

Patrick's pattern of becoming increasingly anxious and demanding in the face of disappointment and loss may be indicative of his anxious-ambivalent attachment pattern, which is also present in his mother. Patrick tries to draw people closer (e.g., his daughter, the therapist) to decrease his own anxiety, but, in so doing, he inadvertently pushes them away (the daughter feels misunderstood; the therapist has no choice but to end the session). This makes him more anxious. He also has difficulty imagining other peoples' internal experiences (mentalization), perhaps because his overwhelming desire to preserve the attachment connection prevents him from considering any needs other than his own.

Linking to attachment styles guides treatment

In psychotherapy, patients repeat their attachment styles with their therapists. Together, the patient and therapist can then observe and identify the attachment style. This can facilitate change in two ways—by making people aware of their attachment patterns and by helping them to attach in new ways.

Becoming aware of attachment styles

Becoming more aware of their characteristic attachment styles and how they evolved enables patients to create new narratives about themselves (Slade, 2008). Consider the following example:

> Jenna had always blamed herself for being an oversensitive, chronically anxious child. In therapy, she learned that the death of her mother's father and her parents' long-term marital difficulties had made her mother anxious during most of Jenna's childhood. She realized that her own anxiety was a reaction to her mother's anxious state. Having a new understanding about the origin of her anxiety helped her to feel more relaxed and increased her empathy for her mother.

Jenna has an anxious-ambivalent attachment style. With a new way of thinking about her life story, Jenna is more able to accept both her own anxiety and her mother's.

Improving affect management

People with a disorganized attachment style can have difficulty with affect regulation, especially during periods of intense emotionality. When this occurs within a therapy session, therapists can help their patients to manage their feelings by describing what is happening and by helping them to think about what might be happening in the minds of both the patient and the therapist (Bateman & Fonagy, 2004). To illustrate this, consider Delma, who has a disorganized attachment style:

> Just as the session was ending, Delma began telling her therapist about her history of sexual abuse. She became more confused and lost track of time. The therapist stated, "This is a hard subject to discuss, particularly when there are only five minutes left to the session." Delma became enraged that the therapist was ending the session abruptly, saying, "You don't care about me . . . I'm not sure I ever want to come back here." The therapist commented, "I see how talking about the abuse disorients you, so much that you feel that I, too, am against you. Can you imagine any other ways of looking at what just happened between us?" This helped Delma to calm down and to consider that the therapist's interruption may have sounded abrupt, but in fact reflected her worry about the patient.

Using attachment theory, the therapist thought about Delma's outburst as the result of her attachment style. She empathized with Delma's experience and realized that Delma was unable to consider that the therapist had an alternate reason to end the session in that way. By asking her to consider other ways of looking at the situation, the therapist was helping Delma to manage her feeling of being hurt by the therapist. Repeating this in therapy can help the patient to process intense feelings more effectively in situations outside of the treatment as well (Bateman & Fonagy, 2004).

Developing a more secure attachment style

Over time, patients can change their attachment styles as they develop a more secure attachment to their therapists. This is thought to occur as therapists repeatedly experience, observe, and describe the way their patients handle feelings. Patients internalize this, gradually learning to have a clearer and more flexible idea of what goes on in their minds, and in the minds of their therapists. In the context of a more secure attachment, patients can develop functions that they were not able to develop as children, such as an increased ability to self-regulate and to modulate affects. Let's consider an example of someone with an anxious-avoidant attachment style who has difficulty experiencing affect:

> *Amy is a 52-year-old gay woman who lives apart from her long-term partner. Her partner complains that Amy is emotionally distant and removed. After 20 years together, they recently got married and Amy says she's tired of putting up so many walls. In treatment, the therapist notices that Amy speaks hesitantly in sessions and often becomes quiet and looks away after she speaks. When the therapist inquires about this, Amy reveals that she is afraid that he doesn't approve of her. She then talks about how harshly critical her mother was. Amy then begins to consider that perhaps the therapist is trying to be helpful and begins to speak more freely.*

Of particular note is the way Amy's attachment style is communicated nonverbally—she turns away. Therapists using techniques from attachment theory are attuned to the nonverbal as well as verbal ways of understanding their patients' attachment patterns. Over time, observing and describing these patterns in the relationship with the therapist enables patients to feel secure enough to consider alternative ways of managing their feelings.

Suggested activity

Can be done by individual learners or in a classroom setting

How would you describe the attachment styles of these adults?

> *Kayla is a 43-year-old woman who married her high school classmate. When her husband suggests that they attend their 25th high school reunion, she says, "Why would I want to do that? Just to see a lot of middle-aged losers? I'd rather go to the gym."*

> *Dante, a 21-year-old college student, had a tumultuous relationship with Cal that ended in a breakup. When he sees Cal in the bookstore after summer vacation, he has the sensation that he is going to throw up, leaves his books in the middle of the aisle, and runs in the opposite direction.*

> *Carolina, a 30-year-old woman who immigrated to the United States from Mexico, talks daily to her mother in Mexico. Carolina and her husband, a White man of European descent who has more limited contact with his family, have been having marital difficulties as her husband criticizes her for devoting too much time to her mother.*

Comment

Kayla likely has an *anxious-avoidant* attachment pattern. Although she remembers past relationships, she does not value them and has a rigid, overly independent stance.

Dante's behavior suggests a *disorganized* attachment pattern. When he sees his ex-boyfriend, he behaves in a bizarre manner.

While Carolina at first appears to have an ambivalent attachment style, talking to a culturally sensitive couples therapist helps both partners understand that Carolina is happy to support her mother, does feel burdened by the responsibility, and appears *securely* attached in her other relationships.

References

1. Ainsworth, M. D. S., Blehar, M. C., Waters, E., & Wall, S. (1978). *Patterns of attachment: A psychological study of the strange situation.* Lawrence Erlbaum Associates.
2. Bateman, A., & Fonagy, P. (2004). *Psychotherapy for borderline personality disorder: Mentalization-based treatment.* Oxford University Press.
3. Bateman, A., & Fonagy, P. (2009). Randomized controlled trial of outpatient mentalization-based treatment versus structured clinical management for borderline personality disorder. *American Journal of Psychiatry, 166*(12), 1355–1364. https://doi.org/10.1176/appi.ajp.2009.09040539
4. Beebe, B., Lachmann, F., & Jaffe, J. (1997). Mother-Infant interaction structures and presymbolic self- and object representations. *Psychoanalytic Dialogues, 7*(2), 133–182. https://doi.org/10.1080/10481889709539172
5. Bouchard, M.-A., Target, M., Lecours, S., Fonagy, P., Tremblay, L.-M., Schachter, A., & Stein, H. (2008). Mentalization in adult attachment narratives: Reflective functioning, mental states, and affect elaboration compared. *Psychoanalytic Psychology, 25*(1), 47–66. https://doi.org/10.1037/0736-9735.25.1.47
6. Bowlby, J. (1958). The nature of the child's tie to his mother. *International Journal of Psychoanalysis, 39,* 350–373.
7. Chen, B.-B., & Chang, L. (2012). Adaptive insecure attachment and resource control strategies during middle childhood. *International Journal of Behavioral Development, 36*(5), 389–397. https://doi.org/10.1177/0165025412445440
8. Coates, S. W. (1998). Having a mind of one's own and holding the other in mind: Commentary on paper by Peter Fonagy and Mary Target. *Psychoanalytic Dialogues, 8,* 115–148.
9. Davis, S. (2007). Racism as trauma: Some reflections on psychotherapeutic work with clients from the African-Carribean diaspora from an attachment-based perspective. *New Directions in Psychotherapy and Relational Psychoanalysis Journal, 1,* 179–199.
10. Dozier, M., Chase-Stovall, K., & Albus, K. E. (1999). Attachment and psychopathology in adulthood. In J. Cassidy & P. R. Shaver (Eds.), *Handbook of attachment: Theory, research, and clinical applications* (pp. 497–519). Guilford Press.
11. Fonagy, P. (1996). The significance of the development of metacognitive control over mental representations in parenting and infant development. *Journal of Clinical Psychoanalysis, 5,* 67–86.
12. Fonagy, P. (2000). Attachment and borderline personality disorder. *Journal of the American Psychoanalytic Association, 48,* 1129–1146.
13. Fonagy, P. (2001). *Attachment theory and psychoanalysis.* Other Press.
14. Fonagy, P., Steele, M., Moran, G., & Higgit, A. (1991). Measuring the ghost in the nursery: A summary of the main findings of the Anna Freud Centre—University College London Parent-Child Study. *Bulletin of the Anna Freud Centre, 14*(2), 115–131.
15. Fonagy, P., & Target, M. (2002). Early intervention and the development of self-regulation. *Psychoanalytic Inquiry, 22*(3), 307–335. https://doi.org/10.1080/07351692209348990
16. Hesse, E. (2008). The adult attachment interview: Historical and current perspectives. In J. Cassidy & P. R. Shaver (Eds.), *Handbook of attachment: Theory, research and clinical applications* (2nd ed., pp. 552–599). Guilford Press.
17. Hesse, E., & Main, M. (2000). Disorganized infant, child, and adult attachment: Collapse in behavioral and attentional strategies. *Journal of the American Psychoanalytic Association, 48*(4), 1097–1127. https://doi.org/10.1177/00030651000480041101
18. Holmes, J., & Slade, A. (2018). *Attachment in therapeutic practice.* Sage Publications.
19. Johow, J., & Voland, E. (2014). Family relations among cooperative breeders. In H. Otto & H. Keller (Eds.), *Different faces of attachment: Cultural variations on a universal human need.* Cambridge University Press.

20. Lyons-Ruth, K. (2002). The two-person construction of defenses: Disorganized attachment strategies, unintegrated mental states, and hostile/helpless relational processes. *Journal of Infant, Child, and Adolescent Psychotherapy, 2*(4), 107–119. https://doi.org/10.10 80/15289168.2002.10486422

21. Lyons-Ruth, K., & Block, D. (1996). The disturbed caregiving system: Relations among childhood trauma, maternal caregiving, and infant affect and attachment. *Infant Mental Health Journal, 17*(3), 257–275. https://doi.org/10.1002/(SICI)1097-0355(199623)17:3<257:: AID-IMHJ5>3.0.CO;2-L

22. Main, M. (1993). Discourse, prediction, and recent studies in attachment: Implications for psychoanalysis. *Journal of the American Psychoanalytic Association, 48*, 209–244.

23. Main, M. (2000). The organized categories of infant, child, and adult attachment: Flexible vs. inflexible attention under attachment-related stress. *Journal of the American Psychoanalytic Association, 48*(4), 1055–1096. https://doi.org/10.1177/00030651000480041801

24. Morelli, A. M., & Henry, P. I. (2013). Afterward: Cross-cultural challenges to attachment theory. In N. Quinn & J. M. Mageo (Eds.), *Attachment reconsidered. Cultural pon a western theory*. Palgrave Macmillan.

25. Otto, H., & Keller, H. (Eds.) (2014). *Different faces of attachment*. Cambridge University Press.

26. Saunders, R., Jacobvitz, D., Zaccagnino, M., Beverung, L. M., & Hazen, N. (2011). Pathways to earned-security: The role of alternative support figures. *Attachment & Human Development, 13*(4), 403–420. https://doi.org/10.1080/14616734.2011.584405

27. Schore, A. (1994). *Affect regulation and the origin of the self*. Lawrence Erlbaum Associates.

28. Schore, A. N. (2001). Effects of a secure attachment relationship on right brain development, affect regulation, and infant mental health. *Infant Mental Health Journal, 22*(1–2), 7–66. https://doi.org/10.1002/1097-0355(200101/04)22:1<7::AID-IMHJ2>3.0.CO;2-N

29. Slade, A. (1996). A view from attachment theory and research. *Journal of Clinical Psychoanalysis, 5*, 12–122.

30. Slade, A. (2000). The development and organization of attachment: Implications for psychoanalysis. *Journal of the American Psychoanalytic Association, 48*(4), 1147–1174. https://doi.org/10.1177/00030651000480042301

31. Slade, A. (2008). The implications of attachment theory and research for adult psychotherapy. In J. Cassidy & P. R. Shaver (Eds.), *Handbook of attachment: Theory, research and clinical applications* (2nd ed., pp. 782–782). Guilford Press.

32. Sroufe, L. A. (2005). Attachment and development: A prospective, longitudinal study from birth to adulthood. *Attachment & Human Development, 7*(4), 349–367. https://doi.org/10.1080/14616730500365928

33. Van Ijzendoorn, M., Schuengel, C., & Bakermans-Krnenburg, M. J. (1999). Disorganized attachment in early childhood: Meta-analysis of precursors, concomitants, and sequelae. *Development and Psychopathology, 11*(2), 225–250. https://doi.org/10.1017/s0954579499002035

34. Vaughn, B., Egeland, B., Sroufe, L. A., & Waters, E. (1979). Individual differences in infant-mother attachment at twelve and eighteen months: Stability and change in families under stress. *Child Development, 50*(4), 971. https://doi.org/10.2307/1129321

35. Waters, E., Merrick, S., Treboux, D., Crowell, J., & Albersheim, L. (2002). Attachment security in infancy and early adulthood: A twenty-year longitudinal study. *Annual Progress in Child Psychiatry and Child Development 2000–2001*, 63–72. https://doi.org/10.4324/9780203449523-4

Putting It Together—LINK to Collaboratively Create Psychodynamic Formulations

Now that you've learned to DESCRIBE, REVIEW, and LINK, let's listen in as two therapists collaboratively create initial psychodynamic formulations with their patients. The first therapist, a 52-year-old White woman, has seen the patient, Mike, for four sessions. We'll hear how the therapist

- Listens to the Mike's initial comments
- DESCRIBES the problems and patterns
- REVIEWS the life story
- LINKS the problems and patterns to the life story by
  - focusing what she's learned from DESCRIBING and REVIEWING
  - choosing ideas about organization.
- Shares a preliminary formulation
- Thinks about how the formulation will guide treatment

Let's meet Mike:

Presentation

Mike is a 32-year-old African-American man who presents to the therapist saying, "My girlfriend thought it would be a good idea for me to talk to someone. Work is getting me down. I'm not doing well there and I don't know why." Mike, who has been working in finance at the same firm since college, reports that he was "doing really well—on track" for several years, but that over the past six months he has received a few "bad reviews" that have made him question whether he's "got what it takes" to really succeed in his field. "I'd say I'm more confused than depressed," he explains. "It used to be fun; now I feel like I'm just going through the motions. And I wake up thinking about it in the middle of the night." He says that his managers have specifically said that he's not aggressive enough about closing deals, and that he needs more of a "killer instinct" if he's going to make it to the "next level." As one of only a handful of people of color at his firm, he says that the past two years have been "challenging" as his coworkers "kind of act like the whole social unrest movement is only important insofar as it affects the market." He says that Jackie, his 30-year-old African-American girlfriend, is a very successful management consultant who is having "no

trouble jumping the management hurdles." "She says I need to get over myself and be the success-
ful man I'm meant to be," he sighs. "So, here I am."

After hearing the presentation, the therapist thinks:

Mike sounds like he's used to having things go really well at work, and that, for the first time,
he's getting negative feedback. I noticed that he said this has confused him. I wonder what's
going on in other aspects of his life.

The therapist then goes on to ask Mike about other aspects of his functioning. Here's
how the therapist DESCRIBES Mike's problems and patterns:

DESCRIBE

Problem

After a lifetime of academic and professional success, Mike has recently—and for the first time—
received negative reviews at work. The reviews suggest that he is not taking an adequately aggressive
approach. This has led to him to feel "down" about work, and to feel that the work is not enjoyable.

Patterns

The therapist then describes Mike's patterns in terms of self, relationships, adapting,
cognition, values, and work and play.

Self

*In terms of **self-perception**, Mike seems to believe that he is smart and hard-working, and that he*
has done well professionally to this point. He describes himself as a loving son, brother, and part-
ner. Given the current situation, it seems that he responds to self-esteem blows with self-blame and
*self-doubt. His **identity** as an African-American man seems ambivalent—Mike is clearly proud of*
how he and his family have done, but he has not been particularly connected to the African-
American community at large.

Relationships

*Mike seems to have a very **secure** relationship with his girlfriend, although he is not clear about*
*why he's unsure about marriage. He seems to have a close **trusting** relationship with his parents,*
however, in talking about his college years, he says that he didn't share some of his difficulties—
particularly those related to racial tensions—because of guilt and shame. ("They sacrificed so
*much for me—they didn't need to hear about problems.") In terms of **mutuality**, he is a ready and*
willing mentor to his younger sister and younger cousins, and expresses interest in his girlfriend
and her career issues. He has friends who tend to be younger and who look to him as an "older
brother." He enjoys his sexual relationship with Jackie, saying, "she knows what she wants," and
feels glad that she expresses her interest in him as he feels that he was "late to the game" in terms
of dating and sexual activity.

Adapting

Mike prides himself on his resiliency, and says that his parents "trained him well" in terms of deal-
ing with stress. He says that his motto is, "Work hard and keep your cool." Despite some stressful

moments in life, he has not had extended periods of depression or anxiety, and so seems to have used **high-benefit coping strategies** *that serve him well. He tends to react to stress* **without extensive emotionality**—*Mike likes to think through problems and treat obstacles as "learning experiences."*

Cognition

Having always done well at school, won scholarships, and graduated with honors, Mike is **academically talented** *and enjoys learning. He describes being adept at running teams and at* **solving problems creatively** *at work. Mike is interested in the feelings of others and is able to imagine how others think, and thus seems able to mentalize. He is proud of his ability to* **manage his emotions** *(which may actually keep him from accessing some unconscious feelings) and of "staying on course" (i.e., not being* **impulsive** *or engaging in risky behaviors).*

Values

Mike values **family**, *which includes his family of origin as well as the family he hopes to have in the future. Being* **financially comfortable** *is important to him: "I want to have enough in the bank so that I don't have to depend on others, and so that I can take care of everyone around me." Mike also wants to be respected by those in his profession. All of this, in addition to his affinity for taking on mentorship roles and pride in being a "straight arrow," suggests his proclivity for* **prosocial** *behavior, and a strong, perhaps even harsh, internal* **sense of right and wrong**.

Work and play

Mike enjoys his work and, prior to the past few months, has enjoyed its challenges. He enjoys spending time with family but often has **difficulty relaxing** *when he has paid time off.*

After several evaluation sessions with Mike, the therapist begins to focus on what Mike has DESCRIBED and says,

"You have so many strengths. You are smart, driven, resilient, connected to your family and Jackie, and from what you've said, you were doing really well at work until the past six months or so. I'm not sure I understand what your managers are referring to, but, assuming you think it's fair criticism, is being aggressive a new issue for you or something you've struggled with before? I'd like to hear more about your life story so that we can get an early idea of what might be getting in the way at work."

The therapist then listens to Mike's life story:

REVIEW

Genetics and prenatal development

Mike is the eldest of two children. He says that his grandparents on both sides of his family moved north in the Great Migration, and that his parents were raised near one another in an industrial city in the Midwest. "We didn't talk about it, but I knew that my grandparents had seen terrible things done to Black people," he describes. "I was taught by my parents—and my maternal grandmother—that we, Black people, have to work harder and pray harder than White people." His parents went to segregated schools and graduated from high school. Without money for college, they married and found solid jobs at which they excelled. "My parents are incredibly strong people. My dad had a few wild friends in high school, but once he met my mother they took care of that row house like their lives depended on it. And it did." He denies depression on either side of the family as well as drug and alcohol use.

Earliest years (birth–age 3)

Mike was born at term when his parents were both in their twenties. Well-liked by his peers, his father had a secure job in the steel mills where he rose to be a local union leader. His mother took meticulous care of the house and was an active member of their church community. He says that stories about his early life indicate that he was an "easy baby" who "never cried." "My mother watched me like a hawk," he says. "I never was anywhere alone. My parents knew the world was dangerous and made sure I knew that from a young age."

Middle childhood (ages 3–6)

"To say that I was the apple of my mother's eye is low-balling it," he says. "They thought I hung the moon. Every photo shows me smiling and well dressed for church." Mike says that his dad would take him with him to union softball games. "I was the team mascot," he recalls. "But I never liked the game. I mostly read picture books in the dugout." His younger sister was born when he was two. "We were both taught to say 'Yes, ma'am,' and 'No ma'am'–I still do it to this day, and it makes people really uncomfortable. No dessert on weekdays, homework right after school, rounds with my mother to bring food to church members who were sick." He says that he knew that his parents loved one another, although it was "not an affectionate family."

Later childhood (ages 6–12)

Mike and his sister attended public school in the neighborhood, which was predominantly African American and Latinx. He excelled immediately, learning to read in kindergarten and scoring extremely well on standardized tests. "My sister did less well, which pained my parents," he said. "My father was very clear—school was the way out and up. He was incredibly proud of me. The only time he was upset with me was when he thought I was what he called 'crowing'. 'Stay in your lane,' he'd say, 'Work hard, but remember that you are no better than anyone else. No reason to call attention to yourself.'" Mike had friends, most of whom were the children of members of the church. "My parents screened my friends incredibly carefully. They were not interested in any infiltration of 'bad influences.'"

Adolescence (ages 13–18)

Thanks to his father's union, Mike was able to enter a program that sent him to an elite prep school for high school. There, for the first time, he was marginalized because of race. "I'm extremely grateful for the opportunity, and the quality of education there was so much better than I would have gotten. But it was tough socially." Occasionally "roughed up" by White boys from his class after school, he "stood tall and took it" and never fought back. He never told his parents about this bullying—he felt that they had sacrificed so much to send him to school that they deserved to be protected from that. One of a handful of "minority guys" at the school, he didn't even try dating and avoided most of the school's social activities. "My parents didn't want me to date in the neighborhood either," he said, "so I was out of luck. More time to study, I guess." He soared academically, earning accolades from his teachers, particularly in the humanities. Simultaneously, his sister had trouble in the local public high school and even had some "questionable" friends. "I spent hours trying to help her with homework," he recalls. With the help of guidance counselors, he won acceptance to a small liberal arts college known to be nurturing to students of color, and, with the help of more union scholarships, he left home for the first time.

Young adulthood (ages 18–23)

His small liberal arts college was "perfect for me and not the real world." He dated for the first time, finding the women "reassuringly sure of themselves—at least they knew what to do." He was often home on weekends, and began to get hired for internships in finance over the summers. "I loved the energy of the offices. I thought they were places where I could really excel. I also loved the apartments we got, and the lunches out. I saw a different kind of life and wanted it. I felt that as long as I had the right suit and made money for the firm, it wouldn't matter if I was Black or White. That was exhilarating." He says that, unless he was home, he stopped attending church but didn't tell his parents.

Later adulthood (ages 23—present)

After graduating with honors, Mike accepted an offer to begin with his firm as an analyst. He excelled with his cohort, worked round-the-clock and was valued by his superiors. He dated—though he had little time—and at 28 met Jackie at a friend's wedding. "I'd never met Black people like her family," he notes. "They were like the rich White people I'd met in high school. Her grandfather went to college and made a lot of money—both of her parents have graduate degrees. She has a kind of self-confidence I didn't know Black people could have." After three years of dating, they have moved in together—although he hasn't told his mother and thinks about proposing all the time. "I don't know why I haven't done it yet. I want to, but something holds me back. I'm confused." His best friend is his White roommate from college, and he routinely throws away offers to join Black-oriented professional networks.

Now the therapist tries to focus on what she has REVIEWED and says to Mike,

"It's clear that your family and community made you feel safe in a world that was clearly dangerous. In general, the strategy they taught you worked—you've done really well. But you've had a few times in your life when it didn't—when you were bullied in high school, and, perhaps, now."

"Look," says Mike. "The person I trusted most in the world taught me to 'keep my cool'. But if there are a few moments in my life I'd like to live again, it would be those afternoons. I sometimes dream about it—taking one perfect Mike Tyson-esque swing and decking the guy. But I would never have been able to face my father. I knew that wasn't the way to go."

This helps the therapist to think about how to LINK Mike's problems and patterns to his life story. Here's how she begins to put it together:

From DESCRIBE, Mike's greatest difficulty seems to be his difficulty with anger and aggression, and this likely relates to his current difficulties at work. From REVIEW, it's clear that he was raised to avoid aggression in order to get along in the White world. So, he has a conflict—he wants to be more aggressive at work to achieve respect and financial rewards, but he avoids aggression because he feels (consciously and unconsciously) that being aggressive as a Black man is dangerous. To LINK these dimensions, I could use a conflict model as the organizing idea about development to help me best understand Mike. But although this conflict may be related to his relationship with his parents—his microsystem—it's clear that it has deep roots in his macrosystem. As a Black man, raised by children of the Great Migration, whose own parents had witnessed atrocities committed by Whites against Blacks, Mike's feeling that being aggressive is dangerous is indelibly connected to the structural racism faced by his family for generations. This also helps me to understand how a man who seems to have been so well nurtured—and to have had such a close relationship to both parents—could have such a deep inhibition about assertion. I think I'm going to use the Ecological Systems model and ideas about intergenerational transmission of trauma to help me understand his feelings about aggression and identity, and I will use the Conflict/Defense model as a secondary theory.

Here's what she writes:

LINK

Mike's greatest area of difficulty is in adapting. In trying to avoid aggression, he has likely inhibited his ability to be assertive, leading to conflicts that are giving him difficulty with work, identity, and perhaps even his relationship. This is most likely related to an unconscious conflict—he wants to be assertive but fears aggression and believes it to be dangerous. This belief, as it relates to being aggressive as a Black person in a White society, is held not only by his parents but by his entire community, and is likely linked to structural racism and the intergenerational transmission of trauma (in his family and community). It may also have been compounded by the particular relationship that Mike had with a father whom he idealized and whom he has much surpassed.

Born into a family and community that experienced the trauma of White violence and systemic oppression, Mike inherited and internalized his parents' fear and wariness of society-at-large. The extremely safe environment that he entered was nurturing while simultaneously being a fortress protecting him from outside dangers. His easy temperament helped to make the family edict to "stay in your lane" a natural fit. He learned to implicitly trust those in his immediate and community environment and to be wary of those beyond.

Middle childhood brought a strengthening of his relationship with his idealized father, while sowing the seeds of the conflict about aggression as his father demonstrated both pride in and anxiety about his gifted son. Mike's father's clear admonition to avoid aggression and "crowing" are likely both about his fears of what happens to aggressive Black men in a White world, as well as to his own unconscious conflicts about having a son surpass him. Mike internalized both of these and they reinforced one another. Mike seems to have been adored by his mother, but also had good boundaries set by the apparent love of his parents for one another. Mike seems to have dealt with (i.e., sublimated) any rivalrous feelings toward his sister through caretaking and mentorship—this has likely been recapitulated in many relationships throughout his life.

Later childhood was a time of growth for Mike, as he quickly found his talents appreciated by teachers and enjoyed learning in all forms. Bookish by nature, he eschewed sports, even though this was a favorite pastime of his father. This may have complicated his ability to connect to aggression as well. Given his parents' protectiveness, he may have had difficulty finding peer relationships during this time, presaging his social difficulties of adolescence.

As opposed to his sheltered but fairly idyllic early life, adolescence was a difficult time for Mike as, for the first time, he faced overt racism and racially inspired violence. The message was complex—the White world was a minefield that was also full of opportunities. The trick was knowing where to step. Trained to avoid aggression at all costs, Mike did not fight. This kept him outwardly safe—and able to continue to idealize his father—but hindered his ability to develop assertion. Living in a predominantly White environment also kept him from developing socially— both in terms of peer and romantic relationships. It is likely that both being in a predominantly White environment, as well as his internal stance in that environment, kept him from forming a strong identity related to the Black community at large. His choice of a small predominantly White college helped him to grow academically, but still did not help him to feel powerful in the face of overt racial aggression.

Mike's attraction to extremely confident women may have been an effort to attach himself to power without actually having to be aggressive, as well as an unconscious attempt to grow powerful by association. This manifested both in his work role, as well as sexually.

The split between his father—seen as strong within the community but weak in the White world— and Jackie's family—seen as strong in the world-at-large—is an externalization of his own internal conflict about aggression, and may serve as the nidus of his confusion about his identity as a Black man.

Mike's wish to be powerful in the White world without being aggressive led him to finance, where he fantasized that hard work, dedication, and loyalty would lead to success. But at a certain point, he had difficulty progressing further, perhaps due in part to racism in the workplace and also to his difficulty with assertion. His conflict about marriage may be related to this as well, as he feels unable to be as powerful as his girlfriend would like him to be, and perhaps also to his fears about being a strong father to Black children in a White world.

Here's how the therapist shares her preliminary formulation with Mike as she recommends psychodynamic psychotherapy:

"You've given me a very vivid picture of your life. I'd like to share with you some preliminary ideas I have that can help us make a plan for therapy. It sounds to me like you may have two competing ideas about being assertive. From your family's history and from your own experience, you learned that our society is a dangerous place for Black people. The message from your family and from your community was that the way to deal with that danger was to, as you say, 'fly under the radar.' But now you're being told being assertive is important. Even necessary. Further, you have some sense that YOU want to be more assertive—and that you even regret not having been more assertive at times in your life. You're aware of some of this, and some is still out of awareness. I think that talking in psychotherapy will be enormously helpful to you—it will allow you to become aware of more of your thoughts and feelings and how they developed. I think that it will help you at work, in your relationships, and in how you feel about yourself. Any thoughts about those ideas?"

"I hear what you're saying and it sounds mostly right," says Mike. *"It's confusing in a way that it didn't used to be. I can't fully wrap my mind around the wanting to be aggressive, but I feel like I have to talk about it. Let's give it a try."*

The therapist wondered how her formulation would change as the treatment progressed. . ..

Now, let's follow as a second therapist, a 45-year-old White man, meets Willa:

Presentation

Willa is a 28-year-old White woman who identifies as heterosexual and supports herself as a graphic designer. She presents to the clinic saying that she is depressed after a "huge fight" with David, her boyfriend of six months. Willa says that she and David had been having difficulty for the last few weeks, precipitated by the announcement that he is interviewing for jobs in another city. Willa says she became "terrified" that David would leave her and began texting and calling him at all hours to "make sure" he still loved her. Three days ago, while they were arguing at David's apartment, Willa says she "refused to leave" until she had David's "guarantee" that they would stay together. She finally left after David threatened to call the police. Since then, she has felt "frantic," has not gone to work, has barely gotten out of bed, and has had very little appetite. She made the call to the clinic after a coworker texted her and suggested that she talk to someone about the situation.

After hearing Willa's initial explanation of what brought her to the clinic, the therapist thinks:

What really jumps out at me is how terrified Willa is that her boyfriend might leave her. Her terror seems to have led her to react so dramatically. I wonder how she functions in other aspects of her life.

The therapist then asks Willa about other aspects of her functioning. Here's how the therapist DESCRIBES Willa's problems and patterns:

DESCRIBE

Problem

Willa has had several days of oversleeping, a poor appetite, and an inability to get out of bed after a tumultuous fight with her boyfriend. These symptoms were not present prior to this episode. The couple has had several weeks of arguing prompted by Willa's fear that her boyfriend might leave her.

Patterns

The therapist then describes Willa's patterns in terms of self, relationships, adapting, cognition, values, and work and play.

Self

*Willa has strengths and difficulties in this area. She believes that she is a good designer and seems to have reasonable **self-perceptions** about her work and creative abilities that are neither grandiose nor self-deprecating. At work, she is generally able to handle **self-esteem threats**, such as having others critique her work, without becoming overly emotional. In her romantic relationships, however, she often responds to self-esteem threats related to rejection with tremendous anxiety and fear. Her **identity** as a designer is strong, but she does not have other strong identifications. She has an urgent feeling that she needs to be married soon and that being a single woman is "not enough."*

Relationships

Willa's personal relationships tend to be marked by **lack of trust**, rapid but shallow **intimacy** followed by estrangement, a **poor sense of self and other** with **lack of empathy**, and lack of **security**. This is particularly true in her romantic relationships. For example, the pressure of her need to be reassured by David prevented her from taking into consideration his feelings, and from considering his way of perceiving the situation.

Adapting

Willa uses different **defenses** in different situations. At work, she uses defenses such as humor and excessive emotionality. In her personal relationships, however, she tends to use **defenses that have a higher cost**, such as splitting, projection, idealization, and acting out. Her style of adapting tends to **emphasize emotions** and to be **inflexible**.

Cognition

Willa graduated with high marks from a prestigious design school. She has been praised for her ability as a graphic designer, and has also scored well on her high-school standardized tests. Thus, she seems to have talent and is likely to be **intelligent**. At work, she collaborates with a team and is able to **solve problems** and to be **creative**. In her romantic relationships, however, she has great difficulty **mentalizing** and is not particularly **self-reflective**. Also in the context of her personal relationships, she has difficulty **managing her emotions**, as was evident in her behavior with David when she was unable to "sit with" her anxiety. Although this leads her to be **impulsive** with her boyfriend (e.g., constant calling and texting), she does not have difficulty controlling her impulses with substances or at work. She does not report difficulty with **sensory regulation**.

Values

From her report, Willa seems to do things, such as paying taxes and taking her turn in a line, which indicate that she has a **system for right and wrong** to which she adheres. This has also been true in her prompt payment for the evaluation sessions. In a later session, she even volunteered that she feels guilty about badgering her boyfriend, although it's hard for her to control her behavior. "He deserves better," she says in one session. She has indicated that she loves **design and esthetics**, and that living in a place that is beautiful is important to her.

Work and play

Willa **supports** herself as a graphic designer. She works hard and has difficulty relaxing on weekends and holidays. She has few friends and tends to spend her **leisure time** cloistered with the man with whom she is currently involved.

After several evaluation sessions with Willa, the therapist begins to focus on what he has DESCRIBED:

"You are a smart, talented, and creative person, but it seems like you're having trouble believing that someone would really want to be with you. That makes you incredibly anxious—and it's that anxiety that brought you here. I'm wondering why that is. I'd like to hear more about your life story to see if it helps us understand why you seem so terrified by the idea of your boyfriend leaving you."

The therapist then listens to Willa's life story.

REVIEW

Genetics and prenatal development

Willa is the youngest of three children born to married parents. She denies any prenatal exposures or birth injuries, and she was a term baby born at seven pounds. Willa says her mother likely had untreated anxiety her whole life—she says she's a "nervous wreck" who thought that everything was a "catastrophe." She does not believe her mother was physically ill during her pregnancy with her or used substances during that time. She thinks other members of her mother's family might have anxiety as well. She does not know her father or her father's family well enough to give this history. She also says her mother has always said she was a difficult baby, who cried a lot, did not want to be left alone, and was "clingy."

Earliest years (birth –age 3)

Although Willa says she has few memories from this time, her older brothers have told her their parents were "constantly fighting." She has vague memories of her father slamming doors and of her mother crying on the couch. Willa says any memories of these years are generally of her brothers excluding her, and she feels she spent much of her time alone. Willa's father, a businessman, left her mother when Willa was three years old and quickly started a new family with a woman with whom he had been having an affair during most of his short first marriage. He moved across the country, and although he continued to send occasional checks, he had little direct contact with Willa and her older brothers. Her earliest memory is of her mother screaming at her on a street corner—she thinks it was because she had momentarily let go of her mother's hand, leading her mother to become afraid that Willa might be hit by a car.

Middle childhood (ages 3–6)

After her father left, Willa says she and her mother became much closer. She developed nightmares and could only sleep if her mother was with her. Willa says, "My brothers teased me mercilessly, saying I was a baby. I wanted to be able to sleep alone, but I couldn't do it." At around age six, her mother started dating a coworker and abruptly insisted Willa sleep in her own bed when the boyfriend began to sleep over. She had trouble separating from her mother every year at the beginning of school—in kindergarten, her mother had to sit in the "coffee room" for weeks—long after all of the other children were just being dropped off. Although she was embarrassed about this, she remembers feeling "panicked" at the thought of being in school without her mother.

Later childhood (ages 6–12)

Willa says she was lonely during later childhood. She had one or two female friends and says, "We walked home from school together, but didn't really do much else." Home life was stressful—her mother remained in an on-again, off-again relationship with the boyfriend who was a heavy drinker. Willa says, "The one thing I remember that was good was that I started drawing. It was something to do after school, and I was good at it." When at home, her mother was anxious, forcing her to wear overly warm clothing and fretting about her homework, but she would frequently forget to pick her up from school and occasionally spent the night with her boyfriend without letting her children know. Willa says, "The boyfriends came first. My mother couldn't really function without a man to help her."

Adolescence (ages 13–18)

Willa began to be noticed in school for her unusual drawing and math skills. A teacher encouraged her to apply for a scholarship to a local summer art program that she attended for several years, and she ultimately won a nationally recognized prize. She says, "Thank goodness for that; it saved me." She reports she had sex for the first time, "younger than most kids; I was probably about 15. The boys were a little older—I always had a boyfriend, but the relationships never lasted very long." She experimented with marijuana and cocaine but found they made her feel uncomfortable and did not continue to use them. She drank fairly heavily during a relationship with a boy who liked alcohol, but stopped when they broke up. Once her brothers had moved out of the house, she rarely saw them; she avoided her mother who had started to drink heavily and was rarely home overnight.

Young adulthood (ages 18–23)

Willa was accepted into a prestigious design school in her home city. Although she had planned to live with her mother, within a few weeks of matriculation she had met and moved in with her first "serious" boyfriend. She felt she had met her "soul mate," but within a few months they were fighting. Throughout her design school years, Willa had serial relationships with men that began "like gangbusters" and then ended tumultuously. Willa did very well in school, won many awards and prizes, and was offered several good jobs on graduation.

Later adulthood (ages 23–present)

Willa now supports herself and feels comfortable at her workplace. She is interested in starting her own firm but fears breaking away from her current colleagues. Her longest romantic relationship lasted almost one year and ended when her boyfriend told her that he was gay. She was "devastated," but then quickly began to date David.

Now, the therapist tries to focus on what he has REVIEWED and says to Willa,

"I'm really getting a picture of a childhood with so many confusing signals about relationships. Your father abandoned the family, and your mother almost smothered you with her anxiety."

Willa immediately breaks in with, "Yeah, she was anxious, but she really abandoned me, too. I couldn't sleep without her and then she unceremoniously tossed me out. It still makes me upset thinking about it, practically like it's happening right now."

This helps the therapist to think about how to LINK Willa's problems and patterns to her life story. Here's how he begins to put it together.

From DESCRIBE, Willa's greatest area of difficulty is her relationships—she needs to be so close to her boyfriends that she ends up emotionally strangling them. From REVIEW, the most problematic part of Willa's history is her overly close but inconsistent relationship with her mother as well as the fact that her father abandoned her. Problematic relationships generally result from problems like these, which makes me think that I could use ideas about attachment to LINK her patterns to her history. Willa was also apparently anxious from birth, and her mother has anxiety as well—this could also be a temperamental trait. So, I should factor in ideas about the impact of early cognitive and emotional difficulties as well—they may be important on their own and in the way that they shaped her early attachments. I think that Willa may also have internalized the societal idea that women cannot function well without men—that they need to be attached to a man to be complete. I should include the effect of culture and society, and I need to make sure that, as a man, I continue to listen for this, and see if I can learn more about these feelings through her feelings about me. Willa also has important strengths, which developed during later childhood and adolescence, that are help-ing her to function in important ways—I need to include that, too. I'll focus on the early development of her attachment problems, and then try to see how that affected her develop-ment throughout her life.

Here's what he writes:

LINK

Willa's area of greatest difficulty is her relationships with others. This is most likely related to her anxious-ambivalent style of attachment, which leads her to become frantic and emotionally dys-regulated when she fears abandonment. This scenario led to her current presentation and has occurred many times in the past. Willa's attachment style may be linked to genetically inherited anxiety, to her internalization of the expectation that women will be mistreated by men in society, and to her inconsistent relationship with her mother during her earliest years.

Temperamentally anxious and fearful of separation, Willa spent her earliest years in an environ-ment filled with violent parental disputes. She experienced her mother as tremendously anxious, frequently tearful, and preoccupied. Thus, it is likely she had difficulty establishing a solid dyadic relationship. Frequently alone and afraid, she never developed basic trust or the capacity for a secure attachment. Her mother's anxiety and preoccupation suggests she was not particularly attuned to Willa—Willa thus had difficulty developing a sense of her own affect states or those of others. This has likely contributed to her adult difficulties with empathy, mentalization, self-regulation, and trust.

Willa entered middle childhood with an anxious attachment style and without having consolidated many crucial capacities. Her developmental trajectory was further hindered by the fact that her father had recently left home—she thus remained locked in her two-person relationship without a desired caregiver to begin to help her feel loved and adored. This role was also not taken up by her older brothers, who had little to do with her. Her mother's abrupt expulsion of Willa from her bed and her replacement by a new boyfriend may have terrified and confused her. This oscillation between extreme closeness and abrupt abandonment likely led to her anxious attachment style. The inconsistency in her relationship with her mother continued into later childhood. Either her mother was overly concerned about her attire, or she was forgetting to pick her up from school. Her school-age separation anxiety may have been related to her temperamental anxiety, but may also have been related to her developing an anxious-ambivalent attachment style. It is likely that her mother's problematic relationship with her alcoholic boyfriend, as well as her own increased drink-ing, worsened her inconsistency and, consequently, Willa's attachment problems. It is also likely that, observing her mother's two relationships, Willa internalized society's general sense that women are dominated and too often mistreated by men.

In school, Willa's difficulty with same-sex peer friendships may have resulted from many fac-tors, including her temperamental anxiety. Her sense of self was weak because of her problematic dyadic relationship and the absence of her father, and was buoyed a bit by her discovery of drawing, which gave her pleasure as well as attention. This talent, the mentorship of her teachers, and her

artistic successes are the features of her life story that helped her most, and that are most responsi-
ble for the self-esteem that she derives from her work.

Willa's precocious sexual relationships were most likely attempts to regain her lost dyadic relation-
ship. They set the stage for the series of intense, short-lived relationships that have characterized
her young adulthood. The continuation of her anxious attachment style as a young adult has ren-
dered her virtually unable to be alone, leading her to emotionally strangle her partners and to, time
after time, destroy the very relationships to which she desperately clings.

Here's how the therapist shares his preliminary formulation with Willa as he recommends psychodynamic psychotherapy:

"You're right—your mother abandoned you, too. I think that your early experiences with both of your parents made you very frightened of abandonment. Even the possibility that it could happen fills you with terror. I think that your mother's experiences may also have taught you that women will generally be mistreated by men. All these things may be contributing to what's happening now with David. I think that psychotherapy could help you to learn more about the way you respond in relationships—that would help you now and in the future, too."

"It's as if the same thing happens to me over and over in my life." says Willa. *"I think I've just felt unlucky, but you're saying that it's a pattern I can learn about. That would be a relief."*

The therapist predicts that Willa will be able to alter her anxious-ambivalent attachment style in the context of the therapeutic relationship. He wondered how his formulation would change as the treatment progressed . . ..

Suggested activity

Can be done by individual learners or in a classroom setting

Now it's time to write a complete psychodynamic formulation of your own. Focus what you've DESCRIBED and REVIEWED, and then select organizing ideas about development that you think will usefully LINK them to form hypotheses about causation. Begin with a summary, and then try to trace the development of the person's major difficulties and strengths throughout their life. Don't forget that you can use many organizing ideas about development in a single formulation. Once again, try to share your work with a peer or a supervisor—talking about the choices you made in constructing your formulation will enhance your learning. You can also role play to practice sharing formulations in treatment.

PART FIVE: Psychodynamic Formulations in Clinical Practice

Introduction

Key concepts

We can create and use psychodynamic formulations in many different clinical situations, including:

- Acute care settings, such as emergency rooms and inpatient units
- Psychopharmacologic treatments
- Psychodynamic psychotherapy

As we learn about our patients, our psychodynamic formulations change.

Psychodynamic formulations can be useful in all clinical settings

Now that we know how to collaboratively create psychodynamic formulations, how and when do we use them? Students and clinicians often erroneously assume that psychodynamic formulations are only useful for psychodynamic psychotherapy, yet nothing could be further from the truth. Psychodynamic formulations help us to understand how and why people think, feel, and behave the way they do, and thus are helpful in every clinical situation. This includes single encounters in emergency rooms, brief therapies on medical or psychiatric inpatient units, psychopharmacologic treatments, and short- and long-term outpatient psychodynamic psychotherapies. In brief clinical situations, our psychodynamic formulations will be based on more limited information and will generally help us to understand the current difficulty. In long-term treatments, our psychodynamic formulations will be based on more extensive information and will help us to understand the broad sweep of a person's development. Regardless of the clinical situation, formulating psychodynamically helps us to understand the impact and development of our patients' conscious and unconscious thoughts and feelings.

Psychodynamic formulations are alive and changing

As we discussed in Part I, creating an initial formulation is extremely useful for many reasons—it helps us to make a treatment recommendation, set goals, and form a therapeutic strategy. However, staying open to new ways of thinking about how and why our patients think, feel, and behave enables us to deepen our formulations throughout our work with them. Psychodynamic formulations are not static—we constantly collaboratively revise them with our patients during our work together.

Let's now consider how we use psychodynamic formulations in many different clinical situations, beginning with acute care settings.

25 Psychodynamic Formulations in Acute Care Settings

Key concepts

Psychodynamic formulations are useful in all mental health treatment settings, including those offering acute care. This includes the following:

- Psychiatric emergency rooms
- Psychiatric inpatient units
- Medical or surgical services

Acute care settings pose special challenges to psychodynamic formulation because of the following:

- The clinician's time with patients is usually limited.
- Patients may be unable to provide a complete history.
- The formulation needs to target the acute problem.
- The formulation needs to include the predictable stresses related to the acute care setting itself.

Even brief, preliminary psychodynamic formulations help us to

- Engage patients
- Make sense of their current and long-term problems and patterns
- Choose the most salient problems and patterns to address
- Predict how patients are likely to respond to help
- Plan acute and ongoing treatment

Christopher, a 26-year-old gay man who is in graduate school and who lives with three friends from college, presents to the emergency room with recurrent bouts of rapid heart rate and difficulty breathing. He is crying, distraught, and frightened that he is going to die. He implores the medical staff to save him. After evaluating his symptoms, the emergency room physician tells Christopher that he is having panic attacks and administers lorazepam. This does little to calm Christopher down, and psychiatry is asked to consult.

Psychodynamic Formulation: An Expanded Approach, First Edition. The Psychodynamic Formulation Collective.
© 2022 John Wiley & Sons Ltd. Published 2022 by John Wiley & Sons Ltd.

If the evaluation of Christopher's presenting problem stopped here, it might be summarized as follows: "26-year-old man with no prior history of mental health problems or treatment presents with new onset of panic attacks." However, even in the setting of the emergency room, it is important to go beyond the presenting problem to ask, "Why did this particular person with this particular life story develop this particular problem at this particular stage of life?" (Gorton, 2000). Here's what happens when the emergency room psychiatrist comes to talk to Christopher:

> After reassuring Christopher that his problem is treatable, the psychiatrist tells him that panic attacks are sometimes precipitated by stress. He asks Christopher whether he can think of anything going on in his life recently that might be causing him stress. "It's sort of mystifying," Christopher responds. "When I finished my dissertation last month, I felt like a huge weight had been taken off my shoulders. My advisor loved it. I felt like anything was possible and I went out celebrating with my boyfriend and roommates." He sighs and adds, "But I don't know if I have what it takes to be an academic. My father says you make peanuts teaching high school and keeps asking me how I'm going to support myself with a PhD in sociology. Please don't tell him I'm here—he's already ashamed of me because I'm gay."

This suggests that Christopher may be suffering from low self-esteem because he feels he lacks his father's respect. This information helps the psychiatrist begin to answer the simple but important question "Why now?" and guides him in planning the best way to alleviate the anxiety that brought Christopher to the emergency room:

> The psychiatrist asks Christopher to say more about his life story. Christopher tells him that he has an older sister who was "born normally" to his parents. His mother desperately wanted a second child, but after a number of miscarriages decided to adopt a newborn. He says, "I've always had this feeling it was more her decision and that my father sort of went along with it to make her happy." Christopher knows nothing about his biological parents or the circumstances of his birth, but does not recall being told about any significant problems in his infancy or childhood. He describes his mother as "wonderful, giving, loving," but no match for his father: "Dad and I used to be close but he's always been a tough act to follow. I did OK in school but didn't get into the prep school or college that everyone in Dad's family attended. I was a good athlete, especially in squash, but Dad was a nationally ranked player in college. And then I came out to him . . . he didn't throw me out but really withdrew. Get the picture?"

At this point, the psychiatrist has a wealth of information about Christopher. It helps him to think about why Christopher is having anxiety now and to suggest acute treatment. It also helps him to understand Christopher's ongoing problems and patterns, and to engage with him in a discussion about possible ongoing therapy. All this will go far beyond the lorazepam dose in helping Christopher understand the way in which he is adapting to his current internal and external environment. The psychiatrist was able to get this information during a short ER consultation and uses it to create this psychodynamic formulation:

> Christopher, a 26-year-old gay man who is a graduate student in sociology, presents to the emergency room with new onset of panic disorder. His panic attacks started in the context of completing his dissertation and beginning to think about future career options. Although he was consciously excited about finishing this work, it is clear that he has been plagued by chronic doubts about his abilities—doubts that have been compounded by his father's tendency to be critical of Christopher's achievements and sexual identity. Christopher yearns for his father's approval but often feels he has

failed to live up to what he believes his father wants him to be. Thus, conflicts about moving ahead at this point may have triggered anxiety and panic. Conflicts between wanting his father's approval/acceptance, and unconscious rage at his father, may also be playing a role.

Christopher also appears to have long-standing difficulties with insecurity and low self-esteem dating back to childhood. While appropriately proud of his academic successes, Christopher is very dependent on his father's opinions, and his view of himself seems to be easily influenced by his father's put-downs. Although he had a close relationship with his mother, it may be that Christopher had difficulty developing a cohesive sense of self because of his father's lack of empathic attunement. Despite feeling loved by his mother, he may also have feelings about having been given up as an infant by parents who never wanted to know him.

The psychiatrist then shares this preliminary formulation with Christopher to collaboratively plan next steps:

"Although you're very excited about having finished your dissertation, it sounds like you might be having anxiety about your next steps. You are clearly worried about your father's feelings about your future, and that might be conflicting with your own good feelings about your achievement. Sometimes, conflicts like these can cause anxiety, and that might be helpful to talk about. What do you think about these ideas? If they resonate with you, it might be that, in addition to medication, psychotherapy might be very helpful for you in the coming months."

Thus, even in acute care settings, psychodynamic formulations provide a vital road map for engaging patients, deciding how best to address their difficulties, and predicting how they are likely to respond to our interventions.

Psychodynamic formulations help in all settings

As in the case of Christopher's brief emergency room visit, psychodynamic formulations can help to guide treatment in all clinical situations, including the following acute care settings:

- Psychiatric emergency rooms (Blackman, 1994; MacKinnon et al., 2006a; Myerson & Glick, 1980; Silbert, 1995; Sulkowicz, 1999; Talbott, 1980).
- Psychiatric inpatient units (Gabbard, 1995; Leibenluft et al., 1993; Wolpert, 1995)
- Medical and surgical services (Barnhill, 2009; Blumenfeld, 2006; Grossman, 1984; Lefer, 2006; MacKinnon et al., 2006b; Muskin, 1990, 1995; Nash et al., 2009; Strain & Grossman, 1975; Viederman, 1983)

Although we often do not have much time during acute care encounters, we can still form preliminary psychodynamic formulations that help us to understand our patients' unconscious thoughts, wishes, feelings, and fears. Even a preliminary psychodynamic formulation can help us to

- Engage our patients
- Answer the "Why now?" question
- Begin to understand the context of the patient's emotional difficulties

- Choose the most important problems and/or patterns to address acutely
- Predict how our patients are likely to respond to the help we offer
- Plan acute and ongoing treatment

Even if it seems the immediate crisis is an expectable episode in a chronic psychiatric illness, it is important to ask ourselves whether what is happening could have been triggered by thoughts or feelings that are out of the patient's awareness. Thinking psychodynamically—wherever we are working—guides us to remember that people are often motivated by unconscious thoughts and feelings. Understanding those motivations can be the key to resolving the problems that bring our patients to treatment (MacKinnon et al., 2006a, 2006b; Nash et al., 2009; Schwartz, 1995; Shapiro, 2012).

When formulating in acute care settings, it is useful to remember that these environments affect all patients in somewhat predictable ways (Schwartz, 1995). For example, coming to an emergency room often confirms a patient's feelings of worthlessness and failure, while simultaneously activating wishes to be rescued by protective caregivers. Locked inpatient units can stimulate fears of being controlled, while medical and surgical units often trigger fears about death and dying. It is important for us to consider these common reactions when collaboratively formulating with patients in these settings.

Challenges of psychodynamic formulation in the acute care setting

Creating psychodynamic formulations in acute care settings presents the clinician with unique challenges, as the time with the patient is limited and they may not hear the patient's entire life story.

The clinician's time with patients is limited

In settings like an emergency room or an inpatient unit, we generally do not have the luxury of learning someone's full life story or waiting for it to unfold over time. Instead, we often have to rely on information obtained in a single interview to formulate an understanding of the salient problems and patterns and to initiate treatment. Still, even with limited information—gathered from the history as well as from our interactions with the patient—it is possible to develop an understanding of the feelings, fantasies, and fears that may contribute to the patient's presenting problems. Consider this example:

> Thelma, a recently widowed woman in her 60's with a long history of depression, is admitted to the hospital for fever, weight loss, and abdominal pain. Her workup reveals chronic myelogenous leukemia, but Thelma refuses further treatment and asks to be discharged, saying, "I've lived long enough." The consulting psychologist acknowledges the medical intern's concern that Thelma may be "too depressed" to make this life-altering decision, but wonders why an otherwise healthy woman would decline treatment that could extend her life for many years. The psychologist

explains to Thelma that her medical doctors have asked him to see her because they are puzzled about why she is refusing relatively benign and potentially lifesaving treatment. Thelma responds, saying, "What's the point?" and begins to cry. Feeling an unexpected sense of loss, the psychologist says quietly, "It doesn't sound like you feel that there is much reason for going on." Thelma looks at him and nods, saying, "Ever since my husband died 2 years ago, I just haven't been able to pick up the pieces and move on. God knows why—he made my life miserable." Asked to say more about her marriage, Thelma says that she was verbally abused and intimidated throughout her 22-year marriage. "Especially when we found out I couldn't have kids, I felt like a failure—like all the mean things he ever said about me were true. I hated him for saying them and dreamed of divorce, but that just made me feel like even more of a sinner. In my family, even lapsed Catholics don't divorce. My girlfriends joke that I married my father. Dad was a mean drunk, always raging at my mother over nothing. It was terrifying—sometimes I was worried he'd kill her. When I was a teenager, he ran off with the church secretary and I never saw him again."

While the psychologist may have numerous goals in the consultation, his first priority is to engage the patient by conveying that he hears and recognizing her immediate concerns (Viederman 1983, 2009). When he echoes Thelma's feelings of futility, she feels understood and shares that she has been depressed since her husband's death, that the marriage was difficult, and that her relationship with her husband recapitulated aspects of her relationship with her father. With these few hints, the psychologist does not continue to probe Thelma's past history, but rather begins to develop a hypothesis that Thelma's treatment refusal may be related to her husband's death. He wonders if resigning herself to dying, when she might otherwise live a normal life span, is related to unconscious guilt about surviving her husband and is exacerbated by her self-critical thoughts about being a "lapsed" and sinful Catholic. The psychologist then uses his psychodynamic ideas to work collaboratively with Thelma:

Thelma goes on to say she has been upset with herself for having wished her husband dead at times—"It wasn't very Christian of me"—and says she feels guilty both about his death and about outliving him. The psychologist suggests to Thelma that she may be blaming herself for something she could not control. He also asks Thelma if she could forgive herself for having had one or two aggressive thoughts about her husband, particularly given the verbal abuse she endured for decades. He files away the information about her abandonment by her father but decides to keep the focus on her current feelings of guilt about her husband, which seem more directly relevant to her decision to refuse medical care. Responding to the psychologist's comment about forgiveness, Thelma smiles for the first time during the conversation. She then asks if it would be possible for the psychologist to be present when she talks to the team about further treatment.

Even in a single encounter, the psychologist learned enough about the patient's unconscious guilt to work collaboratively with Thelma to help her make a life-affirming choice.

The clinician may not be able to hear the whole life story

Patients in acute care settings may be initially unable or unwilling to provide the information necessary for a preliminary·psychodynamic formulation. In this case, it may be necessary to obtain collateral history from relatives, significant others, or outpatient therapists. It is important, however, to remember that the information obtained from other sources may be affected by their feelings about the patient's situation, and thus should be taken with the proverbial "grain of salt"—as in this example:

> *Dennis, a 47-year-old single White man living with his parents, has been hospitalized many times for symptoms of schizophrenia. Now, he is admitted involuntarily to the psychiatric inpatient unit for an acute exacerbation of psychotic symptoms after flushing all of his medications down the toilet. Although he knows that Dennis has often been noncompliant with treatment, the social worker, who emigrated from Pakistan as a child, asks himself what prompted Dennis to stop his medication at this particular time. When he asks Dennis why he thinks that he has been admitted to the hospital now, Dennis glares at him and mutters, "I'm not going to let some terrorist kill my mother." He then puts on sunglasses, turns to the wall and ignores the social worker's questions. The social worker wonders whether Dennis's initial hostility toward him could be related to long-standing anxiety about being controlled and humiliated, exacerbated in the setting of his involuntary admission to a locked ward. In addition, the social worker considers that Dennis' delusions about terrorism may be heightened by his apparent anti-Muslim sentiments. In a quiet voice, the social worker tells Dennis, "I'll try to come back at a better time. I hope we'll be able to talk then. In the meantime, if it's OK with you, I'm going to speak briefly with your mother." Dennis shifts restlessly but doesn't refuse. Looking frustrated and overwhelmed, Dennis's mother tells the social worker, "My son has never accepted that he needs medication. He's always been stubborn as a mule. Even as a teenager, way before he got sick, he was rebellious and difficult." She says that Dennis's father recently suffered a stroke and adds, "I just don't know if I can handle both of them anymore."*

Because of Dennis's paranoia and possible fears about submission and humiliation at the hands of authority figures, the social worker has to rely initially on collateral history obtained from the patient's mother. However, the social worker quickly realizes the mother's history is colored by her distress and frustration and decides that taking a more thorough history from her is unlikely to shed much light on Dennis's noncompliance. Nevertheless, he uses the information she gives him to begin to understand Dennis's current issues. For example, he wonders whether Dennis's current episode of noncompliance could be related to fears of losing his father. This understanding helps him to think about ways to reassure the patient that his father is well taken care of—for example, by arranging for home care for the father. Looking ahead to their next meeting, the social worker also begins to think about ways to circumvent Dennis' suspicion of authority, anxieties about being controlled, and resistance to being interviewed. If he is unable to defuse Dennis's hostility to Muslims, he may offer to reassign Dennis to another member of the team. Although incomplete and gleaned from a family member, the additional information about Dennis's life story helps the social worker to create a brief formulation that will help guide treatment.

The psychodynamic formulation needs to target the acute problem

Because our work with patients in acute care settings is usually time-limited, the formulations we create there should target acute issues. As illustrated in the previous examples, we always have to ask ourselves, "Why now?" In other words, is there a specific, circumscribed crisis that led this particular patient to come to acute care at this particular time? (Gorton, 2000). Even after a brief assessment, we can outline the

- Problem that brought the person to treatment at this time
- Patterns of thinking, feeling, and behaving that are most directly related to the acute crisis

We can then follow up by asking targeted questions about the person's life story that explore possible antecedents of these problems and patterns. Although focused formulations of this kind may feel incomplete, they are vital for helping us to understand our patients and to collaboratively make choices about treatment.

Suggested activity

Can be done by individual learners or in a classroom setting

Consider the following clinical situation:

> Manny is a 76-year-old previously healthy, widowed, retired infectious disease doctor who presents to the emergency room feeling feverish with shortness of breath, chest discomfort, and a pounding headache. He recently returned from a trip to Florida where he had visited his only daughter and grandchildren for the first time since the onset of the COVID pandemic. He was surprised to hear that his vital signs, oxygen saturation, labs, electrocardiogram, and chest x-ray were all normal. Although he had been vaccinated and was conscientious about prevention measures throughout the trip, he was sure he had contracted COVID and seemed almost crestfallen when told that his rapid COVID-19 test was negative. He insisted the test must be a "false negative," and demanded to stay in the emergency room until results of a "more sensitive" test were available. He became irate when told it would be safe for him to follow up with his primary care doctor, contemptuously dismissed the suggestion that his symptoms might be stress-related, and with a tone of condescension, asked the ER doctor where he went to medical school. Psychiatry was asked to consult.

Questions to consider:

- With only this information, what hypotheses might you begin to generate about the specific crisis that brought this man to the emergency room at this time?
- How might you understand his unexpected disappointment that ER staff have not established any clear medical causes for his symptoms and his resistance to their explanations and recommendations?
- What additional information would be helpful to ask him?
- Write a tentative psychodynamic formulation for Manny, targeting the acute issues. Would you share your understanding with him?

Comment

Retired physicians who have also lost a spouse may feel particularly bored, lonely, and rudderless. Often their career has formed a large part of their identity and social interactions and may have left little time for developing outside interests. In addition to these difficulties, Manny may have become even more isolated during the pandemic, cut off from his only daughter, grandchildren, friends, and former colleagues. It is easy to imagine that after a rejuvenating vacation with his family—his first in many months—it must have been depressing and stressful for Manny to return to an empty home with no job and little structure to his day. Although our information is limited, Manny appears to be a proud man who is unaccustomed to acknowledging feelings of depression and loneliness, much less revealing this 'weakness' to others, especially to younger colleagues in the medical profession. He is used to taking care of others rather than admitting his need for help. Physical symptoms may be the only tolerable way for Manny to express emotional distress and to reach out for support.

References

1. Barnhill, J. W. (2009). Overview of hospital psychodynamics. In J. Barnhill (Ed.), *Approach to the psychiatric patient: Case-based essays* (pp. 207–210). American Psychiatric Publishing, Inc.
2. Blackman, J. S. (1994). Psychodynamic techniques during urgent consultation interviews. *The Journal of Psychotherapy Practice and Research, 3*, 194–203.
3. Blumenfeld, M. (2006). The place of psychodynamic psychiatry in consultation-liaison psychiatry with special emphasis on countertransference. *Journal of the American Academy of Psychoanalysis and Dynamic Psychiatry, 34*, 83–92. https://doi.org/10.1521/jaap.2006.34.1.83
4. Gabbard, G. O. (1995). *Psychodynamic psychiatry in clinical practice*. American Psychiatric Publishing, Inc.
5. Gorton, G. E. (2000). Commentary: Psychodynamic approaches to the patient. *Psychiatric Services, 51*, 1408–1409. https://doi.org/10.1176/appi.ps.51.11.1408
6. Grossman, S. (1984). The use of psychoanalytic theory and technique on the medical ward. *Psychoanalytic Psychotherapy, 10*, 533–548.
7. Lefer, J. (2006). The psychoanalyst at the medical bedside. *Journal of the American Academy of Psychoanalysis and Dynamic Psychiatry, 34*, 75–81. https://doi.org/10.1521/jaap.2006.34.1.75
8. Leibenluft, E., Tasman, A., & Green, S. A. (1993). *Less time to do more: Psychotherapy on the short-term inpatient unit*. American Psychiatric Publishing, Inc.
9. MacKinnon, R. A., Michels, R., & Buckley, P. J. (2006a). *The psychiatric interview in clinical practice* (pp. 481–504). American Psychiatric Publishing, Inc.
10. MacKinnon, R. A., Michels, R., & Buckley, P. J. (2006b). The hospitalized patient. In *The psychiatric interview in clinical practice* (pp. 505–520). American Psychiatric Publishing, Inc.
11. Muskin, P. R. (1990). The combined use of psychotherapy and pharmacology in the medical setting. *Psychiatric Clinics of North America, 13*, 341–353.
12. Muskin, P. R. (1995). The medical hospital. In H. J. Schwartz, E. Bleiberg, & S. H. Weissman (Eds.), *Psychodynamic concepts in general psychiatry* (4th ed., pp. 69–88). American Psychiatric Publishing, Inc.
13. Myerson, A. T., & Glick, R. A. (1980). The use of psychoanalytic concepts in crisis intervention. *Psychoanalytic Psychotherapy, 8*, 171–188.
14. Nash, S. S., Kent, L. K., & Muskin, P. R. (2009). Psychodynamics in medically ill patients. *Harvard Review of Psychiatry, 17*(6), 389–397.
15. Schwartz, H. J. (1995). Introduction. In H. J. Schwartz, E. Bleiberg, & S. H. Weissman (Eds.), *Psychodynamic concepts in general psychiatry* (pp. xix–xxi). American Psychiatric Publishing, Inc.
16. Shapiro, E. R. (2012). Management vs. interpretation: Teaching residents to listen. *The Journal of Nervous and Mental Disease, 200*(3), 204–207. https://doi.org/10.1097/NMD.0b013e3182487a3e
17. Silbert, H. (1995). The emergency room. In H. J. Schwartz, E. Bleiberg, & S. H. Weissman (Eds.), *Psychodynamic concepts in general psychiatry* (pp. 49–68). American Psychiatric Publishing, Inc.
18. Strain, J. J., & Grossman, S. (1975). *Psychological care of the medically Ill: A primer in liaison psychiatry*. Appleton-Century-Crofts and Fleschner.
19. Sulkowicz, K. (1999). Psychodynamic issues in the emergency department. *Psychiatric Clinics of North America, 22*, 911–922. https://doi.org/10.1016/S0193-953X(05)70133-7
20. Talbott, J. A. (1980). Crisis intervention and psychoanalysis: Compatible or antagonistic? *Psychoanalytic Psychotherapy, 8*, 189–201.

21. Viederman, M. (1983). The psychodynamic life narrative: A psychotherapeutic intervention useful in crisis situations. *Psychiatry, 46*, 236–246.
22. Viederman, M. (2009). The psychodynamic consultation. In J. W. Barnhill (Ed.), *Approach to the psychiatric patient: Case-based essays* (pp. 183–185). American Psychiatric Publishing, Inc.
23. Wolpert, E. A. (1995). The inpatient unit. In H. J. Schwartz, E. Bleiberg, & S. H. Weissman (Eds.), *Psychodynamic concepts in general psychiatry* (pp. 39–48). American Psychiatric Publishing, Inc.

26 Psychodynamic Formulations in Pharmacologic Treatment

> ## Key concepts
>
> Psychodynamic formulations can help us to optimize psychopharmacologic treatment. In this context, the most helpful psychodynamic formulations target issues related to
>
> - Symptoms
> - Medications
> - Compliance
> - Side effects

Patients who come for mental health care generally seek relief from suffering of some kind. Some may have preferences from the outset about whether or not they want treatment with medication, psychotherapy, or both. Others may not have a particular treatment preference. Increasingly, due to the way mental health care is structured, delivered, paid for (at least in the US), and portrayed in the media, psychiatrists are often called on to just prescribe medication, leaving the talking out of the cure (Mojtabai & Olfson, 2008). Their patients may receive psychotherapy from other mental health professionals—or not at all. Patients who come for medication visits, however, are just as likely to discuss emotionally meaningful topics as are patients in psychotherapy. The pharmacologists they see can listen and respond empathically to what is troubling them (Cabaniss et al., 2017) and can realize that this information, when sensitively elicited and understood, often helps to optimize medication treatment. The realities of today's psychiatric practice, however, often dictate that psychiatrists limit the time of "med check" visits to 15–20 min. How can psychodynamic formulation fit into this treatment modality (Gabbard, 2009; Plakun, 2012)?

Psychodynamic Formulation: An Expanded Approach, First Edition. The Psychodynamic Formulation Collective.
© 2022 John Wiley & Sons Ltd. Published 2022 by John Wiley & Sons Ltd.

A psychodynamic formulation helps guide pharmacologic treatment

A psychodynamic formulation can be a helpful guide even when the treatment is envisioned as primarily pharmacologic. Good formulations help clinicians understand their patient's attitudes toward their illnesses, their medications, and their mental health providers. (Mintz & Belnap, 2011).

For the prescribing provider, the most helpful psychodynamic formulation is concise and problem-focused. Sometimes, the patient has a clear-cut psychiatric diagnosis, few or no comorbid symptoms or conditions, no conflicts about taking medication, good medication response with few or no side effects, and good compliance with the medication regimen. Generally, however, the situation is more complex. The patient may have an unclear diagnosis, multiple stressors or traumas, ambivalent or negative feelings about taking medication, troublesome side effects, or difficulty adhering to medication as prescribed. In these situations, treating clinicians will be well served by taking the time to get to know the patient well enough to collaboratively create a targeted psychodynamic formulation. This will also serve to strengthen the therapeutic alliance, which has been shown to correlate positively with treatment adherence and outcome (Cabaniss et al., 2017; Zeber et al., 2008). For patients who are receiving medication from one clinician and psychotherapy from another (**split treatment**), the willingness of the two clinicians to communicate—including exchanging ideas about the psychodynamic formulation—can be a crucial component of the treatment.

Gathering information for a targeted formulation in pharmacologic treatment

The way in which patients present for the initial consultation will guide the approach to gathering information for the targeted psychodynamic formulation. If a patient presents in crisis—for example, acutely suicidal—the immediate goal will be to ensure patient safety. More extensive history taking can wait. On the contrary, if a patient with long-standing generalized anxiety plans a consultation weeks in advance, we have time to start by getting to know the patient and understanding the "Why now?" of the visit. Of note, some of the data we need for formulation may be obtained by cultivating a good working alliance with the referring clinician, who may be a psychotherapist or a primary care doctor.

Even in a relatively non-urgent situation, however, there may not be time to fully learn the life story, or to explore in depth the patient's current and past relationships. Given the exigencies of the clinical situation, the information gathering must be targeted. So, what type of information is useful to know in order to begin to formulate? Consider this example:

> Alfred, a middle-aged construction worker, tells the pharmacologist he has come for a consultation "because my wife wants me to see you." He says he's been "a bit depressed, but it's no big deal, I get depressed when work isn't going well." He answers questions reluctantly and offers little information. Gazing at the diplomas on the wall, he says in a somewhat sarcastic tone of voice, "So, you went to a lot of schools, you must be pretty smart." The pharmacologist doesn't respond to this, but proceeds to ask questions regarding Alfred's symptoms.

In this example, the pharmacologist might conclude that Alfred has major depression and may decide to prescribe an antidepressant medication. Alfred's provocative comment about the pharmacologist's diplomas, however, suggests that other issues may also be at play, such as vulnerability to self-esteem threats and difficulty trusting others, which could affect the pharmacologic alliance and treatment. Without learning more about Alfred, his sense of self, his relationship with others, and his attitudes toward doctors, medication, and psychiatric diagnoses, there's a good chance that the treatment may not be successful (Skodol et al., 2005, 2011)

When seeing a new patient for the first pharmacology consultation, it's useful to set the frame by explaining the various goals of the visit. For example:

> *Although the main goal of today's visit is to see whether or not medication might be helpful to you, in order to best do that I'll have to get to know you as a person. So I'll be asking some questions about your current life situation as well as your past.*

The following sections discuss important pieces of information that can help clinicians create targeted psychodynamic formulations in psychopharmacologic treatment.

Asking focused questions about the patient's life story

In addition to taking a standard medical and psychiatric history, including a history of trauma, it is useful to know something about the patient's childhood and family of origin. This can be woven into a standard interview, by saying, for example:

> *It would be helpful if you could briefly tell me about yourself and what your family was like when you were growing up. How would people have described you as a child? What were your parents and siblings like? Is there anything important about your childhood or teenage years I should know?*

In particular, it is important to learn about early temperamental patterns, symptoms of cognitive and emotional difficulties, and medication history—both in the patient and in family members.

History of relationships

A useful way to ask about this is with a question such as

> *Tell me about the important people in your life.*

It can be useful to find out if anyone the patient knows is taking, or has taken, medication for a psychiatric disorder. It is also important to find out upon whom the patient relies for support and who might be a source of stress.

Adapting

Understanding how a patient adapts to stress, self-regulates, modulates sensory stimuli, and manages emotions is invaluable for psychopharmacologic treatment. This can help put the concept of medication into a larger context and to suggest nonpharmacologic strategies for managing symptoms. It can also help us to predict a patient's reactions to relapse, side effects, and treatment non-responsiveness. We can ask patients:

> *How do you typically manage stress? How do you generally deal with emotions such as anxiety, anger, or sadness? How well do you feel those coping strategies work?*

Attitudes toward illness

In addition to just getting the facts about our patients' medical and psychiatric history, we can also ask about their experience with illness or treatment, how they understand the current situation or problem, their ideas or theories about what caused or contributed to the current problem, and what they think might be helpful. Questions such as,

> *Sometimes people have ideas about why they are anxious. Do you?*

Or

> *Even though we think of depression as a medical illness, sometimes people with symptoms like yours worry that they have caused their problems. Have you had thoughts like that?*

Understanding our patients' fantasies about their symptoms can be critical to treatment success.

Attitudes toward medication

Articles in the press, direct-to-consumer ads on TV, posts on social media—these are just some of the ways that information about psychiatric medication permeates our culture. It is likely that patients who present to mental health professionals have some pre-existing opinions and feelings about medication, and it's important to ask about these when we start treatment (Drescher, 1995). Patients may know a lot or a little about psychiatric medication, and their feelings about it may range from very negative to quite positive. Often, these attitudes can be elicited by asking whether anyone the patient knows is taking, or has taken, medication for a psychiatric disorder:

> *Liam is referred to a pharmacologist by his therapist for evaluation of depression. During the initial interview, Liam tells the pharmacologist, "My sister has tried several antidepressants and she's had nothing but terrible side effects. I don't have much faith in them."*

Medication may also have specific meanings for patients. Some of these meanings may include a validation that there is something "biological" causing their symptoms, a blow to self-esteem, a "special" form of being taken care of, a means for others (e.g., the psychiatrist) to control their mind or body, or a sense that they have "failed" psychotherapy (Busch & Auchincloss, 1995; Busch & Sandberg, 2007; Frank & Gunderson, 1990)

Attitudes toward the treating clinician

Although we usually do not ask patients directly about their attitudes toward us during a consultation, we look for and note clues about this. Is the patient overly deferential and idealizing? Suspicious and mistrustful? Hostile and argumentative? All of these attitudes signal important information, and our job is to try to understand their causes and sources. They might indicate symptoms of an underlying psychiatric disorder, or they might be long-standing attitudes the patient has toward others in, for example, positions of authority. It's also important to consider that these attitudes might indicate a mistrust of the medical profession rooted in ways the medical profession has, both historically and currently, demonstrated bias against, or mistreatment or abuse of, people of color, women, LGBTQ individuals and other minority groups (Brandon et al., 2005; Drescher, 2015; Hamberg, 2008; Mensah et al., 2021; Saha et al., 2003). These attitudes may have implications for adherence to medication recommendations and can help pharmacologists more effectively engage their patients. (Douglas, 2008).

Constructing a psychodynamic formulation in a psychopharmacologic treatment

The psychodynamic formulation in a psychopharmacologic treatment targets the problems and patterns that affect the patient's feelings, attitudes, and behaviors toward medication. In essence, we want to know

> *Given this person's problems, patterns of relating to self and others, characteristic ways of adapting to stress and conflict, and life story, how can I predict how they will react to pharmacologic treatment?*

Some of the more common patterns and conflicts that may affect a patient's attitudes toward pharmacologic treatment are problems with self-esteem, trust, and dependency. As mentioned earlier, some patients may feel that receiving a psychiatric diagnosis for which medication is recommended constitutes a self-esteem blow. The physical fact of ingesting a pill every day can be experienced as a concrete reminder that one is "defective" or using a "crutch." Patients who have problems with trust may be reluctant to follow the recommendations of a psychiatrist, or to ingest a substance that can cause unpleasant physical sensations or potentially dangerous side effects.

Patients who are reluctant to depend on others may feel that relying on a pill, or on the doctor whom they need to see for the prescription, is a weakness or blow to their sense of independence or self-reliance. Particularly if a medication is helpful, it can be all the more distressing to anticipate a situation in which it is needed but unavailable. Understanding these common fears can help us talk to our patients about them and to find strategies for reducing anxiety and increasing therapeutic alliance.

Here are a few psychodynamic formulations created in psychopharmacologic treatments. Let's start with this formulation for Ivan:

Presentation

Ivan, who is 30 years old, goes to a pharmacologist for evaluation of long-standing anxiety. He has episodic attacks of panic, with shortness of breath and fear he is having a heart attack. He also has a fear of germs and contamination that lead him to spend long amounts of time each day washing his body, belongings, and apartment. This often makes him late to work and has impeded his ability to have a long-standing romantic relationship. He has come now at the recommendation of his psychotherapist, who feels a course of CBT could be aided by medication. Despite his distress, Ivan has not wanted to take medication. He describes his symptoms reluctantly and seems embarrassed when the pharmacologist asks him for details.

DESCRIBE

Problem

Ivan seems to have symptoms of panic disorder and Obsessive Compulsive Disorder (OCD) that interfere with his daily life and romantic relationships.

Patterns

Ivan suffers from a lifelong pattern of low self-esteem. He feels unable to do things other people can do, and he tends to withdraw from relationships when faced with self-esteem threats. Although he is interested in others and able to empathize with them, his relationships have lacked security and intimacy. Since grade school, he has had difficulty with organizing tasks and reading speed, although he has always excelled at math. He enjoys his work as a computer programmer but finds it difficult to relax on weekends and during vacations.

REVIEW the life story

Ivan is the younger of two children whose parents are both highly educated professionals. His older sister always excelled at school and is now a professor. Ivan suffered from a learning disability and struggled academically despite receiving educational support and tutoring. Ivan felt his parents, who highly valued academic achievement, always made him feel as though he was "defective" because of this, and he felt they favored his older, more traditionally successful sister.

Although Ivan first developed symptoms of anxiety in his early teens, he did not disclose this to anyone until his late 20s. Now, in his first significant romantic relationship, he is contemplating moving in with his girlfriend and is terrified about revealing his symptoms to her. Furthermore, he believes "only people who are really ill take psychiatric medication." He feels if he is prescribed medication, it will signify there is "truly" something wrong with him, and it will be one more thing he has to hide from his girlfriend. Also, he has heard some medications used to treat OCD can cause low libido and impotence, and he is unwilling to consider a medication that might have that side effect.

LINK problems/patterns to life story

Ivan's low self-esteem may be related to his experience of his parents' attitudes toward him and his academically more successful sister, as well as to the difficulty he encountered in school. He has kept his symptoms a secret as a way to manage shame. He views medication as further evidence that there is something wrong with him, and this may influence his willingness to adhere to pharmacologic treatment. Ivan worries about potential sexual side effects of medication; therefore, if such symptoms were to develop, he might view them as a further, perhaps intolerable, blow to self-esteem.

This formulation helps the pharmacologist realize that in discussing a treatment plan with Ivan, it will be important to keep in mind Ivan's sensitivity about matters of self-esteem and his tendency not to reveal potentially shameful information about himself.

Now consider this formulation for Estee:

Presentation

Estee is a 45-year-old mother of two whose husband died of cancer a year and a half ago. She comes for a consultation with a psychopharmacologist, at the suggestion of a friend who has benefited from medication for depression. Estee has felt "under a lot of pressure" since her husband's death, has had trouble sleeping and concentrating, and feels "down" and often short-tempered. This is causing friction with her children at home and with colleagues at work. She has also fallen behind on professional obligations. She attributes these symptoms to her difficult life situation—that is, raising and supporting two children on her own. She tells the pharmacologist she's not sure if anyone, or anything, can help her and that she should just "pull [herself] together and get over it." When asked her thoughts about medication, Estee says, "I wouldn't want to take anything that I could get addicted to." After the psychopharmacologist discusses the likelihood that an antidepressant medicine could help her feel and function better, Estee says, "Well, let's say that I do feel better – then what? Would I have to stay on the medicine for the rest of my life in order to function? I wouldn't want that."

DESCRIBE

Problem

Estee has symptoms of depression in the context of a major loss, the death of her husband. She is ambivalent about considering medication treatment.

Patterns

Estee has generally had good self-esteem and has a stable sense of identity. Throughout her life she has had close friendships, characterized by empathy and intimacy, although she tends to prefer to rely on herself rather than on others. She feels that, before her husband's illness, she had a mutually satisfying relationship with him. She likes her work, believes she does well at it, and, in the past, has enjoyed getting together with friends and reading.

REVIEW the life story

Estee grew up in a chaotic family, the oldest of four children. Her mother was addicted to alcohol and prescription drugs, and by the time Estee was an early adolescent, her mother spent most of the time in her own bedroom. Her father was often away on business and was emotionally distant when home. Through most of her teenage years, Estee was responsible for caring for her younger siblings and helping to run the household. Despite all of this, Estee excelled at school and won a scholarship to a good college. After graduating she embarked on a successful career. She married in her mid-30s and had two children within a few years. She describes her late husband as a kind, loving, and trustworthy man, but says, "In the end, I couldn't depend on him; he got cancer and died."

LINK problems/patterns to life story

Although Estee appears to have considerable strengths, such as motivation, self-reliance, and resilience, which have helped her to establish a secure and successful life as an adult, she has had lifelong difficulty depending on others. Her early life history is notable for the lack of parental support, both emotional and practical, and her assumption of adult caregiving responsibilities while still in her teens. It is likely that her childhood experience of her parents as unreliable and undependable affected her attitude toward depending on others, a situation she mistrusts and avoids if possible. This attitude will likely influence her stance toward psychotropic medication and the clinician who prescribes it. Even if she agrees to try medication, and particularly if it helps her symptoms of depression, Estee may remain highly ambivalent about remaining on medication.

Being able to formulate a theory about how Estee's fears of dependency developed over her lifetime and currently influence her decision making about medication may help Estee disentangle present-day choices from long-standing patterns of emotion and behavior.

Suggested activity

Can be done by individual learners or in a classroom setting

Consider a patient with whom you work who is taking medication. Write a few sentences describing (or discuss with a colleague) two ways that their life story could affect their experience of their pharmacologic treatment. Pay particular attention to their attitudes toward you, as either the therapist, the prescriber, or both.

References

1. Brandon, D., Isaac, L., & LaVeist, T. (2005). The legacy of Tuskegee and trust in medical care: Is Tuskegee responsible for race differences in mistrust of medical care? *Journal of the National Medical Association, 97*(7), 951–956. PMID: 16080664

2. Busch, F. N., & Auchincloss, E. L. (1995). The psychology of prescribing and taking medication. In H. J. Schwartz, E. Bleiberg, & S. Weissman (Eds.), *Psychodynamic concepts in general psychiatry* (1st ed., pp. 401–416). American Psychiatric Publishing, Inc.

3. Busch, F. N., & Sandberg, L. S. (2007). *Psychotherapy and medication: The challenge of integration.* Analytic Press.

4. Cabaniss, D. L., Cherry, S., Douglas, C. J., & Schwartz, A. (2017). *Psychodynamic psychotherapy: A clinical manual* (2nd ed.). Wiley Blackwell.

5. Douglas, C. J. (2008). Teaching supportive psychotherapy to psychiatric residents. *American Journal of Psychiatry, 165*, 445–452. https://doi.org/10.1176/appi.ajp.2007.07121907

6. Drescher, J. (1995). Psychotherapy, medication and belief. *Issues in Psychoanalytic Psychology, 17*(1), 7–28.

7. Drescher, J. (2015). Ethical issues in treating LGBT patients. In J. Sadler, C. W. van Staden, & K. W. M. Fulford (Eds.), *Psychodynamic concepts in general psychiatryoxford handbook of psychiatric ethics* (pp. 180–192). Oxford University Press.

8. Frank, A. F., & Gunderson, J. G. (1990). The role of the therapeutic alliance in the treatment of schizophrenia: Relationship to course and outcome. *Archives of General Psychiatry, 47*(3), 228–236. https://doi.org/10.1001/archpsyc.1990.01810150028006

9. Gabbard, G. O. (2009). Deconstructing the "med check." *Psychiatric Times, 26*(9). http://www.psychiatrictimes.com/display/article/10168/1444238

10. Hamberg, K. (2008). Gender bias in medicine. *Women's. Health, 4*(3), 237–243. https://doi.org/10.2217/17455057.4.3.237

11. Mensah, M., Ogbu-Nwobodo, L., & Shim, R. (2021). Racism and mental health equity: History repeating itself. *Psychiatric Services.* Published January 12, 2021, https://doi.org/10.1176/appi.ps.202000755

12. Mintz, D., & Belnap, B. A. (2011). What is psychodynamic psychopharmacology? An approach to pharmacologic treatment resistance. In E. Plakun (Ed.), *Treatment resistance and patient authority: The Austen Riggs reader.* W.W. Norton & Co. p. 42–65

13. Mojtabai, R., & Olfson, M. (2008). National trends in psychotherapy by office-based psychiatrists. *Archives of General Psychiatry, 65*(8), 962–970. https://doi.org/10.1001/archpsyc.65.8.962

14. Plakun, E. (2012). Treatment resistance and psychodynamic psychiatry: Concepts psychiatry needs from psychoanalysis. *Psychodynamic Psychiatry, 40*(2), 183–210.

15. Saha, S., Arbelaez, J., & Cooper, L. (2003). Patient-physician relationships and racial disparities in the quality of healthcare. *American Journal of Public Health, 93*, 1713–1719. https://doi.org/10.2105/AJPH.93.10.1713

16. Skodol, A. E., Gunderson, J. G., Shea, M. T., McGlashan, T. H., Morey, L. C., Sanislow, C. A., Bender, D. S., Grilo, C. M., Zanarini, M. C., Yen, S., Pagano, M. E., & Stout, R. L. (2005). The collaborative longitudinal personality disorders study (CLPS): Overview and implications. *Journal of Personality Disorders, 19*, 487–504. https://doi.org/10.1521/pedi.2005.19.5.487

17. Skodol, A. E., Grilo, C. M., Keyes, K., Geier, T., Grant, B. F., & Hasin, D. S. (2011). Relationship of personality disorders to the course of major depressive disorder in a nationally representative sample. *American Journal of Psychiatry, 168*, 257–264. https://doi.org/10.1176/appi.ajp.2010.10050695

18. Zeber, J., Copeland, L. A., Good, C. B., Fine, M. J., Bauer, M. S., & Kilbourne, A. M. (2008). Therapeutic alliance perceptions and medication adherence in patients with bipolar disorder. *Journal of Affective Disorders, 107*, 53–62. https://doi.org/10.1016/j.jad.2007.07.026

27 Psychodynamic Formulations in Long-Term Psychodynamic Psychotherapy

---

Key concepts

When we first see patients, we create initial psychodynamic formulations that help us to

- Make treatment recommendations
- Conceptualize therapeutic strategy

In long-term psychodynamic psychotherapy, we continuously revise the formulation as we learn more about patients from

- How they see themselves in their outside lives
- New information that emerges about their life stories
- How they react to us in the context of the treatment

Formulations change over time

One of the most exciting and gratifying aspects of long-term psychodynamic psychotherapy is that it enables us to get to know patients very well over time. Week after week, we learn about our patients through what they say and how they behave. We learn about how they react to good and bad news, excitement and stress, victories and losses. We learn about how they think and how they feel, how they love and how they hate. As our alliance with them grows, they tell us more about their lives. We use this information to revise our initial formulation over time as we understand our patients more fully.

In this chapter, we will focus in detail on one psychodynamic psychotherapy to understand how a therapist's understanding of a person evolves during long-term treatment.

Psychodynamic Formulation: An Expanded Approach, First Edition. The Psychodynamic Formulation Collective.
© 2022 John Wiley & Sons Ltd. Published 2022 by John Wiley & Sons Ltd.

Initial presentation

Sofia, a 34-year-old Latinx woman comes to see a 42-year-old African-American male therapist. The mother of a 4-year-old son, she is seeking help with stress related to managing her divorce and starting a new relationship. Sofia, who is expressive, warm, and personable, says, "I really hope you can help me. I'm finally ready to try once and for all to figure this stuff out." She tells the therapist she and her now ex-husband, Matt, a White man, separated 2 years ago after she found out he was having an affair with a colleague. Sofia says Matt was prone to angry outbursts, and she thinks that leaving him was the right decision. She adds that she never felt accepted by his family, who frequently made disparaging comments about their son needing to learn Spanish or about her making empanadas for Christmas. Explaining that co-parenting has been difficult, Sofia states, "My ex-husband travels a lot for work and, although he says he wants to co-parent, he often cancels visits with our son at the last minute." Sofia says her son is the "one good thing that came out of the marriage," and that she is relieved that he seems to be holding up well.

When the therapist asks about her life story, he learns that Sofia grew up in what she calls a "tight knit family" that supports one another both emotionally and financially when necessary. She says that she is particularly close to her mother, but that she is estranged from her older sister. "She's very judgmental," Sophia explains.

Sofia currently works as a software programmer and has recently been promoted to a position in which she supervises a team of about 10 people. When a colleague remarked that this promotion was because of "affirmative action," Sofia felt she was able to "brush that comment off." She says that she enjoys her work and adds, "Thank goodness for my job. I think it keeps me sane."

Sofia explains she has begun a new relationship with Douglas, a 40-year-old African-American man who works at her company. She says that although he is still married, Douglas is separated from his wife and has hired a divorce lawyer. She says that, in many ways, her relationship with Douglas is an improvement over her relationship with her ex-husband. She thinks Douglas is kinder and more thoughtful than Matt, and that he is more able to talk about his feelings and less likely to fly off the handle. She also notes it is a little easier to be in a relationship with someone who is also a member of a minority group. Sofia says she wants to stay in this relationship, but she is increasingly anxious about Douglas's friendship with an ex-girlfriend who is now their colleague. She says she becomes intensely jealous whenever he mentions this colleague and she remarks, "I'm afraid I'm going to sabotage this relationship." She also worries about Douglas's safety, saying that, if he is more than a few minutes late, she imagines he has been in a car accident or the target of discriminatory behavior at the hands of the police. When the therapist asks her about her past psychiatric history, she says she had several years of binging and purging in her early 20s that "went away on its own after I met my husband."

After the therapist's first interview with Sofia, he conceptualizes her presenting **problems and patterns** in the following way:

DESCRIBE

Problem

Sofia is adjusting to being divorced. She wonders why she chose to marry a man who turned out to be so difficult and did not share her values (e.g., having a close-knit family, enjoying her cultural background, and being a hands-on parent). In addition, she has become increasingly worried and jealous in her relationship with a new boyfriend.

Patterns

Self

Sofia has a relatively positive sense of her capabilities, particularly at work. She has a strong sense of her identity as a Latinx woman. In the context of her relationships, however, she is less secure and more vulnerable to self-esteem threats.

Relationships

Relationships are clearly the area in which Sofia has the most difficulty. Throughout her life, she has chosen to have relationships with people she is not fully able to trust, thus limiting the degree of intimacy, security, and mutuality she is able to experience. In her marriage, she chose to be with someone she now describes as angry and difficult and who did not help to ease her discomfort with his family. She is currently with a man who is not yet divorced and whose friendship with another woman makes her jealous. Her difficulty with relationships also seems to predate her marriage, because she is estranged from her older sister.

Adapting

Sofia tends to react quickly and somewhat impulsively. She is an emotional person who easily expresses anger. At vulnerable times in her life (e.g., going to college, being on her own as a young adult), she has turned to action-oriented ways of handling her feelings (e.g., binging and purging). Of note, Sofia is able to handle her emotions far more effectively at work than in her personal relationships.

Cognition

Sofia's cognitive functioning is an area of strength. She performed well in school and has continued to advance at work. In addition, she has a good capacity for self-reflection. For example, she realizes that her jealousy about Douglas could sabotage the relationship.

Values

Sofia values close family relationships as well as hard work, fairness, and loyalty. Her cultural background is important to her, and she wants to transmit aspects of it to her son. She has a sense of right and wrong, and she values doing things for others.

Work/Play

Sofia has found a satisfying career in which she is doing well. She enjoys being a parent and is relatively comfortable with her work/personal life balance.

Based on this, the therapist asks himself this focus question after his first interview with Sofia:

Why does Sofia have such difficulty with romantic relationships?

He hypothesizes that there are likely developmental explanations for this pattern, and as he reviews Sofia's history in his second session, he keeps this question in mind.

REVIEW the life story

Sofia grew up relatively well-off in Central America. She says she met normal developmental milestones and performed well in school. Her earliest memories are of her mother as warm and attentive. She describes her father as controlling and sometimes prone to angry outbursts, especially when things weren't going well at work. Sofia says she "shut down" during these times, and her mother "tried her best to protect me but would ultimately give in to my father."

When Sofia came to the United States to go to college, she had a difficult adjustment and missed her family. She felt very alone as she did not have any extended family here. She worried how her mother would manage at home without her. Sofia spoke to her mother almost every day, saying, "My mother says she wouldn't have gotten through that time without me." Sofia excelled academically and found mentors in her college professors, including one who spoke Spanish. Sofia's parents later immigrated to the United States, and they remain married. She says that, once here, her father, who had a secure job in their country of origin, struggled to keep a job and that he has likely had affairs. Sofia is the middle of three sisters, each separated by four years. She reports that, as children, the girls were close. Sofia feels she was "always my father's favorite . . . that drove my older sister crazy. I was better in school than she was, and that went a long way with my father." As adults, the oldest sister and Sofia had a falling-out. Sofia says, "my sister never approved of my relationship with Matt, so I couldn't bear talking to her."

Sofia says she has several close male friends but finds that for some reason her friendships with women "don't tend to last." She had a later start to dating as she didn't feel she could connect to many of the male students at her mostly White, small-town college. She had two serious relationships prior to meeting her husband; she says, "They were a lot like him—actually, they were probably worse. I seem to like intense, strong-minded men who aren't so good for me in the long run."

LINK

After their first two sessions, the therapist organizes his thoughts about the most important aspects of Sofia's psychology. Here is his thought process as he writes his initial formulation:

When I describe Sofia's problems and patterns, the area that stands out is relationships—that's where she's having the most difficulty. She repeatedly gets involved with people about whom she becomes jealous. Although she seems to be moving in the right direction—she says she is happier in the relationship with Douglas than she was with her husband—this pattern has repeated. She has many strengths—she has a good work history, enjoys being a parent, and is self-reflective.

What about her life story? She seems to have had a secure attachment to her mother, but it sounds like things got more complicated in middle childhood. Being her father's favorite in the context of her parents' contentious relationship could not have been easy. It sounds like a trouble spot. Perhaps she had difficulties with triadic relationships; I think I could link her relationship problems to her trouble in middle childhood using ideas about conflict and defense as an organizing idea. Her difficulties during this period may have contributed to her problems in romantic relationships later in life.

Sofia's problems likely also link to the effects of culture and society. She immigrated to the United States to attend college and found it difficult to make a connection with male students at her school. She didn't start dating until she moved to a larger city after graduation. For the first few years in the United States, she felt alone. When her parents moved here, she watched them strug-gle to make ends meet and wanted to help support them. She ultimately married a man who could not relate to her experience as a bicultural immigrant. While she is in a happier relation-ship now, she worries about how her boyfriend is treated in a racist society, although she feels that, as a member of a minority group himself, Douglas can understand her experience more than her ex-husband could.

Initial psychodynamic formulation

The therapist uses these points to develop his thinking about Sofia and writes the following formulation.

Sofia has a strong positive sense of herself as evidenced by her confidence and enjoyment in her work and parenting. Her vulnerability to self-esteem threats is predominantly in relationships with other people. For example, Sofia could not tolerate her sister's criticism, and therefore, cut-off contact with her.

Most significantly, Sofia's greatest difficulties are in the area of her intimate relationships. She thought that in marrying a man from a different culture, she was choosing someone different from her father. Yet, she now wonders about that choice. The trouble Sofia has in relationships often involves three people: herself, her partner, and a rival. This suggests that her difficulties with men could be related to problems with the three-person relationships of middle childhood. Sofia was her father's favorite—but she was the favorite of a man who was abusive to her mother. She may seek men like her father because she unconsciously continues to crave the admiration she felt for him. In addition, she now realizes that in attempting to escape from her father's anger, she may have also been rejecting her culture, and that she may have chosen a man who did not share many of her values.

Use of the formulation

In the beginning of treatment

The therapist's initial formulation suggests that Sofia has unresolved unconscious conflicts related to three-person relationships. He decides to recommend twice-a-week psychodynamic psychotherapy that will encourage further exploration of her unconscious conflicts, perhaps in the context of the transference. He says to Sofia:

"Your divorce has been a major event in your life, and I can see that it is making you rethink a lot of things. I appreciate that you are noticing patterns in your relationships. I think you are asking a very important question when you wonder why you tend to get involved with difficult, angry men. This is something we can try to figure out together in psychotherapy. You're aware of a lot about yourself—this will be helpful in this process. However, I think you have thoughts and feelings that are out of awareness and are driving some of your choices. In therapy, we'll try to get as much access as we can to how your mind works and what you feel on a deeper level, so that we can learn about what affects your decisions and choices. We can learn about your internal world from your thoughts and feelings about yourself, about people in your life, and even about me."

Sofia begins twice-weekly psychotherapy, is able to talk in sessions, and is enthusiastic about treatment. As she engages in therapy, she talks less about her ex-husband and more about her relationship with Douglas. In particular, she frequently mentions Douglas's ex-girlfriend with whom she fears he will reunite—despite the fact he has reassured her there is no longer anything between them. Sofia confesses she has begun to check Douglas's computer for evidence of communication with his ex-girlfriend but so far has found nothing.

After a few months of treatment

Months go by and the therapist begins wondering how Sofia's jealous and competitive feelings might emerge in her transference to him. Because three-person relationships appear to be central to Sofia's difficulties, the therapist has been listening for hints about whether Sofia is curious about who else is in his life. About six months after starting therapy, right before the therapist is going away for a planned two-week vacation, Sofia has the following dream:

> Sofia: *It was winter and snow was all around. I knocked on the door of a beautiful house. YOU answered the door! I said, "Hi, I'm here for the party." And you said, "Sorry, I think you got the date wrong." Then I heard a woman calling in the background, saying, "Who is it honey?" And I felt so bad and started sobbing. That was the end of the dream.*

The therapist thinks about the meaning of his upcoming vacation and wonders if perhaps Sofia is imagining with whom he will be. He says:

> Therapist: *I wonder if my going away has something to do with this dream. Was there something about hearing the woman's voice in the dream that was upsetting to you?*

> Sofia: *No, it wasn't that. It was that I had gotten the day wrong. I was so disappointed. I felt like I was being turned away into the cold.*

The therapist's first response is to think that Sofia is not quite ready to talk about her feelings of jealousy related to him. He considers pursuing Sofia's feelings about the woman but notices that talking about "being turned away into the cold" has seemed to shake her up. Following her affect, he decides to ask about this:

> Therapist: *What about being turned away into the cold? Does that remind you of anything in particular?*

> Sofia: *I felt so very sad. That house—it reminded me of the one I lived in when I was little in my country, before my father started having trouble at work and we had to move to a smaller house. I think he was very angry because he was not promoted, and a White guy who was less deserving than he was promoted instead. It was definitely discrimination because my father was from an indigenous background, but there was no way to speak up about those things where he worked. It reminds me of my work colleague thinking I was promoted only because of affirmative action and not because I am qualified. I remember there was this one winter, I was probably about 5 years old. I was so cold, we couldn't go out. There was nothing to do. I was so lonely.*

Therapist:	Lonely?
Sofia:	I don't know if I ever told you, but my mother got very depressed after my younger sister was born. The thing is, her mother, the grandmother I never met, died a few months before my sister was born. No one ever talks about it now, but I think my mother might even have had to go to a hospital (she starts to cry).
Therapist:	It sounds like that was a very difficult time for you and your family.
Sofia:	Yes, actually, now I'm thinking about it, I don't know if my mother was ever really the same after that. Maybe that's why she had such a hard time when I went away to college.

The therapist mulls over this addition to Sofia's life story. He thinks more about what she has been discussing in recent weeks. He realizes that while she initially focused on her jealousy about Douglas's relationship with his ex-girlfriend, Sofia is now more preoccupied with details like how long it takes Douglas to respond to her text messages, how many times they see each other in a week, and whether he remembers details about her life. The therapist finds himself shifting his formulation toward considering Sofia's experience of her two-person relationships. He also notes how much culture and society have influenced her development both as a child and as an adult. He makes a note to explore this with Sofia in further sessions. In the next session, the last before the therapist's vacation, Sofia starts by saying she's having a terrible time sleeping and that she is feeling very anxious. The therapist decides to change his focus to see if this information confirms his new viewpoint:

Therapist:	I wonder if your trouble sleeping and anxiety might be related to my going away for two weeks.
Sofia:	Why are you going away anyway? What if something happens to you while you're gone? I feel like I might totally fall apart. It seems like we are just getting started. Why do you have to go away right now? And what if something happens to you and you're not able to come back to work?
Therapist:	You know, I wonder if this could have something to do with what we were talking about last time, about your mother's depression and when you felt so lonely without her, and then so worried about her when you went away to college. That must have been very scary.
Sofia	Huh . . . Maybe. I've been thinking a lot about it since our last meeting. I can't remember my mother being around much at all during those years. You know, my son is almost the same age I was back then. He needs me so much right now. How did I cope? I'm always there for him. And I don't just leave for vacation.

Sofia's response confirms the therapist's evolving thoughts about her. He thinks:

Sofia's reactions to me and the degree of anxiety she feels about my upcoming absence now seem less about jealousy or competitiveness, and more about worrying about me and being taken care of by me. It's interesting the way this vacation brought out that early memory about both her mother's depression and her father's painful experience of discrimination at work. Both her *reaction to me and this new information seem to confirm my thought that I had focused too much on her three-person relationships and not enough on her early dyadic relationship with each of her parents. This is helping me to focus more on how preoccupied and stressed by grief and the difficulties of discrimination and systemic oppression her parents were during her childhood. I think I'll revise the formulation, now using attachment as an organizing idea about development to link the problems/patterns to the life story. Middle childhood relationships are also likely to have been problematic, but at this point in the treatment, it seems that thinking about attachment will help me more in trying to understand her.*

He revises his formulation as in the following.

Revised formulation from later in treatment

Sofia has a strong positive sense of herself as evidenced by her confidence and enjoyment in her work and as a parent. Her vulnerability to self-esteem threats is predominantly in relationship to other people. For example, Sofia could not tolerate her sister's criticism, and therefore, cut off contact with her. Her greatest difficulties are in the area of her intimate relationships. It is likely that this is linked to difficulties which she had in her earliest relationships. Her mother, who was depressed from the time Sofia was aged 3 or 4 years, was likely unable to attend to her daughter's needs. There may even have been a period of separation. Her father suffered discrimination at work, leading to a sense of insecurity in relationship to the world around the family. This likely led Sofia to develop an anxious attachment. This attachment style was compounded by her father's volatility and mother's submissive distress. This attachment style was useful in that she provided badly needed support for her mother. In addition, the frequent contact with her mother gave Sofia support she needed as well. This led to Sofia's having difficulty developing certain central functions, including an ability to self-regulate and to modulate affect. As a child, her anxious attachment style may have been the most adaptive response to her mother's depression and need for her support. As an adult, however, her preoccupied/anxious attachment style may make her unable to tolerate any absence from her partners, leading to continuous fears of abandonment and loss. Sofia has also experienced losses associated with immigration, including initial separation from her family as a young adult that may have also primed her for these fears. In addition, her difficulty with self-regulation may have led to her binging and purging behavior, as well as to her tendency to act impulsively. Her middle childhood relationships were undoubtedly affected by her attachment style as well—she may have clung more desperately to her volatile but doting father, given her mother's emotional unavailability. This may have made it more difficult to identify with her mother and may have affected her current ability to connect to women.

Using the revised formulation

The therapist shares with Sofia his thought that this is an important phase in her therapy, which, although difficult, will help them to understand her relationships. He reassures Sofia that there's a covering therapist whom she can call in his absence, that he will take care to be safe while he is away, and that they will resume discussing these issues when he returns. Sofia seems calmer and wishes the therapist a good vacation.

When the therapist returns, he focuses on further understanding the period of Sofia's development during the time of her mother's depression, as well as during the time when she began college. They also discuss Sofia's memory that, as a child, she suffered stomach aches that caused her to miss many days of kindergarten, leaving her home with her mother who sat for long periods without talking. Sofia then talks more about her marriage, stating, "You know, I think I sort of drove him crazy, always asking him when he'd be home. I used to get so mad if he was even 10 minutes later than he said he'd be." The therapist helps Sofia to realize that she worries about her partner's safety whenever he is away from her, and that this is central to her relationship difficulties. As Sofia talks more about Douglas, it becomes clear that her feelings about his ex-girlfriend are less about jealousy and competition, and more about wanting his full attention and worrying about whether he is safe. The therapist is then able to help Sofia understand this as a carryover from her feelings of longing for her mother. Over time, Sofia learns to trust that the therapist cares about her and that he will reliably return from absences to resume their work together. This trust ultimately carries over to Douglas, whom Sofia tells that letting her know when he will return is more about his safety in an unsafe world than her jealousy about prior relationships. This enables them to develop a closer, more mutually satisfying relationship. Additionally, as the therapist (like Douglas) is African American, he wonders if Sofia may have fears about *his* safety and imagines that this may soon come up in the therapy.

In all of these situations, the formulation was central to the way the therapist planned and conducted the treatment. But how is the patient involved? When do we share our formulations? That is the subject of Chapter 28.

Suggested activity

Can be done by individual learners or in a classroom setting

Think about a patient with whom you have been working for over six months. Can you think of two things that have you learned about the patient recently that might lead you to rethink your initial formulation? Write a few sentences about each, and about your revised formulation.

28 Collaborative Formulations in Clinical Practice

Key concepts

Throughout treatment, we share our evolving ideas about the formulation with our patients. This helps us to

- Collaboratively create our initial formulation
- Recommend treatment and set early goals
- Create a life narrative
- Offer explanations and perspective throughout the therapy
- Prepare for ending therapy

Timing is important when sharing ideas about formulation.

- Before we share our ideas about formulation, we should anticipate our patients' reactions.
- After we share our ideas about formulation, we should monitor our patients' responses.

"I wonder," says a therapist during a session, "whether your intense feelings of envy at your friend's wedding could be related to feelings you had about your little sister."

In psychodynamic psychotherapy, we call that intervention an **interpretation**. Thinking in terms of formulation, each interpretation is really a little piece of formulation—a nascent hypothesis—that the therapist floats out to the patient to see how it will land. The patient's response helps to shape and hone the therapist's ideas. This back-and-forth, which continues throughout the treatment, is the **collaborative process of formulation**.

Just as we do not always make interpretations during the treatment, we must think about how and when to engage in this collaborative process. When working with patients, we constantly make choices about whether or not to share our hypotheses and, when we do share, on what to focus. In this chapter, we review some principles for considering how and when to engage in collaborative formulating with our patients.

Psychodynamic Formulation: An Expanded Approach, First Edition. The Psychodynamic Formulation Collective.
© 2022 John Wiley & Sons Ltd. Published 2022 by John Wiley & Sons Ltd.

How do we decide how and when to engage in collaboratively formulating with our patients?

No patient needs to get a single-spaced typewritten formulation. Rather, we share **parts** of our formulations as they are relevant to what we are discussing in the treatment. We can use the same **choosing principles,** which we use for deciding when and how to intervene, to help us to think about how and when to share our formulations (Cabaniss et al., 2017). These principles are

- Focus on material that is closest to the surface
- Follow the affect
- Listen to your countertransference

Is the patient trying to make connections between their current life and the past? Are they newly receptive to ideas about a lifelong pattern? Would the patient benefit from considering the potential impact of social factors or discrimination on their daily life or recent events? These could be good reasons to share parts of the formulation. On the other hand, moments of strong feelings about here-and-now situations, difficulties considering connections between the past and present, and points of weakened alliance are not likely to be opportune moments for collaborative formulation. Each situation is unique, and the choosing principles are our guides.

Notice that we are talking about sharing "parts" of our formulations. Sharing our hypotheses about the developmental origins of a person's problems and patterns should help to deepen the process, not to overwhelm or intellectualize it. Short segments of formulation that are directly related to what is uppermost in the patient's mind are most likely to have a therapeutic effect. Sharing formulations can backfire if we say too much, are not attuned to the patient's current feeling, or try to impose hypotheses on patients who are not open to new views about themselves. Patients with self-esteem problems and/or long-standing, difficult interpersonal relationship patterns may experience even the most gently worded formulations as being critical. As therapists, we must be aware of this possibility and carefully monitor our patient's reactions to the pieces of formulation we share. Consider this example:

> Audrey is 80 years old when she presents for help with feelings of loneliness and depression. She has two sons who are married with established families of their own and who live across the country. She says now that airplane travel is more difficult for her, she doesn't see them as much as she'd like. She feels alone and is upset that her children live so far away. She worries they do not love her. She no longer calls them because she feels she is intruding into their lives, which makes her feel even more alone and isolated. As she tells her story, she reports she has suffered multiple abandonments in her life. Her mother was depressed and hospitalized on and off throughout her childhood and adolescence. Her husband died from lung cancer in his 40s, leaving her to raise her sons alone. Although she was occasionally drawn to other men over the years, she never married again because she did not want to risk having another ill husband. She was independent, frugal with her small teacher's salary, kept to herself, asked little of her children as they grew up, and acted as if family ties were unimportant. She believed that one's children should "live their own lives."

The therapist formulates that Audrey has an avoidant attachment style, stemming from her experience with a depressed, emotionally unavailable mother. The therapist notes that Audry has tried to live without relying on others and seems to expect little from her family. Now, she feels abandoned and hurt by her sons, but acts as if she is not interested in making contact. The therapist shares this formulation with Audrey, saying, "Ever since your husband died you have acted as if you are fine on your own and expect little from your children. While they have grown up nicely, this approach has given them the signal that you do not need very much from them. I think you may have developed this strategy in childhood as an approach to your mother's depression. You had to be independent then. You used it again after your husband passed away. But it seems that it is no longer working for you, because now you actually would like more connection with your children and their families."

After the therapist speaks, Audrey says, "You're right, I have really messed this all up, and they do not like me or wish to be with me. I have raised selfish children. I guess I deserve to die alone."

In this case, the patient experienced the therapist's shared formulation as further evidence of her own bad feelings about herself. While this was not the therapist's intention, hearing the patient's reaction to the formulation helped the therapist to experience firsthand the way the patient contributes to her negative self-perception. Even when we carefully consider how and when to share our formulations, we will not always get it right, but if we listen to our patients' reactions, it will always help us to deepen the treatment.

Situations in which collaborative formulation is particularly helpful

Several treatment situations exist in which collaborative formulation is particularly helpful. We discuss them next.

Making treatment recommendations

In all health fields, explaining the rationale for the recommended treatment is a crucial part of **informed consent** (Cabaniss et al., 2017). When we recommend psychodynamic psychotherapy, it often involves helping patients understand that unconscious factors may play a role in their difficulties—that is, sharing part of our initial formulation. For example:

Ever since bringing his youngest daughter to college 2 weeks ago, Bryan, who is in his mid-40s, has been unable to sleep. He states that he was looking forward to the "empty nest" so he could take a trip with his wife and socialize more with friends, but that he is too exhausted to do much of anything. When he tells his life story, he reports that his parents were in an unhappy marriage and waited to separate until after he went to college. He feels lucky that he loves his wife.

Toward the end of the session, the therapist, who is also a psychiatrist, offers Bryan some advice about sleep hygiene and gives him a prescription for a sleeping pill, offering the appropriate instruction on its safe use. In addition, the therapist says:

Even though you have been looking forward to this time with your wife, it sounds like you have some feelings about your daughter leaving home. It is possible that the feelings you have about your own parents' divorce are affecting your ability to transition into this next phase of your life. I think that talking about this in psychotherapy will help you to understand what you are going through. That should help your current symptoms and give you insights to help you to enjoy what you have ahead.

In this example, the therapist hypothesizes that taking his daughter to college has

- caused Bryan to activate unconscious feelings about his parents' divorce, and
- that this is affecting his ability to sleep.

The therapist describes the problem (difficulty with loss and moving forward), reviews the patient's life story (parental divorce at a similar time of life), and uses ideas about the impact of early relationships, conflicts, and defenses to hypothesize that Bryan is defending against experiencing the loss of his daughter because it reminds him of a painful loss from his past. The therapist keeps this more technical version of the formulation in his mind, while translating it into straightforward language to which the patient can relate. This enables Bryan to get a better sense of his current situation, as well as a clear idea of why the therapist is recommending psychotherapy.

Generating a life narrative

For many patients, being able to construct a narrative of how they came to be the way they are can be very therapeutic. It can often help them to gain perspective, particularly at difficult moments of their lives. Collaboratively formulating with our patients can help them to create and revise their life narratives (Viederman, 1983). We continue on with Bryan:

As the psychotherapy sessions continue, it becomes clear that, after his parent's divorce, Bryan's mother was very unhappy and took a long time to make a new life for herself. In college, Bryan remained dedicated to his mother, making frequent trips home to keep her company. He recapitulates this pattern in his current life, often denying his own difficulties in order to be strong for others. For example, he has supported his depressed wife for years, and he is the parent who helps his daughter when she is overwhelmed by schoolwork. This further information suggests that Bryan may be having difficulty dealing with his feelings about his daughter's transition because he continues to feel that he needs to be positive and to support others.

The therapist now has a new idea about the way Bryan uses defenses to adapt to loss that goes beyond the initial formulation. He thinks that sharing this aspect of the formulation with Bryan may help him to understand his trouble with grieving. The therapist says:

One reason why you may be having trouble moving on to the next phase of your life is that you are actually very sad that your daughter has left home. You are usually the one called on to "look at the bright side"—whether that was to help your mother after the divorce or to help build your wife's and daughter's confidence. You are the upbeat one, so you naturally want to think about what fun you can have traveling with your wife, rather than pause to allow yourself to be sad that your daughter has left. All your life you have helped others manage their pain, but now YOU are in pain and you don't know how to depend on someone emotionally to work this through. In some ways, this therapy is a first step at learning how to do this.

In response, Bryan comments:

> *You're right—that's the story of my life. I learned to be that way in my relationship with my mother, and I've repeated it in my relationship with my wife and my daughter. It's a nice way to be, and I'm sure that I'll always help them in that way, but I think that it has made it difficult for me to be sad now.*

By sharing his ideas about formulation, the therapist helps Bryan revise his life narrative, which helps Bryan to understand his past, his present, and his future.

Fostering insight during treatment

By offering a developmental perspective, sharing our formulations can also help patients who face difficult insights about themselves in therapy. Think about Nadine, who feels guilty during a therapy session when she realizes that she has been overly harsh with her daughter. The therapist says,

> *I know that you feel bad about your behavior, but it sounds like you learned from your mother to have very high standards, and that you were never allowed any flexibility. It was the only model you knew.*

This simple formulation, which traces a current problem to an early relationship template, links Nadine's current behavior toward her daughter to her mother's behavior toward her. It helps Nadine to understand a possible etiology of her behavior, and to recognize why she is so hard on herself. These insights can help to lessen Nadine's guilt, making her more able to work on these issues in treatment and helping her to improve her relationship with her daughter.

Offering formulations that acknowledge realities related to structural racism and cultural bias can also affect a patient's view of themselves. Consider Prakash, a South Asian man in his 30s who is a very successful small business owner, and who is in psychotherapy to understand challenges relating to cultural differences with his White romantic partner. While he has made real progress sorting out the marital issues, he comes to a psychotherapy session more despondent after a trip abroad to a conference where he was detained at the airport, questioned, and searched extensively by immigration officials. He states, "I can't believe I still let this kind of thing get me down; I should be over it by now." The therapist might reflect back to him:

> *It is really so disturbing that racial stereotypes persist in settings like airports. It is understandable that this recent experience has been deeply troubling and has lowered your mood, even though it is not the first time this has happened.*

Sharing the formulation that Prakash's change in mood was connected to the very real experience of prejudice supports the patient's experience of reality and lessens his self-blame. The patient responds by saying that he knows this kind of thing is still rampant, but that he feels he should not let himself be brought down by this behavior. The therapist might respond with a developmentally based formulation:

> *You have always strived to be immune from cultural bias, perhaps because your parents put such a premium on not letting discrimination deter you in life. While you have attained significant success in dealing with racial stereotyping, an emotional component can still become activated when you are experiencing an incident like this one.*

Preparing the patient for ending therapy

Ending therapy is another time when sharing formulations can be helpful. During the ending phase of therapy, it is often helpful to give patients explanatory summaries they can take with them, reminding them of what they have learned. Often, these summary statements help patients to mark the work they have done and to feel more confident about confronting the future. Consider Bryan, whose daughter just left for college and who learned in therapy that he is more comfortable helping others than taking care of himself. After benefitting enormously from the treatment, Bryan is ready to end therapy. In one of the final sessions, his therapist decides to share some of the formulation with him, saying,

> *As we've learned, your most comfortable stance with other people has been to be the strong one. You developed this approach to manage your own sadness in childhood when your parents were unhappy with each other, and again later when they divorced. You continued this strategy to help your mother after your father left, to help your wife with her depression, and to support your daughter with her academic challenges. While this approach "worked" for many years, it interfered with your ability to lean on others when you were in need. When you first came to see me, you were sad but didn't know it—you experienced it as an inability to sleep. Our therapy was the first time you really sought help for a problem of your own, and your ability to enable yourself to work with me has really helped you. In recent months, you've been much more able to communicate your needs to your wife, and even to some friends. Going forward, this will help you enormously. It's possible that in the future, you may have another situation in which you have some kind of symptom—it could be insomnia again, or something else. If this happens, you are welcome to return to therapy. However, you might also consider what we've learned together and ask yourself whether you are in need of support from the people around you.*

This formulation helps Bryan to consolidate what he has learned and to think about possible problem spots that might arise in the future. In this way, our psychodynamic formulations remain with our patients, reminding them of their work with us and helping them with new situations and transitions for the rest of their lives.

References

1. Cabaniss, D. L., Cherry, S., Douglas, C. J., & Schwartz, A. R. (2017). *Psychodynamic psychotherapy: A clinical manual* (2nd ed.). Wiley Blackwell.
2. Viederman, M. (1983). The psychodynamic life narrative: A psychotherapeutic intervention useful in crisis situations. *Psychiatry, 46,* 236–246.

End Note

Lived experience
and genetics, shape conscious
and unconscious mind.

Together, create
the narratives that help us
learn about ourselves.

The Psychodynamic Writing Collective
January 1, 2022

Appendix A – An Educator's Guide to Using *Psychodynamic Formulation*: An Expanded Approach

As we mentioned in the Introduction, we do not teach psychodynamic formulation all at once. Our aim is to help students feel that collaboratively creating psychodynamic formulations is an automatic and natural part of treating all patients, rather than an onerous task that they will only perform once in their lives. Thus, we teach this process in a gradual way that allows students to consolidate learning without feeling overwhelmed.

Setting the stage for formulating

We believe that psychodynamic formulations—and for that matter, all formulations—can only be truly helpful if they are collaboratively created with our patients, and if they take into consideration the way that biological, psychological, and cultural/social factors influence people throughout their lives. Thus, we suggest that educators consider beginning the process of teaching psychodynamic formulation with conversations about the following topics:

Working collaboratively – Psychodynamic (and other) formulations are not carved-in-stone explanations that we (therapists) create independently and bestow upon our patients. They are ever-changing hypotheses that we collaboratively create with our patients. As therapists, we have ideas we share with our patients, and their thoughts and responses help us to form ideas about the lifelong mental development of the people with whom we are privileged to work. We encourage you to talk about this process with your students, perhaps providing examples of this type of approach, or even engaging in exercises in which give and take is necessary for understanding a situation.

Taking a biopsychosocial approach – Our conscious and unconscious minds are affected throughout our lives by our biology (genetics, intrauterine experience, epigenetics, and temperament), our psychology (early experiences with caregivers), and our culture/society

Psychodynamic Formulation: An Expanded Approach, First Edition. The Psychodynamic Formulation Collective.
© 2022 John Wiley & Sons Ltd. Published 2022 by John Wiley & Sons Ltd.

(community groups, laws, policies, and cultural values). Take some time early in training to think about the ways each of these factors affect patients. This can be done with short writing exercises about any patient with whom your trainees are working—it does not have to be a patient in psychodynamic psychotherapy.

Development and lived experience – Consider beginning the process of teaching about formulation with the idea that development continues throughout life, and that the implicit and explicit values of our culture and society shape the conscious and unconscious minds of our patients. Consider offering examples from your own work with patients that highlight the ways adult experience shapes conscious and unconscious thoughts about the self, relationships, and adapting. Readings from outside the field about racism, sexism, and other forms of social biases can set the stage for these important conversations.

Bias – Help your students examine their own biases before they begin considering the formulations of their patients. Do they have a sense of their own cultural identities? Can they think about how this might affect the way they think about their patients? Are they already thinking that some coping mechanisms are "better" or more "mature" than others? Can they use the ADDRESSING (Age, Developmental and other Disabilities, Religion, Ethnic and Racial identity, Sexuality, Socio-economic status, Indigenous background, Nationality, Gender) framework (Hays, 2016) when thinking about their patients? Are they aware of the assumptions they are inevitably making based on their own and their patients' backgrounds? Having these conversations at the beginning of this learning process will help students to consider this an essential part of all the formulations they co-create throughout their careers.

These topical conversations can be introduced before formal training in psychodynamics begins—they are central to work with patients across all psychotherapeutic modalities.

Teaching the describe/review/link method for formulating

Learning to construct psychodynamic formulations is a multistep process we call the Describe/Review/Link method. It requires student to learn how to

- DESCRIBE problems and patterns
- REVIEW life stories
- LINK problems and patterns to the life story
- Use psychodynamic formulations to guide treatment

Each of these steps requires different kinds of learning and is appropriate for different phases of training. Here are some suggestions about how to teach each of these steps in a mental health training program:

Early in training

DESCRIBE

Early in training is a good time to begin to learn to DESCRIBE patients. Whether or not junior trainees are seeing patients in psychodynamic psychotherapy, junior trainees are seeing **patients** if they are in a clinical training program. Many trainees are used to thinking about making Diagnostic and Statistical Manual of Mental

Disorders (DSM) diagnoses—having them begin to think beyond disorders is the first step toward getting them to think psychodynamically. You can begin by teaching them the difference between the **Problem** and the **Person**. Next, try introducing the six patterns—SELF, RELATIONSHIPS, ADAPTING, COGNITION, VALUES, and WORK AND PLAY. Chapters 6–11 are appropriate for this teaching. In a four-year psychiatry residency, we teach this material in our PG-II year (suggested time frame: four to eight weeks).

Suggested activities

1. **Problem/Person exercise**
   Have students do a writing exercise in which they describe the **Problem** and the **Person** for one of their patients (no longer than a page). They can select any patient whom they have seen recently.
2. **DESCRIBE "putting it together" exercise**
   Have students describe the six patterns: SELF, RELATIONSHIPS, ADAPTING, COGNITION, VALUES, and WORK/PLAY for one of their patients. Encourage them to write each section separately, addressing each variable. Share the work in class so that students are exposed to a range of patients. Encourage group discussion on how to **focus** what they have described to home in on major difficulties.
3. **Interview patients in class**
   Have students generate DESCRIBE sections in small groups.

REVIEW

Next, trainees can learn to REVIEW, which involves more than simply teaching development. They must be taught how to ask their adult patients about their life stories. This involves helping students correlate certain developmental periods with particular adult problems and patterns. Chapters 12–17 are appropriate for this teaching. In a four-year psychiatry residency, we teach this in the PG-III year (suggested time frame: four to eight weeks).

Suggested activities

1. **REVIEW "putting it together" exercise**
   Have students write a REVIEW section for one of their patients (no longer than one page). As with the DESCRIBE exercise, try to have them use the headers so they include all phases of development. Share the work among students. Group discussion can help students to **focus** on key points in development.
2. **DESCRIBE+REVIEW exercise**
   Students can now begin to combine two sections together for the same patient.
3. **Vignettes**
   Instructors can write vignettes about common adult presentations and have students work in groups during class to think about when patients might have had difficulty during life.

Later in training

LINK

Once students have learned to DESCRIBE and REVIEW, it's time to teach LINKING. First, introduce the organizing ideas about development:

Organizing ideas about development

Although mental health trainees are often champing at the bit to learn about "theory," learning it too early can lead to intellectualization in formulation and treatment. Therefore, we wait until slightly later in training to introduce this (during the PG-III year). Again, learning in this area involves more than just becoming familiar with the different organizing ideas; it also requires guidance about how to choose the ones that will be most useful for explaining certain clinical situations. Chapters 19–24 are appropriate for this teaching (suggested time frame: eight weeks).

Suggested activities

Choosing ideas about development

1. **Group work**
   With vignettes or videos of psychotherapy sessions, use group discussion to consider how clinical situations might be understood using different ideas about development.
2. **Individual work**
   Have students write up a short clinical situation using two different ideas about development.

Writing and sharing formulations

You can use the model outlined in the Introduction to Part Four for this teaching. The skills involved are learning to focus on what they have DESCRIBED and REVIEWED, asking a focus question, choosing organizing ideas for linking, and writing a chronological narrative. The examples in Chapters 18–24 can serve as guides, as can the "Putting It Together" example from Part Four. This teaching is best reserved for more senior trainees—we teach it late in the PG-III year (suggested time frame: four to eight weeks). This section can culminate in writing and sharing full formulations

Suggested activities

1. **Focusing DESCRIBE and REVIEW**
   Offer students sample DESCRIBE and REVIEW segments and have them identify the areas they think could be the focus.
2. **Forming questions**
   Have students describe patient presentations and ask the group to suggest focus questions that they would like to answer with a psychodynamic formulation.
3. **"Putting it together"**
   Have students write DESCRIBE, REVIEW, and LINK sections for one of their patients. Involve their supervisors in this project. Have the students read each other's work. In class, students can discuss the choices they made about focusing and choosing ideas about development. This helps the groups to learn about different ways of LINKING and exposes them to more psychodynamic formulations.
4. **Sharing formulations**
   Use role play to help students learn how to share their initial formulations in treatment. Working in pairs, with one student playing the therapist and the other playing the "patient", students can discuss what they might share with a patient, try it out in role play, and then hear how the "patient" thought it sounded.

Using formulations to guide treatment

Once students have written their own psychodynamic formulations, they can begin to think about how to use them to guide treatment. For this, it is important to enlist the help of their clinical supervisors. Chapters 1–5 and 25–28 are appropriate for this teaching. Areas to emphasize include goal setting and making treatment recommendations, using psychodynamic formulations in different clinical settings, ending treatment, and revising formulations over time. This teaching can begin in the middle of training and continue forever.

Suggested activities

1. **Have a faculty development workshop**
   Bring your clinical supervisors together to discuss writing and using psychodynamic formulations in training. Consider doing some of the above exercises with the supervisors so that they can have a sense of what and how the students are learning.
2. **Learn about formulating in other treatment modalities**
   Have educators from other treatment areas (e.g., psychopharmacology and other psychotherapies) teach together so students can learn about different ways of formulating—often for the same patients.

Reference

1. Hays, P.A. (2016) Addressing cultural complexities in practice (3rd ed). American Psychological Association.

Appendix B – DESCRIBE, REVIEW, LINK—An Outline

DESCRIBE (Six Domains of Function)

1. Self
   - Self-perception
     - Identity
     - Fantasies about the self
   - Self-esteem
     - Vulnerability to self-esteem threats
     - Internal responses to self-esteem threats
     - Use of others to regulate self-esteem
     - Responses to external effects on self-esteem

2. Relationships
   - Trust
   - Sense of self and other
   - Security
   - Intimacy
   - Mutuality

3. Adapting (Defense Mechanisms)
   - Current benefit and cost
   - Emotionality
   - Flexibility and range

Psychodynamic Formulation: An Expanded Approach, First Edition. The Psychodynamic Formulation Collective.
© 2022 John Wiley & Sons Ltd. Published 2022 by John Wiley & Sons Ltd.

4. Cognition
   - Basic cognitive abilities
   - Higher (Executive) Functions
     - Emotional regulation
     - Impulse control
     - Judgment
     - Sensory stimulus regulation
     - Decision Making and Problem-Solving
   - Reflective (Metacognitive) Functions
     - Reality testing/Sense of reality
     - Self-reflection
     - Mentalization

5. Values
   - Sense of right/wrong
     - Right/Wrong System
     - Harshness
     - Flexibility
   - Right/wrong behavior
     - Consistency with sense of right/wrong
     - Consistent with one's family/culture
     - Prosocial behavior
   - Personal values
     - Types (e.g., education, family, money)
     - Consistent with/divergent from those around them

6. Work and Play
   - Consistent with developmental level/talents/limitations
   - Comfortable/satisfying/pleasurable
   - Adequate for care of self and dependents
   - Culturally sanctioned
   - Limited because of restricted access

REVIEW

- What we're born with
- Earliest years
- Middle childhood
- Later childhood
- Adolescence
- Adulthood

LINK

- Trauma
- Early cognitive and emotional difficulties
- Effect of culture and society
- Conflict/defense
- Self
- Relationships
- Attachment

Recommended Reading

Recommended Reading: Part One

Chapters 1–5

1. Cabaniss, D. L., Cherry, S., Douglas, C. J., & Schwartz, A. R. (2011). *Psychodynamic psychotherapy: A clinical manual*. Wiley-Blackwell.
2. Campbell, W. H., & Rohrbaugh, R. M. (2006). *The biopsychosocial formulation manual*. Routledge.
3. Compton, M. T., & Shim, R. S. S. (Eds.) (2015). *The social determinants of mental health*. American Psychiatric Association Publishing.
4. Eels, T. D. (Ed.) (2007). *Handbook of psychotherapy case formulation*. Guilford Press.
5. Friedman, R. S., & Lister, P. (1987). The current status of psychodynamic formulation. *Psychiatry, 50*(2), 126–141.
6. Gabbard, G. O. (2009). *Textbook of psychotherapeutic treatments* (1st ed.). American Psychiatric Publishing.
7. Hays, P. A. (2016). *Addressing cultural complexities in practice* (3rd ed.). American Psychological Association.
8. Kassaw, K., & Gabbard, G. O. (2002). Creating a psychodynamic formulation from a clinical evaluation. *American Journal of Psychiatry, 159*, 721–726.
9. MacKinnon, R. A., & Yudofsky, S. C. (1986). *The psychiatric evaluation in clinical practice*. J.B. Lippincott Company.
10. McWilliams, N. (1999). *Psychoanalytic case formulation*. Guilford Press.
11. Perry, S., Cooper, A. M., & Michels, R. (1987). The psychodynamic formulation: Its purpose, structure, and clinical application. *The American Journal of Psychiatry, 144*, 543–550.
12. Shim, R. S. S., & Vinson, S. Y. (Eds.) (2021). *Social (in)justice and mental health*. American Psychiatric Association Press.
13. Summers, R. F., & Barber, J. P. (2010). *Psychodynamic therapy: A guide to evidence-based practice*. Guilford Press.
14. Tummala-Narrra, P. (2016). *Psychoanalytic theory and cultural competence in psychotherapy*. American Psychological Association.

Psychodynamic Formulation: An Expanded Approach, First Edition. The Psychodynamic Formulation Collective.
© 2022 John Wiley & Sons Ltd. Published 2022 by John Wiley & Sons Ltd.

Recommended Reading: Part Two

Chapter 6

1. Eng, D. L., & Han, S. (2000). A dialogue on racial melancholia. *Psychoanalytic Dialogues, 10,* 667–700.
2. Erikson, E. H. (1968). *Identity, youth, and crisis.* Norton.
3. Fanon, F. (1967). *Black skin, white masks.* Grove Press.
4. Hong, C. (2020). *Minor feelings: An Asian American reckoning.* One World.
5. Kernberg, O. F. (1970). Factors in the psychoanalytic treatment of narcissistic personalities. *Journal of the American Psychoanalytic Association, 18,* 51–85.
6. Kohut, H., & Wolff, E. S. (1978). The disorder of the self and their treatment, an outline. *International Journal of Psychoanalysis, 59,* 413–414.
7. Sandler, J., Holder, A., & Meers, D. (1963). The ego ideal and the ideal self. *Psychoanalytic Study of the Child, 18,* 139–158.
8. Wilkerson, I. (2020). *Caste: The origins of our discontents.* Random House.

Chapter 7

1. Beebe, B., & Lachman, F. M. (1988). The contribution of mother-infant mutual influence to the origins of self and object representation. *Psychoanalytic Psychology, 5,* 305–337.
2. Bowlby, J. (1958). The nature of the child's tie to his mother. *International Journal of Psychoanalysis, 39,* 350–373.
3. Bowlby, J. (1982). *Attachment, Vol. 1 of attachment and loss.* Basic Books.
4. Greenberg, J. R., & Mitchell, S. A. (1983). *Object relations in psychoanalytic theory.* Harvard University Press.
5. Slade, A. (2008). Attachment theory and research: Implications for the theory and practice of individual psychotherapy with adults. In J. Cassidy & P. R. Shaver (Eds.), *Handbook of attachment: Theory, research and clinical applications* (pp. 762–782). Guilford Press.
6. Stern, D. N. (1985). *The interpersonal world of the infant.* Basic Books.

Chapter 8

1. Freud, S. (1862). The neuro-psychoses of defense. In Strachey, J (ed). The Standard Edition of the Complete Psychological Works of Sigmund Freud, Volume III (1893–1899), Early Psycho-Analytic Publications. Hogarth Press. (Originally published in 1894).
2. Gabbard, G. O. (2005). *Psychodynamic psychiatry in clinical practice* (4th ed.). American Psychiatric Publishing, Inc.
3. Kernberg, O. F. (1976). *Object-relations theory and clinical psychoanalysis.* Aronson.
4. Shapiro, D. (1973). *Neurotic styles.* Basic Books.
5. Vaillant, G. E. (1977). *Adaptation to life how the best and the brightest came of age* (1st ed.). Little, Brown & Co.

Chapter 9

1. Allen, J. G. (2006). Mentalizing. In J. G. Allen & P. Fonagy (Eds.), *Practice in handbook of mentalization-=Based treatment* (pp. 3–30). Wiley.

2. Clarkin, J. F., Howieson, D. B., & McClough, J. (2008). The role of psychiatric measures in assessment and treatment. In R. E. Hales, S. C. Yudofsky, & G. O. Gabbard (Eds.), *American psychiatric publishing textbook of psychiatry* (5th ed., pp. 73–112). American Psychiatric Publishing, Inc.

3. Coltart, N. E. (1988). Assessment of psychological mindedness in the clinical interview. *British Journal of Psychiatry, 153*, 819–820.

4. Folstein, M. F., Folstein, S. E., & McHugh, P. R. (1975). 'Mini-mental state'. A practical method for grading the cognitive state of patients for the physician. *Journal of Psychiatric Research, 12*, 189–198.

5. Fonagy, P. (1991). Thinking about thinking: Some clinical and theoretical considerations in the treatment of a borderline patient. *International Journal of Psychoanalysis, 72*, 639–656.

6. Friedman, C. (2017). Defining disability: Understandings of and attitudes towards ableism and disability. *Disability Studies Quarterly, 37*(1). Available at http://dsq-sds.org/article/view/5061/4545

7. Goldstein, G. (2010). Cognitive assessment with adults. In J. C. Thomas & M. Hersen (Eds.), *Handbook of clinical psychology competencies* (pp. 237–260). Springer.

8. Hall, J. A. (1992). Psychological-mindedness: A conceptual model. *American Journal of Psychotherapy, 46*(1), 131–140.

9. Hehir, T. (2002). Eliminating ableism in education. *Harvard Educational Review, 72*(1), 1–32.

10. Lichter, D. G., & Cummings, J. L. (2001). *Psychiatric and neurological disorders*. Guilford Press.

11. Roberts, A. C., Robbins, T. W., & Weiskrantz, L. (2002). *The prefrontal cortex: Executive and cognitive functions*. Oxford University Press.

12. Semerari, A., Carcione, A., Dimaggio, G., Falcone, M., Nicolò, G., Procacci, M., & Alleva, G. (2003). How to evaluate metacognitive functioning in psychotherapy? the metacognition assessment scale and its applications. *Clinical Psychology & Psychotherapy, 10*(4), 238–261. https://doi.org/10.1002/cpp.362

13. Stoute, B. J. (2019). Racial socialization and thwarted mentalization: Psychoanalytic reflections from the lived experience of James Baldwin's America. *American Imago, 76*(3), 335–357.

14. Taylor, G. J. (1995). Psychoanalysis and empirical research: The example of patients who lack psychological-mindedness. *Journal of the American Academy of Psychoanaylsis, 23*, 263–281.

Chapter 10

1. Gibbs, J. C. (2019). *Moral development and reality* (4th ed.). Oxford University Press.
2. Jensen, L. A. (Ed.) (2015). *Moral development in a global world: Research from a cultural-developmental perspective*. Cambridge University Press.

Chapter 11

1. Brown, S. (2009). *Play: How it shapes the brain, opens the imagination, and invigorates the soul*. Penguin Books.
2. DeLamater, J. (2012). Sexual expression in later life: A review and synthesis. *The Journal of Sex Research, 49*(2–3), 125–141.
3. Paluska, S. A., & Schwenk, T. L. (2000). Physical activity and mental health. *Sports Medicine, 29*(3), 167–180.
4. Terr, L. (1999). *Beyond love and work: Why adults need to play*. Touchstone.

Recommended Reading: Part Three

Chapter 12

1. Burmeister, M., McInnis, M. G., & Zöllner, S. (2008). Psychiatric genetics: Progress amid controversy. *Nature Reviews Genetics, 9*(7), 527–540.
2. Dunkel Schetter, C., & Tanner, L. (2012). Anxiety, depression and stress in pregnancy: Implications for mothers, children, research, and practice. *Current Opinion in Psychiatry, 25*(2), 141–148.
3. Eisenberg, N., Spinrad, T. L., & Knafo-Noam, A. (2015). Prosocial development. In M. E. Lamb & R. M. Lerner (Eds.), *Handbook of child psychology and developmental science: Socioemotional processes* (pp. 610–656). Wiley.
4. Hyman, S. (2000). The genetics of mental illness: Implications for clinical practice. *Bulletin of the WHO, 78*(4), 455–463.
5. Jawaid, A., Roszkowski, M., & Mansuy, I. M. (2018). Transgenerational epigenetics of traumatic stress. *Progress in Molecular Biology and Translational Science, 158*, 253–278.
6. Minnes, S., Lang, A., & Singer, L. (2011). Prenatal tobacco, marijuana, stimulant, and opiate exposure: Outcomes and practice implications. *Addiction Science & Clinical Practice, 6*(1), 57–70.
7. Monk, C., Lugo-Candelas, C., & Trumpff, C. (2019). Prenatal developmental origins of future psychopathology: Mechanisms and pathways. *Annual Review of Clinical Psychology, 15*, 317–344.
8. Riley, E. P., Infante, A., & Warren, K. R. (2011). Fetal alcohol spectrum disorders: An overview. *Neuropsychology Review, 21*(2), 73–80.
9. Shang, S., Wu, N., & Su, Y. (2017). How oxytocin receptor (OXTR) single nucleotide polymorphisms act on prosociality: The mediation role of moral evaluation. *Frontiers in Psychology, 8*, 396.
10. Yehuda, R., & Lehrner, A. (2018). Intergenerational transmission of trauma effects: Putative role of epigenetic mechanisms. *World Psychiatry, 17*, 243–257.

Chapter 13

1. Ainsworth, M. D. S., Blehar, M. C., Waters, E., et al. (1978). *Patterns of attachment: A psychological study of the strange situation.* Erlbaum.
2. Bateman, A., & Fonagy, P. (2006). Mentalizing and borderline personality disorder. In J. G. Allen & P. Fonagy (Eds.), *Handbook of mentalization based treatment* (pp. 185–200). Wiley.
3. Beebe, B., & Lachmann, F. (2002). *Infant research and adult treatment: Co-constructing interactions.* Analytic Press.
4. Davies, D. (2011). *Child development: A practitioner's guide.* Guilford Press.
5. Hirschfeld, L. A. (2008). Children's developing conceptions of race. In S. M. Quintana & C. McKown (Eds.), *Handbook of race, racism, and the developing child* (pp. 37–54). Wiley.
6. Main, M. (1995). Recent studies in attachment: Overview, with selected implications for clinical work. In S. Goldberg, R. Muir, & J. Kerr (Eds.), *Attachment theory: Social, developmental and clinical perspectives* (pp. 407–474). Analytic Press.
7. Oppenheim, D., Emde, R. N., Hasson, M., & Warren, S. (1997). Preschoolers face moral dilemmas: A longitudinal study of acknowledging and resolving internal conflict. *The International Journal of Psychoanalysis, 78*(5), 943–957.
8. Winnicott, D. W. (1965). *The maturational processes and the facilitating environment.* Hogarth Press.

Chapter 14

1. Freud, S. (1953). Three essays on the theory of sexuality. In: Strachey, J (ed). The Standard Edition of the Complete Psychological Works of Sigmund Freud, Volume VII (1901–1905): A Case of Hysteria, Three Essays on Sexuality and Other Works. Hogarth Press. (Originally published in 1905). Hogarth Press. (Originally published in 1905).
2. Isay, R. (1989). *Being homosexual: Gay men and their development*. Farrar Strauss Giroux.
3. Lewes, K. (1988). *The psychoanalytic theory of male homosexuality*. Simon and Schuster.
4. Roiphe, H., & Roiphe, A. (1985). *Your child's mind*. St. Martin's Press.
5. Sophocles. (1982). *The three theban plays*. Penguin Books.

Chapter 15

1. Erikson, E. H. (1995). *Childhood and society*. Vintage.
2. Piaget, J. (1929). *The child's conception of the world*. Harcourt.
3. Tatum, B. (2017). *Why are all the black kids sitting together in the cafeteria?* (Revised ed.). Basic Books.

Chapter 16

1. Beardslee, W. R., & Valliant, G. (2008). Adult development. In A. Tasman, J. Kay, J. A. Lieberman, et al. (Eds.), *Psychiatry* (3rd ed., pp. 181–195). Wiley.
2. Bienenfeld, D. (2008). Late life. In A. Tasman, J. Kay, J. A. Lieberman, et al. (Eds.), *Psychiatry* (3rd ed., pp. 196–202). Wiley.
3. Drescher, J. (2002). Invisible gay adolescents: The developmental narratives of gay men. *Adolescent Psychiatry, 26,* 73–94.
4. Erikson, E. (1963). *Childhood and dociety* (2nd ed.). W.W. Norton & Co.
5. Pruitt, D. (1999). *Your adolescent*. HarperCollins.
6. Shapiro, T., & Amso, D. (2008). School-age development. In A. Tasman, J. Kay, J. A. Lieberman, et al. (Eds.), *Psychiatry* (3rd ed., pp. 150–160). Wiley.
7. Towbin, K. E., & Showalter, J. E. (2008). Adolescent development. In A. Tasman, J. Kay, J. A. Lieberman, et al. (Eds.), *Psychiatry* (3rd ed., pp. 161–180). Wiley.
8. Vaillant, G. (1977). *Adaptation to life*. Harvard University Press.

Chapter 17

1. Vaillant, G. E. (2003). *Aging well: Guideposts to a happier life*. Warner.

Recommended Reading: Part Four

Chapter 18

1. Fonagy, P., Gergely, G., Jurist, E., et al. (2002). *Affect regulation, mentalization and the development of the self*. Other Press.
2. Frankl, V. (1959). *Man's search for meaning*. Beacon Press.

3. Herman, J. (1992). *Trauma and recovery*. Basic Books.
4. Kellerman, N. (2009). *Holocaust trauma: Psychological effects and treatment*. iUniverse, Inc.
5. Menakem, R. (2017). *My grandmother's hands: Racialized trauma and the pathway to mending our hearts and bodies*. Central Recovery Press.
6. Shengold, L. (1989). *Soul murder: The effects of childhood abuse and deprivation*. Fawcett Columbine.
7. Terr, L. D. (1991). Childhood traumas: An outline and overview. *American Journal of Psychiatry, 148*, 10–20.
8. van der Kolk, B. (2014). *The body keeps the score: Mind, brain and body in the transformation of trauma*. Penguin Books.
9. Yovell, Y. (2000). From hysteria to posttraumatic stress disorder: Psychoanalysis and the neurobiology of traumatic memories. *Neuropsychoanalysis, 2*, 171–181.

Chapter 19

1. Andrews, G., Pine, D. S., Hobbs, M. J., et al. (2009). Neurodevelopmental disorders: Cluster 2 of the proposed meta-structure for DSM-V and ICD-11. *Psychological Medicine, 39*(12), 2013–2023.
2. Bernard, S. (2009). Mental health and behavioural problems in children and adolescents with learning disabilities. *Psychiatry, 8*, 387–390.
3. Buitelaar, J., Kan, C., & Asherson, P. (2011). *ADHD in adults: Characterization, diagnosis, and treatment*. Cambridge University Press.
4. Costello, E. J., Mustillo, S., Erkanli, A., et al. (2003). Prevalence and development of psychiatric disorders in childhood and adolescence. *Archives of General Psychiatry, 60*, 837–844.
5. Kim-Cohen, J., Caspi, A., Moffitt, T. E., et al. (2003). Prior juvenile diagnoses in adults with mental disorder: Developmental follow-back of a prospective-longitudinal cohort. *Archives of General Psychiatry, 60*(7), 709–717.
6. Sachdev, P., Andrews, G., Hobbs, M. J., et al. (2009). Neurocognitive disorders: Cluster 1 of the proposed meta-structure for DSM-V and ICD-11. *Psychological Medicine, 39*(12), 2001–2012.
7. Soloman, M., Hessl, D., Chiu, S., et al. (2009). Towards a neurodevelopmental model of clinical case formulation. *Psychiatric Clinics of North America, 32*(1), 199–211.

Chapter 20

1. Baldwin, J. (1962). *The fire next time*. Vintage.
2. Banaji, M. R., & Greenwald, G. A. (2016). *Blind spot*. Bantam Books.
3. Coates, T. (2015). *Between the world and me*. One World.
4. Compton, M. T., & Shim, R. S. (2015). *The social determinants of mental health*. American Psychiatric Association Publishing.
5. Diangelelo, R. (2018). *White fragility*. Beacon Press.
6. Dimeb, M. (2011). *With culture in mind*. Routledge.
7. Drescher, J. (1998). *Psychoanalytic therapy and the gay man*. Routledge.
8. Fanon, F. (1952). *Black skin, white masks*. Grove Press.
9. Grier, W. H., & Cobbs, P. M. (1968). *Black rage*. Basic Books.
10. Hays, P. A. (2016). *Addressing cultural complexities in practice*. American Psychological Association.

11. Magee, M., & Miller, D. (1997). *Lesbian lives: psychoanalytic narratives old and new.* Routledge.
12. Moane, G. (2011). *Gender and colonialism.* Palgrave/MacMillan.
13. Shim, R. S., & Vinson, S. Y. (Eds.) (2021). *Social (in)justice and mental health.* American Psychiatric Association Publishing.
14. Tatum, B. D. (2017). *Why are all the black kids sitting together in the cafeteria?* Basic Books.

Chapter 21

1. Brenner, C. (1974). *An elementary textbook of psychoanalysis* (Revised and Expanded ed.). Anchor Books.
2. Freud, A. (1937). *The ego and the mechanisms of defense.* Hogarth Press.
3. Gottlieb, R. M. (2012). Classical psychoanalysis: Past and present. In *Textbook of psychoanalysis* (2nd ed.). American Psychiatric Publishing, Inc.
4. Mitchell, S. A., & Black, M. J. (1995). *Freud and beyond.* Basic Books.

Chapter 22

1. Fairbairn, W. R. D. (1954). *An object-relations theory of personality.* Basic Books.
2. Fonagy, P., & Target, M. (2003). *Psychoanalytic theories: Perspectives from developmental psychology.* Brunner-Routledge.
3. Greenberg, J., & Mitchell, S. (1983). *Object relations in psychoanalytic theory.* Harvard University Press.
4. Kernberg, O. F. (1976). *Object relations theory and clinical psychoanalysis.* Aronson.
5. Kernberg, O. F. (1987). An ego-psychology object relations approach to the transference. *Psychoanalytic Quarterly, 57,* 481–504.
6. Klein, M. (1948). *Contributions to psychoanalysis, 1921–1945.* Hogarth Press.
7. Sullivan, H. S. (1953). *The interpersonal theory of psychiatry.* W.W. Norton & Co.
8. Winnicott, D. W. (1958). *Collected papers.* Basic Books.

Chapter 23

1. Fonagy, P., & Target, M. (2003). *Psychoanalytic theories: Perspectives from developmental psychology.* Brunner-Routledge.
2. Kohut, H. (1971). *The analysis of the self.* The University of Chicago Press.
3. Kohut, H. (1977). *The restoration of the self.* The University of Chicago Press.
4. Kohut, H. (1979). The two analyses of Mr. Z. *International Journal of Psychoanalysis, 60,* 3–27.
5. Kohut, H., & Wolf, E. S. (1978). The disorders of the self and their treatment: An outline. *International Journal of Psychoanalysis, 59,* 413–425.
6. Kohut, H., & Goldberg, A. (Eds.) (1984). *How does analysis cure?* The University of Chicago Press.
7. Mitchell, S., & Black, M. (1995). *Freud and beyond: A history of modern psychoanalytic thought.* Basic Books.
8. Stolorow, R. D. (1975). Toward a functional definition of narcissism. *International Journal of Psychoanalysis, 56,* 179–185.

9. Winnicott, D. W. (1990). *The maturational process and the facilitating environment: Studies in the theory of emotional development*. Routledge.
10. Winnicott, D. W. (1991). *Playing and reality*. Routledge.

Chapter 24

1. Bowlby, J. (1958). The nature of the child's tie to his mother. *International Journal of Psychoanalysis, 39*, 350–373.
2. Fonagy, P. (2001). *Attachment theory and psychoanalysis*. Other Press.
3. Holmes, J., & Slade, A. (2018). *Attachment in therapeutic practice*. Sage Publications Ltd.
4. Otto, H., & Keller, H. (Eds.) (2014). *Different faces of attachment: Cultural variations on a universal human need*. Cambridge University Press.
5. Slade, A. (2000). The development and organization of attachment: Implications for psychoanalysis. *Journal of the American Psychoanalytic Association, 48*, 1147–1174.
6. Stern, D. N. (1985). *The interpersonal world of the infant*. Basic Books.

Recommended Reading: Part Five

Chapter 25

1. Barnhill, J. W. (2018). *Approach to the psychiatric patient: Case-based essays* (2nd ed.). American Psychiatric Publishing, Inc.
2. Leibenluft, E., Tasman, A., & Green, S. (1993). *Less time to do more: Psychotherapy on the short-term inpatient unit*. American Psychiatric Association Publishing.
3. MacKinnon, R. A., Michels, R., & Buckley, P. J. (2006). *The pinterview in clinical practice*. American Psychiatric Publishing, Inc.
4. Schwartz, H. J., Bleiberg, E., & Weissman, S. H. (1995). *Psychodynamic concepts in general psychiatry*. American Psychiatric Publishing, Inc.

Chapter 26

1. Busch, F. N., & Auchincloss, E. L. (1995). The psychology of prescribing and taking medication. In H. Schwartz, E. Bleiberg, & S. Weissman (Eds.), *Psychodynamic concepts in general psychiatry* (pp. 401–416). American Psychiatric Publishing, Inc.
2. Busch, F. N., & Sandberg, L. S. (2007). *Psychotherapy and medication: The challenge of integration*. Analytic Press.
3. Roose, S. P., Cabaniss, D. L., & Rutherford, B. R. (2012). Combining psychoanalysis and psychopharmacology: Theory and technique. In G. O. Gabbard, B. E. Litowitz, & P. Williams (Eds.), *Textbook of psychoanalysis* (2nd ed., pp. 319–332). American Psychiatric Publishing, Inc.
4. Tutter, A. (2006). Medication as object. *Journal of the American Psychoanalytic Association, 54*, 781–804.

Chapter 27

1. Bateman, A., Brown, D., & Pedder, J. (2010). *Introduction to psychotherapy: An outline of psychodynamic principles and practice* (4th ed.). Tavistock/Routledge.
2. Perry, S. W., Cooper, A., & Michels, R. (1987). The psychodynamic formulation: Its purpose, structure and clinical applications. *American Journal of Psychiatry, 144,* 543–550.
3. Summers, R. F., & Barber, J. P. (2010). *Psychodynamic therapy: A guide to evidence-based practice.* Guilford Press.

Index

Psychodynamic Formulation: An Expanded Approach, First Edition. The Psychodynamic Formulation Collective.
© 2022 John Wiley & Sons Ltd. Published 2022 by John Wiley & Sons Ltd.